CURRENT TOPICS IN

EXPERIMENTAL ENDOCRINOLOGY

Volume 4

THE ENDOCRINOLOGY OF PREGNANCY AND PARTURITION

CONTRIBUTORS

T. Chard
J. K. Findlay
Henry G. Friesen
Anna-Riitta Fuchs
Arnold Klopper
Ulrich A. Knuth
Robert E. Oakey
Premila Rathnam
Brij B. Saxena
Rodney P. Shearman
Francesca Stewart
C. H. Tyndale-Biscoe

EDITORIAL BOARD

Current Topics in
EXPERIMENTAL ENDOCRINOLOGY

Edited by

L. MARTINI
DEPARTMENT OF ENDOCRINOLOGY
UNIVERSITY OF MILAN
MILAN, ITALY

V. H. T. JAMES
ST. MARY'S HOSPITAL
MEDICAL SCHOOL
UNIVERSITY OF LONDON
LONDON, ENGLAND

VOLUME 4

THE ENDOCRINOLOGY OF PREGNANCY AND PARTURITION

1983

ACADEMIC PRESS
A Subsidiary of Harcourt Brace Jovanovich, Publishers
New York London
Paris San Diego San Francisco São Paulo Sydney Tokyo Toronto

ACADEMIC PRESS, INC.
111 Fifth Avenue, New York, New York 10003

United Kingdom Edition published by
ACADEMIC PRESS, INC. (LONDON) LTD.
24/28 Oval Road, London NW1 7DX

Library of Congress Catalog Card Number: 70–187922

ISBN 0–12–153204–6

PRINTED IN THE UNITED STATES OF AMERICA

83 84 85 86 9 8 7 6 5 4 3 2 1

CONTENTS

CONTRIBUTORS ix
PREFACE xi

Pregnancy and Parturition in Marsupials

Francesca Stewart and C. H. Tyndale-Biscoe

I. Introduction 2
II. Hormones and Their Measurement 6
III. Estrous Cycle 8
IV. Pregnancy 11
V. Parturition 22
VI. Conclusions 29
References 30

The Endocrinology of the Preimplantation Period

J. K. Findlay

I. Introduction 36
II. Steroids 39
III. Endometrial Proteins 46
IV. Prostaglandins 50
V. Histamine 59
VI. Conclusions 60
References 61

Prolactin and Pregnancy

Ulrich A. Knuth and Henry G. Friesen

I. Introduction 70
II. Effect of Prolactin on the Ovary 70
III. Prolactin in Normal Pregnancy 71
IV. Influence of Prolactin on Pregnancy-Specific Events 81
V. Prolactin as a Marker in Pathological Pregnancy 84
VI. Lactation 85
VII. Prolactin-Secreting Tumors during Pregnancy 88
VIII. Summary and Future Research 90
References 91

Human Chorionic Gonadotropin in Early Pregnancy

Brij B. Saxena and Premila Rathnam

I. Introduction 98
II. Chemistry and Biosynthesis 98
III. Measurement of hCG 105
IV. Secretory Patterns of hCG during the Reproductive Cycle 110
V. Role of hCG in Early Pregnancy 118
VI. Role of hCG in Abnormal Conditions 118
VII. Interaction of hCG with "Receptor" Site 121
References 122

Specific Pregnancy Proteins

Arnold Klopper

I. Introduction 128
II. Schwangerschaftsprotein 1 (SP_1) 129
III. Pregnancy-Associated Plasma Protein A (PAPP-A) 147
IV. Pregnancy-Associated Plasma Protein B (PAPP-B) 155
V. Placental Protein 5 (PP5) 156
VI. Other Pregnancy-Associated Proteins 159
VII. Envoy 160
References 160

Human Placental Lactogen

T. Chard

I. Introduction 168
II. Nomenclature 168
III. Placental Lactogenic Hormones in Other Species 169

IV. Placental Lactogen and Other Placental Proteins 169
V. Synthesis 169
VI. Immunochemical Nature 172
VII. Biological Nature 173
VIII. Biological Functions 174
IX. Control Mechanisms 176
X. Metabolism and Clearance 177
XI. Levels in Different Biological Fluids 178
XII. Assay of hPL in Blood 179
XIII. Maternal Levels in Normal Pregnancy 179
XIV. Interpretation of Biochemical Tests of Fetoplacental Function 180
XV. Maternal Levels in Complications of Pregnancy 181
XVI. Clinical Use of hPL—Conclusions 186
References 187

Estrogen and Progesterone Production in Human Pregnancy

Robert E. Oakey

I. Introduction 194
II. Nomenclature 194
III. Biosynthesis of Estrogens 196
IV. Control of Estrogen Production 197
V. Estrogens in Plasma in Relation to the Onset of Labor 211
VI. Biosynthesis of Progesterone 213
VII. Control of Progesterone Production 215
VIII. Progesterone in Plasma in Relation to the Onset of Labor 218
IX. Conclusions 219
References 223

The Role of Oxytocin in Parturition

Anna-Riitta Fuchs

I. Introduction 231
II. Indirect Evidence of a Role for Oxytocin 233
III. Direct Evidence of a Role for Oxytocin 241
IV. Control of Uterine Sensitivity 249
V. Interaction of Oxytocin with Prostaglandins 256
VI. Conclusions 260
References 260

Threatened Abortion

Rodney P. Shearman

I. Definition 268
II. Incidence 268

III. Natural History 268
IV. Etiology 271
V. Clinical Features 273
VI. Management 282
VII. Threatened Abortion and the Intrauterine Device (IUD) 284
References 285

INDEX 287

CONTRIBUTORS

Numbers in parentheses indicate the pages on which the authors' contributions begin.

T. CHARD (167), Departments of Reproductive Physiology and Obstetrics and Gynaecology, St. Bartholomew's Hospital Medical College, London EC1A 7BE, England

J. K. FINDLAY (35), Medical Research Centre, Prince Henry's Hospital, Melbourne, Victoria 3004, Australia

HENRY G. FRIESEN (69), Department of Physiology, University of Manitoba, Winnipeg, Manitoba R3E OW3, Canada

ANNA-RIITTA FUCHS (231), Department of Obstetrics and Gynecology, Cornell University Medical College, New York, New York 10021

ARNOLD KLOPPER (127), Department of Obstetrics and Gynecology, University of Aberdeen, Aberdeen AB9 2ZB, Scotland

ULRICH A. KNUTH (69), Department of Physiology, University of Manitoba, Winnipeg, Manitoba R3E OW3, Canada

ROBERT E. OAKEY (193), Division of Steroid Endocrinology, Department of Chemical Pathology, School of Medicine, University of Leeds, Leeds LS2 9LN, England

PREMILA RATHNAM (97), Department of Obstetrics and Gynecology, Cornell University Medical College, New York, New York 10021

BRIJ B. SAXENA (97), Department of Medicine, Cornell University Medical College, New York, New York 10021

RODNEY P. SHEARMAN (267), Department of Obstetrics and Gynecology, University of Sydney, and Division of Obstetrics and Gynecology, Royal Prince Alfred Hospital, Sydney, Australia

FRANCESCA STEWART[1] (1), CSIRO Division of Wildlife Research, Lyneham, A.C.T. 2602, Australia

C. H. TYNDALE-BISCOE (1), CSIRO Division of Wildlife Research, Lyneham, A.C.T. 2602, Australia

[1] Present address: ARC Institute of Animal Physiology, Animal Research Station, Cambridge CB3 OJQ, England.

PREFACE

Volume 3 of this series, published in 1978, marked a change in policy by the editorial board, and aimed at bringing together a number of contributors to discuss a single topic in endocrinology. For the reader, it was felt that this approach offered a more useful perspective, enabling him to review fairly extensively a major area in what is now a rapidly growing and rather wide discipline. This policy has been retained, and Volumes 4 and 5 are written by a number of contributors who have dealt with various aspects of one of the most important areas of endocrinology—pregnancy and parturition. The two volumes are to some extent complementary because of the inevitable overlap of these topics.

In this volume, Stewart and Tyndale-Biscoe have dealt with pregnancy and parturition in marsupials, and the vital role of the corpus luteum. Findlay has reviewed the endocrinology of the preimplantation period, looking at the variety of hormones and other agents and their involvement in the implantation process. Prolactin is a hormone whose importance continues to attract study because of the extraordinary breadth of potential actions; Knuth and Friesen review recent work in this field in relation to pregnancy. Saxena and Rathnam have surveyed the extensive literature on chorionic gonadotropin, in both normal and abnormal pregnancy, adding much of their personal data.

An area of growing importance, the chemistry and role of specific proteins in pregnancy, is considered in detail by Klopper, who points out the need to properly understand the physiological function of these proteins. Chard reviews placental lactogen, particularly in relation to abnormal pregnancy and the clinical usefulness of placental lactogen measurements. Oakey has considered the problems of steroid production by the fetal–placental unit and the complex mechanism of biosynthesis.

Like many of the other authors, he reminds us of the problems still outstanding in spite of the considerable volume of investigational work in this field. Oxytocin is a hormone of major significance in normal pregnancy, and also as an agent for induction of labor, and Fuchs reviews current ideas on its physiological role and mechanism of action. Finally, Shearman addresses the important issues surrounding the problem of threatened abortion, a matter of concern and interest to both clinical scientists and physicians.

It is hoped that the breadth of coverage given by these articles will enable the reader to follow current advances, and to obtain more insight into controversial areas, which need and merit further research. To the many authors who prepared their articles so carefully, the editors express their warm appreciation.

L. MARTINI
V.H.T. JAMES

CURRENT TOPICS IN

EXPERIMENTAL ENDOCRINOLOGY

Volume 4

THE ENDOCRINOLOGY OF PREGNANCY AND PARTURITION

PREGNANCY AND PARTURITION IN MARSUPIALS

Francesca Stewart[1] *and C. H. Tyndale-Biscoe*

CSIRO DIVISION OF WILDLIFE RESEARCH
LYNEHAM, AUSTRALIA

I. Introduction 2
II. Hormones and Their Measurement 6
III. Estrous Cycle 8
A. Follicular Development and Ovulation 8
B. Progesterone Levels 10
C. The Corpus Luteum 10
IV. Pregnancy 11
A. Relevant Anatomy 11
B. Conception 13
C. Cleavage 15
D. Maintenance of Pregnancy 15
E. Embryonic Diapause 17
V. Parturition 22
A. Overview 22
B. Role of the Corpus Luteum 23
C. Role of the Pituitary 26
D. Role of the Fetus and/or Placenta 27
E. Mammary Gland Development 28
VI. Conclusions 29
References 30

[1] Present address: ARC Institute of Animal Physiology, Animal Research Station, 307 Huntingdon Road, Cambridge CB3 OJQ, England.

Current Topics in Experimental Endocrinology, Vol. 4

ISBN 0-12-153204-6

I. Introduction

Comparatively little is known about the endocrinology of reproduction in marsupials and very few of the 249 known species have been studied in any detail. This is probably because, until quite recently, marsupials were considered to be little more than a curiosity. However, recent interest in their reproduction in its own right, a realization of the general importance of the modes of reproduction they have evolved, and an appreciation of the economic and ecological importance of these species have all led to a reawakening of interest in marsupial reproduction (Renfree, 1981). As a result, a number of new and often unexpected insights have been generated in recent years.

Because many readers may not be familiar with the different species of marsupial which have been investigated, Table I lists the common and generic names of the species considered in this article. The common names will be used throughout the text.

The discovery, in 1954, of embryonic diapause in two island-dwelling marsupials, the quokka from Rottnest Island, Western Australia (Sharman, 1954, 1955a) and the tammar wallaby from Garden Island, Western Australia (Sharman, 1955b) stimulated considerable interest in the reproduction of marsupials which, until then, had been largely neglected. A series of comprehensive reviews provide the interested reader with a summary of the mainly descriptive work which followed during the 1960's (Sharman, 1959, 1965c, 1970; Waring *et al.,* 1966; Sharman *et al.,* 1966). As a result of these studies, it was possible to make a number of broad generalizations regarding the reproductive patterns exhibited by marsupials.

Most marsupials are polyestrous. All species ovulate spontaneously and have active corpora lutea which induce a distinct luteal phase. Pregnancy is brief, is accommodated within a single estrous cycle, and subsequent cycles are suppressed during the relatively long period of lactation.

Four broad patterns of reproduction can be distinguished according to the relationship between length of gestation, estrous cycle, and the pattern of lactational inhibition of reproductive activity (Tyndale-Biscoe, 1982). However, all but a few species exhibit one or other of the two basic patterns illustrated in Fig. 1. In the first pattern of reproduction (Fig. 1a), which is found in the majority of species, the females are polytocous or monotocous and the gestation period is considerably shorter than the estrous cycle. Parturition coincides with the decline of the corpora lutea and proestrous, estrous, and ovulation are suppressed during lactation. The best known examples of this group are the polytocous American opossum (Hartman, 1923; Reynolds, 1952) and the monotocous Australian brushtail possum (Pilton and Sharman, 1962).

Table I
The Generic and Common Names of Marsupials Considered in This Article

	Generic name	Common name
American		
Family Didelphidae	*Didelphis virginiana*	American opossum
	Philander opossum	Four-eyed opossum
Australian		
Family Dasyuridae	*Dasyurus viverrinus*	Eastern quoll (native cat)
	Antechinus stuartii	Brown antechinus
	Sminthopsis crassicaudata	Fat-tailed dunnart
Family Peramelidae	*Isoodon macrourus*	Northern brown bandicoot
	Perameles nasuta	Long-nosed bandicoot
Family Phalangeridae	*Trichosurus vulpecula*	Brushtail possum
Family Burramyidae	*Cercartetus concinnus*	Western pygmy-possum
Family Macropodidae	*Bettongia lesueur*	Burrowing bettong
	Macropus eugenii	Tammar wallaby
	M. fuliginosus	Western grey kangaroo
	M. giganteus	Eastern grey kangaroo
	M. parma	Parma wallaby
	M. parryi	Whiptail wallaby
	M. rufogriseus	Red-necked wallaby (Bennett's wallaby)
	M. rufus	Red kangaroo
	Setonix brachyurus	Quokka
	Wallabia bicolor	Swamp wallaby
Family Tarsipedidae	*Tarsipes spencerae*	Honey possum

The second pattern (Fig. 1b) is found in most of the kangaroos (Macropodidae) (see Tyndale-Biscoe *et al.*, 1974). The females are monotocous and polyestrous and the gestation period is almost the same length as the estrous cycle. Postpartum estrus and ovulation occur, but growth and development of the newly formed corpus luteum is suppressed during lactation (Fig. 1b). If conception occurs at the postpartum estrus, the embryo remains in a state of diapause as a unilaminar blastocyst until the corpus luteum resumes activity. This pattern has been investigated in the quokka, the tammar wallaby, the red-necked wallaby, the red kangaroo, and the burrowing bettong. The swamp wallaby closely resembles these except that it shows a prepartum estrus and ovulation. Four macropods, the Eastern grey kangaroo, the Western grey kangaroo, the parma wallaby, and the whiptail wallaby, show an intermediate pattern in that gestation is several days shorter than the estrous cycle so that postpartum estrus and ovulation does not occur. To this extent, these species resemble those in the first group.

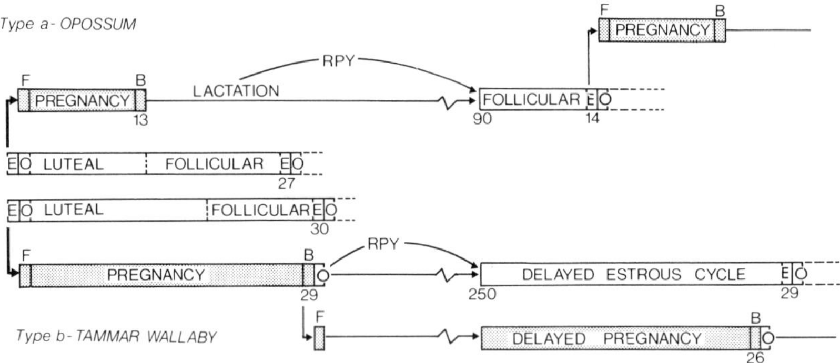

Fig. 1. Diagrammatic representation of the two commonest patterns of reproduction in marsupials. (a) The American opossum is polyestrous with a cycle of 27 days. Estrus (E) is followed by ovulation (O) and a luteal phase of about 13 days. This passes into a follicular phase of about 14 days culminating in the next estrus. Fertilization (F) occurs 1 day after estrus and pregnancy is accommodated within the luteal phase with birth (B) on day 13. The follicular phase and subsequent estrus and ovulation are supressed until the end of lactation (90 days) or until the pouch young are removed (RPY). (b) The tammar wallaby has an estrous cycle of 30 days and pregnancy is 29 days. Estrus occurs immediately after birth and postpartum ovulation 1 day later. During lactation the new corpus luteum is inhibited and, if fertilization occurred, the embryo enters diapause. Corpus luteum activity resumes at the end of lactation or after RPY. If the female is pregnant, the embryo resumes development and birth and postpartum estrus occurs 26 days after RPY—3 days sooner than in the nonpregnant female.

However, all but the Western grey kangaroo can undergo estrus during lactation resulting in the corpus luteum becoming quiescent and the embryo entering diapause.

The third pattern of reproduction is found in the bandicoots (Peramelidae). In this instance the gestation period of 12.5 days is shorter than the luteal phase and so the corpora lutea remain large throughout most of lactation. However, the corpora lutea will regress if the pouch young are experimentally removed (Gemmell, 1981). These species also have a well-developed chorioallantoic placenta, which is retained in the uterus after parturition. The best know examples of this group are the long-nosed bandicoot and the brown bandicoot.

The fourth pattern which is rare and not well understood is seen only in the honey possum and the pigmy possums (Burramyidae). These species display gestation periods of 60–80 days sometimes, but not exclusively, associated with lactation (Renfree, 1980a; Clark, 1968).

More detailed experimental studies of marsupial reproduction became possible during the 1970s as a result of the successful maintenance of a number of species in captivity. This led to a better understanding of many physiological aspects of marsupial reproduction. Species which have proven amenable to captivity include the tammar wallaby, the quokka, the American opossum, two species of bandicoot, the fat-tailed dunnart, and the brushtail possum. The tammar wallaby has proven particularly successful in this respect, which is fortunate because it also has one of the most interesting patterns of reproduction. For this reason, this species has been employed in the majority of laboratory studies. Successful hypophysectomy experiments have enabled the role of the pituitary gland to be examined (Hearn, 1973, 1974, 1975) and a range of biochemical assay methods has been employed to study placental function (Renfree, 1973a, b, 1975; Renfree and Tyndale-Biscoe, 1973b). The aspects of reproduction which have attracted most attention are the control of embryonic diapause, seasonal breeding, and maternal recogniton of pregnancy. Much of this work has been reviewed extensively in recent years (Tyndale-Biscoe, 1973, 1979, 1983; Renfree, 1980b; Amoroso *et al.*, 1980; Tyndale-Biscoe and Hinds, 1981) and so will not be discussed at length here.

This article will concentrate on a number of new developments in the area of marsupial pregnancy and parturition which have arisen largely as a result of the development of adequate assay techniques for the measurement of reproductive hormones in these species. The hormones themselves and the difficulties encountered in measuring them will be discussed first. This will be followed by a brief description of the estrous cycle. Pregnancy and parturiton will then be considered, with emphasis being placed on several of the more recent findings which bear on the endocrine control of these events.

Since most of the experimental work reviewed here has been carried out on the tammar wallaby, this species will be used to provide a basis for discussion, with results from other marsupials being introduced where appropriate. It is therefore pertinent to consider the salient features of the reproductive pattern of the tammar wallaby before proceeding. The tammar wallaby is polyestrous and monovular, with an estrous cycle of 30 days and a gestation period of 29 days (Merchant, 1979). The estrous cycle is not interrupted by pregnancy and so birth is followed almost immediately by a postpartum estrus. The embryo conceived at this postpartum estrus enters diapause in response to the suckling stimulus of the new born pouch young and/or lactation. This embryo will normally remain in diapause as a dormant blastocyst for about 11 months unless lactation is interrupted, in which case it will reactivate (see Fig. 1b). The tammar wallaby is also a seasonal breeder and is responsive to changes in photoperiod during the nonbreeding season. In their natural habitat on Kangaroo Island, South Australia, the quiescent blastocysts reactivate at the Summer solstice and all the young are born within a week or two of one another in January–February (Berger, 1966; Renfree and Tyndale-Biscoe, 1973a).

II. Hormones and Their Measurement

A major problem encountered with the measurement of marsupial reproductive hormones is that the levels of protein and steroid hormones in the peripheral circulation often appear to be unusually low when compared to the levels generally encountered in eutherians. While, in the case of the protein hormones, this may be partly due to a low cross-reactivity of the marsupial hormones to antibodies prepared against eutherian hormones, it is unlikely that this is an adequate explanation for the results obtained for the steroid hormones. The levels of the latter are extremely variable and also very low in many marsupials. For example, basal levels of progesterone in the tammar wallaby are of the order of 200 pg/ml plasma and rise to a maximum of only 1 ng/ml during the luteal phase of the estrous cycle and pregnancy (Sernia *et al.,* 1980; Hinds and Tyndale-Biscoe, 1982a). These levels are apparently due to a high metabolic clearance rate as well as a low rate of production when compared to eutherian species (Sernia *et al.,* 1980). Progesterone levels in polyovular marsupials are generally higher than those in monovular species (see for example, Fig. 6). However, apart from the tammar wallaby, the only monovular marsupials in which progesterone levels have been measured successfully are the brushtail possum (Thorburn *et al.,* 1971; Shorey and Hughes, 1973a,b) and the quokka (Cake *et al.,* 1980), while the only polyovular marsupials in which progesterone levels have been measured are the Northern brown bandicoot (Gemmell, 1979, 1981) and the American opossum (Harder and Fleming, 1981). Circulating estrogen concentrations also appear to be low in both the mono- and polyovular species although, again, the only two species in which it has been measured are the tammar wallaby (Renfree and Heap, 1977; Flint and Renfree, 1982) and the American opossum (Harder and Fleming, 1981).

The measurement of protein reproductive hormones in marsupials has proven even more difficult and a lack of highly purified marsupial protein hormones has hampered attempts to set up homologous radioimmunoassays or related types of assay. The first attempt to measure gonadotropin hormones was made by Hearn (1972, 1974) who raised an antiserum against a partially purified tammar wallaby pituitary extract. Although this assay was unable to distinguish between follicle stimulating hormone (FSH) and luteinising hormone (LH), a preovulatory peak in plasma gonadotropin concentration was detected. This suggested that the assay was likely to be more sensitive to LH than for FSH. When these experiments were undertaken, it was thought that marsupials may have possessed a single gonadotropin which had both FSH-like and LH-like biological activity. However, subsequent studies have indicated that this is unlikely to be so. For example,

Farmer and Papkoff (1974) were able to effect a partial separation of red kangaroo FSH-like and LH-like activities. A later, more comprehensive study (Gallo, *et al.*, 1978) was able to demonstrate unequivocally that there were two hormones present, although it was suggested that wallaby LH still appeared to show some intrinsic FSH-like activity. Receptor binding methods offered another approach to this problem. These assays indicated the presence of specific FSH-like and LH-like receptors on marsupial gonadal cells which had very similar properties to their eutherian counterparts (Stewart *et al.*, 1981). Furthermore, these methods indicated that the FSH-like activity detected in marsupial LH was probably due to contamination rather than to the hormone having any dual binding activity such as that seen, for example, in pregnant mare serum gonadotropin (PMSG; Stewart *et al.*, 1976).

The low yields obtained when attempting to purify these hormones and the incomplete separation of the two marsupial gonadotropins has made the development of homologous assays for LH and FSH difficult. Therefore, a number of heterologous assay systems have been investigated. Two radioimmunoassays for LH, one originally developed for the ovine and bovine hormones (Niswender *et al.*, 1969) and the other for rat LH (Welschen *et al.*, 1975), have been validated for the measurement of LH in the tammar wallaby (Sutherland *et al.*, 1980; Tyndale-Biscoe and Hearn, 1981). However, only one heterologous radioimmunoassay has been validated for marsupial FSH (Evans *et al.*, 1980) and, while this assay was able to detect FSH levels in ovariectomized females and in both intact and castrated male tammar wallabies (Catling and Sutherland, 1980), it was not sufficiently sensitive to detect FSH in intact females (Evans *et al.*, 1980). Similar results have been obtained with radioreceptor assays using both rat and marsupial receptors (Stewart *et al.*, 1981) where the LH, but not the FSH assays, were able to detect hormone levels in tammar wallaby blood. It would therefore appear that the marsupial gonadotropins and their receptors are similar to their eutherian counterparts, although there may be some minor antigenic differences between the hormones. Peripheral FSH levels also appear to be unusually low in the tammar wallaby.

Attempts have also been made to assay for prolactin in marsupials, mainly as a result of the suggestion (Tyndale-Biscoe and Hawkins, 1977) that this hormone may have a role in inhibiting the corpus luteum and in maintaining embryonic diapause. An homologous assay for grey kangaroo prolactin has been described (Farmer *et al.*, 1981), but, while this assay appeared to be quite specific for purified fractions of Eastern grey kangaroo and tammar wallaby prolactin, it could not detect prolactin in plasma from either species. Several heterologous assays for prolactin using antisera raised to ovine or bovine prolactin have been tested without success (Farmer *et al.,* 1981; Hinds and Tyndale-Biscoe, 1982b) but recently, an assay developed by McNeilly and Friesen (1978) for rabbit prolactin has been applied successfully to the measurement of prolactin levels in tammar wallaby plasma (Hinds and Tyndale-Biscoe, 1982b).

Prostaglandin F2α, detected by assay of its major metabolite, 13,14-dihydro-15-keto-prostaglandin F2α (PGFM) has been found in appreciable quantities at parturition in the bandicoot (Gemmell *et al.,* 1980) but was only elevated above basal levels in tammar wallabies immediately after parturition (Tyndale-Biscoe *et al.,* 1982) and was not elevated in brushtail possums at any stage (G. Jenkin, personal communication).

In summary, although the marsupial hormones appear to be basically very similar to their eutherian counterparts, some may differ functionally (Tyndale-Biscoe and Hinds, 1981). This will become apparent in the following sections on the estrous cycle, pregnancy, and parturition.

III. Estrous Cycle

The length of the estrous cycle in marsupials is similar to that generally observed in eutherians and ranges from 21 days in the burrowing bettong (Tyndale-Biscoe, 1968) to 45 days in the Eastern grey kangaroo (Poole and Catling, 1974). Most herbivorous marsupials, including the macropodids, are monovular and ovulation is thought to occur on alternate ovaries during successive cycles (Tyndale-Biscoe, 1983). Among the polyovular species there is a range of ovulation rates, with the opossums shedding 20 or more eggs at each ovulation (Hartman, 1921; Hill, 1918) while other species, such as the bandicoots (Lyne and Hollis, 1979) and pigmy possums (Burramyidae), shed 6 or less (Clark, 1967)

A. Follicular Development and Ovulation

Hypophysectomy experiments in the tammar wallaby have demonstrated that the pituitary gland has an important role in maintaining ovarian function. Both follicular development and ovulation were blocked after removal of the pituitary (Hearn, 1973, 1974) and 60 days after the operation the ovaries had decreased in size to about half their initial weight and contained no follicles greater than 0.5 mm in diameter (Hearn, 1975). Although attempts to measure peripheral levels of FSH have been unsuccessful (Section II), there seems to be little doubt that this hormone is responsible for follicular development in this and other marsupials (Evans *et al.,* 1980).

Figure 2 summarizes the relationship between estrus, mating, and ovulation in the tammar wallaby. Estrus lasts about 8 hours and, during this time, mating may take place several times. About 8 hours after the onset of estrus there is a sharp peak of pituitary LH (Sutherland *et al.*, 1980). This peak lasts for about 8 hours and ovulation takes place 20 to 40 hours later (Sutherland *et al.*, 1980). Thus, the endocrine control of ovulation in marsupials appears to conform to the pattern observed in eutherians.

The formation of the corpus luteum has been studied in a number of marsupials and most authors agree that only the granulosa cells of the follicle, and not the thecal cells, become luteinized to form the corpus luteum (Tyndale-Biscoe, 1983).

Mitoses are observed in marsupial corpora lutea during the first few days after ovulation, in the same way as is commonly found in eutherians. Subsequent growth of the marsupial corpus luteum to its full size derives from hypertrophy of the luteal cells which is the same as in eutherians. There is, however, an interesting feature found in marsupials in which embryonic diapause occurs and this relates to the growth of the corpus luteum when it is reactivated after a period of quiescence which may be as long as 11 months. In the three species which have been studied in detail, the quokka (Tyndale-Biscoe, 1963a), the red kangaroo (Sharman, 1965a), and the tammar wallaby (Sharman and Berger, 1969), the luteal cells undergo a transient period of cell division 4 to 6 days after reactivation of the dormant corpus luteum and

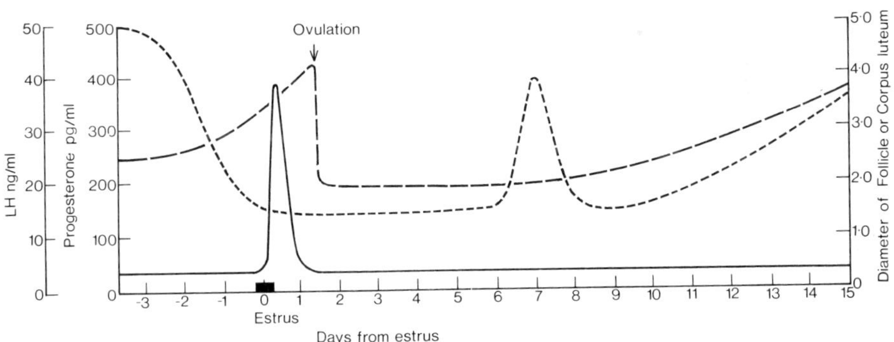

Fig. 2. The time relationship (days) between the decline in plasma progesterone (----), estrus, the preovulatory LH peak (——), and ovulation (↓) in the tammar wallaby. Ovarian events are shown as the mean diameter (mm) of the preovulatory follicle until its collapse at ovulation and then as the mean diameter of the newly formed corpus luteum (----). Note the transient peak of progesterone on day 7 postestrus without a corresponding change in size of the corpus luteum but the correlation of both subsequently. (Based on data in Hinds and Tyndale-Biscoe, 1982a; Sutherland *et al.*, 1980; Tyndale-Biscoe and Rodger, 1978; Tyndale-Biscoe *et al.*, 1982.)

blastocyst. This phenomenon will be discussed in more detail in Section IV,E).

B. Progesterone Levels

Cook and Nalbandov (1968) were the first to identify progesterone as the main steroid synthesized by marsupial luteal tissue *in vitro*. Peripheral progesterone levels were subsequently measured in several species throughout the estrous cycle and the profiles as well as the peak levels varied considerably. Levels in the brushtail possum (Thorburn *et al.*, 1971; Shorey and Hughes, 1973a) were hardly distinguishable from anestrus levels during the first week after ovulation. These levels rose to a maximum of 4.5 ng/ml at day 12 of the estrous cycle and had declined to basal levels by day 20. These values have recently been independently confirmed by radioimmunoassay (L. A. Hinds, R. T. Gemmell, and J. Curlewis, personal communications). A similar pattern was observed in the American opossum which is polyovular, but in this case somewhat higher peak values (around 16 ng/ml) were observed (Harder and Fleming, 1981). On the other hand, the tammar wallaby had extremely low levels and a quite different profile (Lemon, 1972). During the first half of the cycle progesterone was barely detectable (at less than 200 pg/ml), although a small but significant peak of about 500 pg/ml occurred at around day 6 (Hinds and Tyndale-Biscoe, 1982a). The likely significance of this peak is discussed in Sections IV,D,1 and IV,E. Progesterone levels then rose steadily to a maximum of about 1 ng/ml at day 20, followed by a rapid decline to basal levels just prior to estrus at day 28. There are no data on progesterone levels during the estrous cycle of bandicoots, but Gemmell (1981) considered it unlikely that they would be different from the levels observed during pregnancy (see Fig. 6).

C. The Corpus Luteum

Although LH appears to stimulate ovulation in the tammar wallaby (Sutherland *et al.*, 1980), the corpus luteum, once formed, does not appear to depend on a luteotrophic stimulus for progesterone secretion. In the tammar wallaby, quiescent corpora lutea will reactivate and follow a normal life span in the complete absence of the pituitary gland (Hearn, 1974) and the rate of progesterone secretion by luteal tissue *in vitro* is unchanged by incubation with LH (Sernia *et al.*, 1980). These observations are supported by the finding that the corpora lutea of the tammar wallaby and the red kangaroo appear to be devoid of LH receptors, even though follicular and testicular tissues from the same species possess abundant LH receptors

(Stewart and Tyndale-Biscoe, 1982). However, some preliminary evidence suggests that this latter phenomenon may be restricted to the Macropodidae, since receptors for LH were found on the corpora lutea of brushtail possums (Stewart and Tyndale-Biscoe, 1982). In the possum the corpora lutea grow and maintain pregnancy after adenohypophysectomy, but the peak level of progesterone was then less than in sham-operated controls (Tyndale-Biscoe, Horn, and Hinds, unpublished results).

The fixed life span of the corpus luteum is not prolonged by hysterectomy in either the American opossum (Hartman, 1925a) or the brushtail possum (Clark and Sharman, 1965). This suggests that the marsupial corpus luteum is not under the influence of a uterine luteolysin. Irradiation of the ovaries of the possum also failed to prolong the life of the corpus luteum, from which Cook *et al.* (1977) concluded that estrogen from the ovarian follicles was not luteolytic. However, as illustrated in Fig. 1a, the presence of a fetus hastens the decline of the corpus luteum and the onset of estrus and ovulation in the tammar wallaby (Merchant, 1979). This will be discussed in Section V,D.

The corpus luteum also seems to provide a negative feedback to the pituitary during the early phase of the estrous cycle. Ablation of the corpus luteum during the first 12 days of the estrous cycle in the tammar wallaby resulted in premature estrus and ovulation 9 to 18 days later (Tyndale-Biscoe and Hawkins, 1977) but after day 12 did not. Likewise Gemmell (1981) has observed that removal of the corpus luteum and young in the bandicoot immediately after parturition leads to premature ovulation 10 days later. Progesterone is the major product of the corpus luteum (Renfree *et al.,* 1979) but, since its output only begins to rise coincident with follicle growth after day 12, it is unlikely that progesterone could be the inhibitory agent. Ovarian cortex transplanted into ovariectomized tammars reversed the rise in plasma LH and FSH that otherwise occurs after ovariectomy (Evans *et al.,* 1980; Tyndale-Biscoe and Hearn, 1981). These observations imply that estrogen rather than progesterone may be the inhibitor and the finding of estrogen in phenolic extracts of marsupial corpora lutea by Renfree and Heap (1977) may be significant in this regard.

A further point of interest with respect to marsupial corpora lutea is their relaxin content which will be considered further in Section V.

IV. Pregnancy

A. Relevant Anatomy

Although their name is derived from it, not all marsupials possess a "marsupium" or pouch and so it is not this anatomical feature which actually distinguishes Marsupialia from other mammals. However, one striking and distinguishing feature of marsupials is the relationship between their urinary and genital ducts. In marsupials the urinary ducts pass mesially to the genital tracts, whereas those of eutherians pass laterally (Sharman, 1965c, 1970; Tyndale-Biscoe, 1973). The marsupial female reproductive tract therefore consists of two separate uteri which open into a median vaginal cul-de-sac by way of entirely separate cervical canals (Fig. 3). There are also three vaginas. In addition to the median vagina, there are two lateral vaginas through which the spermatazoa travel at insemination (Fig. 3). Many male marsupials have a bifurcated glans penis, the right and left prongs apparently being placed in the corresponding lateral vaginal canals during copulation (Sharman, 1970). All three vaginas merge with the urinary ducts to form the urogenital sinus, which leads to a single outlet, the cloaca. Birth takes place through the median vagina which is always occluded with connective tissue prior to the first birth. In some species this birth canal remains patent after the first birth, but in others the connective tissue reforms after each birth. The remainder of the reproductive organs of marsupials generally resemble their eutherian counterparts.

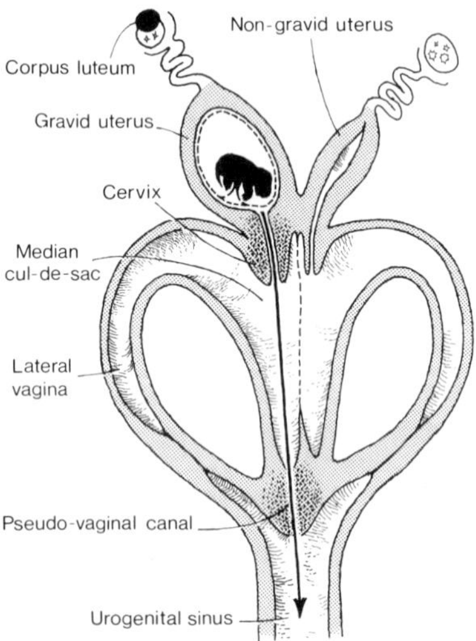

Fig. 3. Diagram of the urogenital tract of the female marsupial to show the two uteri each with a separate cervix opening into the vaginal cul-de-sac. From this chamber, two lateral vaginas pass around the ureters to join the urogenital sinus posteriorly. At copulation semen traverses these two canals but at parturition the fetus passes through the median pseudovaginal canal formed *de novo* at this time.

B. Conception

The length of estrus varies from a few hours in the kangaroos and wallabies to several days in the monoestrous marsupials such as Antechinus. In the tammar wallaby, estrus lasts for about 8 hours and mating takes place many times with several different males (Tyndale-Biscoe and Rodger, 1978). As a result, the lateral vaginas increase in size enormously and become distended with semen and vaginal secretions. This was originally thought to be an adaptation for sperm storage, but subsequent studies have shown that this is not the case because sperm do not remain in the macropodid or didelphid reproductive tract for more than a few days (Sharman, 1955a,b; Tyndale-Biscoe and Rodger, 1978; Godfrey, 1975). However, sperm are retained for long periods in the median vaginas of bandicoots (Lyne, 1976).

In those species in which postpartum mating occurs, copulation takes place within a few hours, or at most days, of birth. Furthermore, in these species there is an unequal distribution of spermatozoa between the two uteri. In quokka reproductive tracts examined soon after mating, abundant spermatozoa were found in the uterus associated with imminent ovulation, but virtually none in the parturient uterus. This was thought to be indicative of a differential transport of sperm in favor of the ovulating side (Tyndale-Biscoe, 1963a). More extensive studies in the tammar wallaby have indicated that this effect is probably due to a failure of sperm transport in the recently pregnant side of the tract, rather than to an attraction of sperm to the ovulating side (Tyndale-Biscoe and Rodger, 1978). This may arise as a consequence of the continued flow of secretions through the recently pregnant uterus. The uneven distribution of spermatozoa between uteri is established at the level of the cervix and, on the ovulation side, provides a reservoir of spermatozoa for 24 hours after copulation, by which time ovulation is about to occur (Tyndale-Biscoe and Rodger, 1978).

Ovulation is spontaneous in all the marsupials studied to date and there is no evidence that copulation or other stimuli are necessary for the shedding of eggs.

The surface layers of marsupial eggs are unusual (see Fig. 4). In addition to the zona pellucida, which is common to all mammalian eggs, the marsupial egg is surrounded by a mucin layer secreted by the oviduct and in which the sperm become trapped (Hughes, 1974). While such a layer is not unknown in eutherians, it is comparatively rare. The composition of the mucin layer is analogous to that seen on rabbit eggs and consists chiefly of acidic mucopolysaccharides (Hughes and Shorey, 1973). As the egg passes through the lower segment of the oviduct, a third outer shell membrane is laid down (Fig. 4). This keratinous shell is unique to the marsupials and is

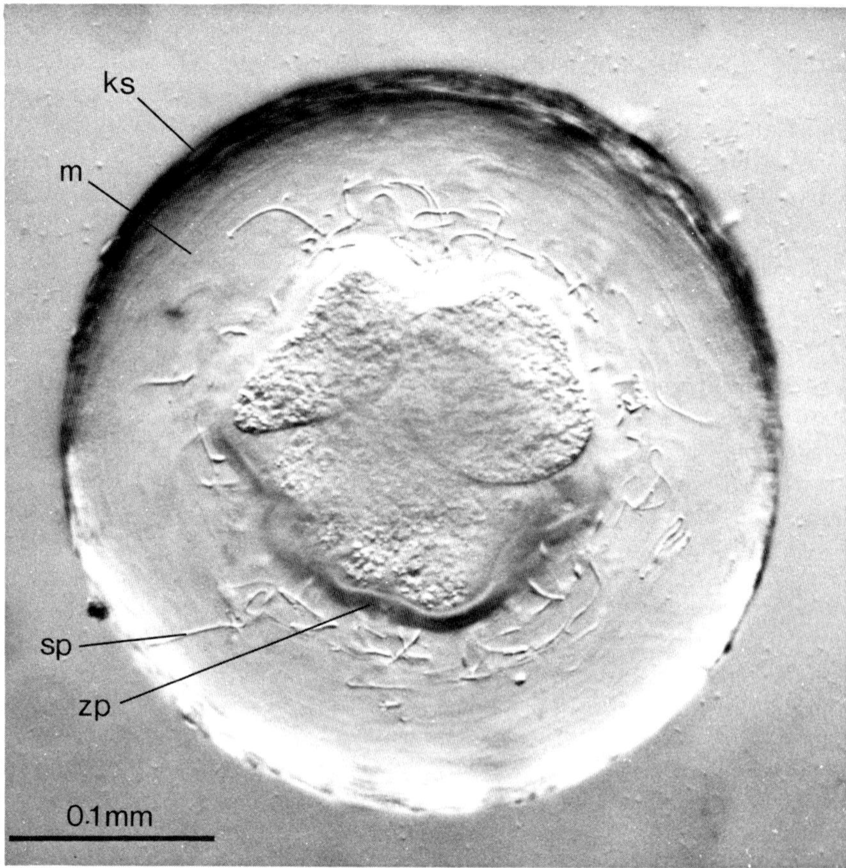

Fig. 4. Photograph of a living four cell egg collected from the uterus of an Eastern grey kangaroo (diameter 0.29 mm), to show the outer keratin shell membrane (ks), the mucin layer (m) containing numerous sperm (sp), and the zona pellucida (zp) investing the cleaving egg; three of the four cells are visible. Scale = 0.1 mm.

thought to be analogous to the basal layer of the leathery shell of monotreme and reptile eggs. It is secreted by cells of the lower segment of the oviduct and uterus and is resistant to enzyme digestion (Hughes, 1974). It may play a role in protecting the blastocyst during diapause. This shell has somewhat unusual properties, being inelastic and yet capable of great dilation.

Tubal transport is rapid and in the four species adequately studied, it has been shown that the fertilized egg takes about a day to reach the uterus (Renfree and Tyndale-Biscoe, 1978). This is rapid compared to eutherians where eggs generally take several days to cover this distance.

C. Cleavage

In many marsupials the rate of cleavage of the fertilized ovum is unusually slow and it has been suggested that this may be related to the occurrence of embryonic diapause (Tyndale-Biscoe, 1979). For example, blastocyst formation takes 8 days in the tammar wallaby (which displays embryonic diapause) but only 4 days in bandicoots (Lyne and Hollis, 1977) and the American opossum (McCrady, 1938), neither of which displays embryonic diapause. Selwood (1981) has shown that the cleavage rate in the brown antechinus is even slower than in the tammar and this species also displays a delay in development (Selwood, 1980). Consequently, there does appear to be a link between cleavage rate and embryonic diapause but it remains to be tested rigorously.

In addition to the slow rate of cleavage, the preattachment phase of pregnancy is relatively long in marsupials and, since embryonic diapause (when present) occurs during this phase, it is often extended to encompass a considerably longer interval of time than the attachment phase. By contrast, expansion and organogenesis are both very rapid and it takes only a few days for the blastocyst to develop into a fully formed neonate, which is capable of climbing unaided into its mother's pouch (Hughes, 1974; Renfree and Tyndale-Biscoe, 1978).

D. Maintenance of Pregnancy

1. The Corpus Luteum

Little is known about maintenance of pregnancy in the polyovular marsupials, but, in the monovular species, such as the macropods, the single corpus luteum appears to provide all the progesterone that is necessary to maintain active pregnancy. Furthermore, it is during the first week of pregnancy that the corpus luteum appears to be most important, even though the peripheral progesterone concentration is quite low at this time. Experiments in the tammar wallaby, brushtail possum, and quokka have all demonstrated that, although the corpus luteum is essential for the first few days of gestation, ovariectomy or lutectomy after days 7 or 8 does not influence fetal development to full term. However, parturition fails in these animals (Tyndale-Biscoe, 1963b, 1970; Sharman, 1965b; Sharman and Berger, 1969; Young and Renfree, 1979). Similarly, quiescent blastocysts transferred to tammar wallabies immediately after ovariectomy on day 8 of the estrous cycle reactivate and develop normally (Tyndale-Biscoe, 1970). Exogenous progesterone will also initiate reactivation and maintain pregnancy in the absence of an active corpus luteum (Renfree and Tyndale-Biscoe, 1973a; Clark, 1968). Thus, once the luteal phase is established, the endometrium appears capable of maintaining embryo development without further stimulation by the corpus luteum.

Recent studies involving the *in vitro* incubation of corpora lutea and measurement of peripheral progesterone levels have yielded some interesting results with regard to luteal function during early pregnancy in macropods. Tammar wallaby corpora lutea collected on day 5 of the estrous cycle or pregnancy secreted significantly more progesterone *in vitro* than those collected on days 0, 9, and 16 (Hinds *et al.,* 1983). This transitory period of enhanced luteal activity was subsequently supported by the observation of a sharp peak in peripheral progesterone levels at day 5, 6, or 7 after reactivation of the corpus luteum in both pregnant and nonpregnant animals (Hinds and Tyndale-Biscoe, 1982a; Figs. 2 and 6). A similar peak has been demonstrated at around day 5 of pregnancy in the quokka, but, unlike the tammar wallaby, this peak was absent in three nonpregnant animals and Cake *et al.* (1980) concluded that this pulse was initiated by the embryo in some way. This is not the case in the tammar wallaby and further work is needed to clarify this point in the quokka. This pulse of steroidogenesis coincides with a surge of mitotic activity in the luteal cells of both species (Tyndale-Biscoe, 1963a; Sharman and Berger, 1969) and, since it gives rise to the only significant increase in peripheral progesterone levels during the first week of pregnancy, it probably represents the essential contribution which the corpus luteum makes to the maintenance of early pregnancy. Its possible role in the reactivation of quiescent blastocysts is discussed in Section IV,E. In all species examined plasma progesterone increased to reach a maximum in the latter part of pregnancy (see Fig. 6).

2. The Placenta

Because gestation is so short in marsupials and because pregnancy appeared to have little or no endocrine influence on the mother, marsupials were long considered to be aplacental (Sharman, 1970). However, this is certainly not the case and, while most marsupial placentas are termed "primitive" (in that the only fetal component involved is the yolk sac membrane) there is at least one family, the Peramelidae (bandicoots), in which a functional chorioallantoic placenta is formed (Hill, 1897).

Attempts have been made to infer an evolutionary sequence between the metatherian and eutherian placental types, but it is fairly obvious that both the yolk sac and chorioallantoic placentas of marsupials have evolved independently from those of Eutheria. First, the marsupial yolk sac placenta is unique in that the yolk sac membrane completely surrounds the allantois and apparently carries out the respiratory functions which, in eutherians, are performed by the allantois (Renfree, 1973b, 1980b). Second, the bandicoot chorioallantoic placenta displays a remarkable feature which distinguishes it completely from all other placentas when, during the last few days of its 12.5 day gestation, the trophoblastic layer disappears completely, apparently by a process involving fusion between fetal and maternal cells (Padykula and Taylor, 1976, 1977).

There is little doubt that the trophoblastic attachment seen in both the yolk sac and the chorioallantoic placentas of marsupials is not merely a means of anchoring fetal to maternal tissues.

Initially, it was believed that the increase in weight of the gravid compared to nongravid uterus was due simply to the bulk of the embryo occupying it. However, subsequent studies in the tammar wallaby revealed a considerable increase in endometrial mass of the gravid uterus (Renfree, 1972; Renfree and Tyndale-Biscoe, 1973a). It was suggested that this could be due to either an immunological response or to a hormone of fetal or placental origin (Renfree, 1972). The most likely hormone to cause such a reaction is progesterone and, although the yolk sac placenta has a low synthetic ability *in vitro* (<2% conversion of pregnenelone to progesterone for the quokka and tammar wallaby; Bradshaw *et al.,* 1975; Renfree and Young, 1979), it actively metabolizes other steroids (Heap *et al.,* 1980). The low steroidogenic activity of the placenta *in vitro* is in accord with the observation that peripheral levels of progesterone are not elevated during pregnancy in the tammar wallaby (Hinds and Tyndale-Biscoe, 1982a) or quokka (Cake *et al.,* 1980).

Therefore, although the endocrine activity of the marsupial placenta may be limited and effective only at the local level, it may well play an important endocrine role in maintaining pregnancy.

E. Embryonic Diapause

Embryonic diapause in marsupials is restricted almost entirely to the macropodids. The only nonmacropodid marsupials in which diapause has been observed are the Western pigmy-possum (Clark, 1967) and the honey possum (Renfree, 1980a), whereas the only macropod in which it has not been found to date is the Western grey kangaroo (Poole, 1975). Embryonic diapause generally arises because the presence of a newborn young in the pouch prevents development of the zygote past the blastocyst stage. This can take place only when the gestation period and the estrous cycle are of similar length so that conception takes place immediately after (or, in rare instances, immediately before) parturition. When, as is found in most nonmacropodid marsupials, the gestation period is much shorter than the estrous cycle, lactation is well established, and this prevents the postpartum estrus.

Less commonly, embryonic diapause can be initiated and controlled by seasonal factors as well. This is observed in Bennett's wallaby and in the tammar wallaby, where embryos can enter diapause without the presence of a suckling young in the pouch, provided that conception takes place in the Winter months (July–December in the Southern Hemisphere). This phenomenon is termed "seasonal quiescence" to distinguish it from the more general "lactational quiescence" (Sharman and Berger, 1969; Tyndale-Biscoe *et al.*, 1974).

It is important to realize that macropodid marsupials can enter a state of reproductive quiescence whether or not they are actually carrying a blastocyst. In the absence of a blastocyst, quiescence still manifests itself in characteristic changes in the corpus luteum which are discussed below.

Apart from a variety of hormonal treatments and surgical procedures described below, the dormant blastocyst can be reactivated in a number of ways. Removal or death of the suckling pouch young during lactation or departure of the pouch young at the end of lactation will cause reactivation during lactational quiescence, while, in the tammar wallaby, a change in photoperiod will initiate reactivation during the period of seasonal quiescence (Sadleir and Tyndale-Biscoe, 1977).

During quiescence, peripheral progesterone levels remain at less than 200 pg/ml (Tyndale-Biscoe and Hinds, 1981) but 7 days after reactivation there is a short transient peak (Fig. 2). When tammar wallabies were experimentally induced to reactivate during seasonal quiescence by altering the photoperiod, the same transient peak occurred about 7 days after the change in photoperiod (L. A. Hinds and R. von Ottolander, personal communication). The occurrence of the transient peak at the time when the corpus luteum is essential for pregnancy to continue suggests that it may have a role in reactivation, but this has yet to be tested experimentally.

Maintenance of Diapause

The maintenance of embryonic diapause in marsupials is more a matter of suppression of reactivation rather than an active process of maintenance. It would appear that development of the embryo past the blastocyst stage is prevented by a lack of uterine secretions which, in turn, are not being produced or released because of a lack of progesterone. Low levels of progesterone are maintained by a tonic suppression of the corpus luteum and some recent work suggests that this inhibitor may be prolactin (Tyndale-Biscoe and Hawkins, 1977; Tyndale-Biscoe and Hinds, 1981).

The endocrine control of embryonic diapause has been investigated in detail only in the tammar wallaby, which exhibits both lactational and seasonal forms of control. Since there appear to be significant differences between the mechanisms controlling these two types of diapause, they will be considered separately.

a. Lactational Quiescence. Sharman (1965b) established in the red kangaroo that the proximate stimulus that maintains quiescence is the frequency of suckling. He concluded that this was mediated by oxytocin, since injection of oxytocin prolonged quiescence after the removal of young (Sharman, 1965a). This idea was followed up by Renfree (1979) who denervated the suckling mammary glands of tammar wallabies. The operation did not influence the subsequent course of lactation, but it did remove the inhibition upon the corpora lutea, which resumed growth and supported pregnancies. Hearn (1974) had shown that the pituitary was involved, since corpora lutea resumed growth immediately after hypophysectomy, but his results did not differentiate between the two parts of the pituitary. Repeating Sharman's (1965a) experiment in tammar wallabies, Tyndale-Biscoe and Hawkins (1977) were able to delay corpus luteum development with both oxytocin and prolactin, but only prolactin was effective after hypophysectomy. From these several results it would appear that suckling increases prolactin secretion from the pituitary which, in turn, inhibits corpus luteum growth and/or the rate of progesterone secretion. The observation that tammar wallaby corpora lutea contain high concentrations of prolactin receptors (Sernia and Tyndale-Biscoe, 1979) but no LH receptors (Stewart and Tyndale-Biscoe, 1982) (see Fig. 5), led to the proposal that prolactin might act directly on the corpus luteum to suppress progesterone secretion. *In vitro* studies by Sernia *et al.* (1980) and Hinds *et al.* (1983) have failed to show any effect of prolactin or LH on steroidogenesis by luteal tissue and so the conclusion must be that prolactin inhibits the growth of the corpus luteum, and that the change in the total mass of luteal tissue is sufficient to account for the rise in peripheral progesterone concentration.

Experiments using bromocriptine, a specific inhibitor of prolactin secretion, have added further weight to the proposal that prolactin is the inhibitor of luteal function. A single injection of bromocriptine during lactational quiescence caused reactivation followed by the birth of a second pouch young which, in some cases, was able to attach itself to one of the unoccupied teats in the pouch (Tyndale-Biscoe, 1979; Tyndale-Biscoe and Hinds, 1981). However, the newborn young did not survive for very long, probably due to the presence of the much larger first-born young in the pouch. Subsequent determination of prolactin levels in these animals demonstrated that the action of prolactin and also possibly the action of bromocriptine appeared to be quite different in the tammar wallaby to that observed in eutherian mammals. First, prolactin levels were low in females during the early stages of lactation and were indistinguishable from nonlactating animals (Hinds and Tyndale-Biscoe, 1982b). Second, the injections of bromocriptine which gave rise to reactivation produced no change in prolactin levels (Tyndale-Biscoe and Hinds, 1983). This has led to the suggestion that, in marsupials, bromocriptine may act directly on the corpus luteum rather than as an inhibitor of prolactin secretion.

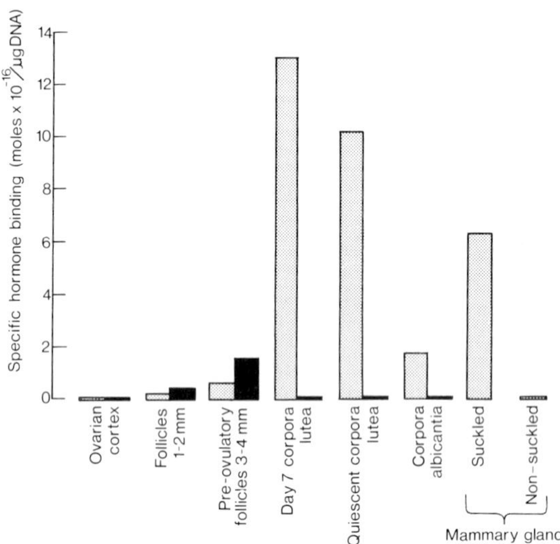

Fig. 5. Specific hormone binding (expressed as moles $\times$ $10^{-16}/\mu g$ DNA) for prolactin (hatched columns) and luteinizing hormone (solid columns) in ovarian tissues, corpora lutea, and mammary glands of the tammar wallaby. Note the absence of LH receptors and abundance of prolactin receptors in corpora lutea. Also the difference in receptor concentration between suckled and nonsuckled mammary glands in the same animals. (Data from Stewart and Tyndale-Biscoe, 1982.)

b. Seasonal Quiescence. As in lactational quiescence, removal of the pituitary will cause reactivation during seasonal quiescence (Hearn, 1974). Similarly, daily injections of prolactin after hypophysectomy will delay the reactivation (Tyndale-Biscoe and Hawkins, 1977). However, unlike the situation in lactational quiescence, the sham hypophysectomy operation (which was always performed as a control) often leads to reactivation during seasonal quiescence (Tyndale-Biscoe and Hawkins, 1977). The reason for this difference is unknown. This and several other differences between the two types of quiescence suggest that the underlying control mechanisms are different in each case.

Peripheral prolactin levels are considerably higher during seasonal quiescence compared to lactational quiescence, but doses of bromocriptine as high as 125 to 1250 times greater than that which was effective in the anestrous ewe (Niswender, 1974; McNeilly and Land, 1979) had no effect on the corpus luteum and did not significantly alter the circulating prolactin levels in tammar wallabies (Tyndale-Biscoe and Hinds, 1983). This again indicated that, in marsupials, bromocriptine does not appear to inhibit prolactin secretion.

Under natural conditions, reactivation takes place in the tammar wallaby around the Summer solstice. The observation that peripheral prolactin levels dropped from around 50–100 to less than 20 ng/ml at the Summer solstice provides further strong circumstantial evidence for a role of prolactin in maintaining quiescence. However, bromocriptine was again ineffective at this time, even though 2 months later it produced reactivation in the same animals (then in lactational quiescence) when peripheral prolactin levels were similar (Tyndale-Biscoe and Hinds, 1983). Therefore, the lack of response to bromocriptine during seasonal quiescence was almost certainly not due to the higher prolactin levels generally present at this time.

One possibility was that the concentration of prolactin receptor sites on the cells of the corpus luteum might vary through the year and hence influence the response to varying levels of prolactin. However, no difference could be detected in receptor concentration between 3- and 8-month-old corpora lutea nor between corpora lutea taken during lactational or seasonal quiescence (Stewart and Tyndale-Biscoe, 1982). It has been recognized for some time that involvement of photoperiod in seasonal quiescence, with its onset at the Winter solstice and its close at the Summer solstice, implicates the pineal gland. Kennaway and Seamark (1976) reported a significant difference in the level of hydroxyindole methyltransferase in pineals of female tammar wallabies collected three nights after the Summer solstice and, more recently, Renfree *et al.* (1981) showed that excision of the superior cervical ganglia in female tammar wallabies before the Winter solstice (which presumably denervated their pineal glands) abolished the nocturnal rise in plasma melatonin and abolished seasonal quiescence. It is not known what effect this treatment had on prolactin levels. Table II summarizes the several factors known to influence quiescence in the tammar wallaby.

c. Conclusions. The maintenance of embryonic diapause in marsupials is rather complex and many aspects are poorly understood. Although the

Table II
Factors Leading to Reactivation during Lactational and Seasonal Quiescence in the Tammar Wallaby

Lactational quiescence (summer to winter solstice)	Seasonal quiescence (winter to summer solstice)
Removal of pouch young	Decrease in photoperiod
Denervation of suckled mammary gland	Denervation of pineal gland
Hypophysectomy	Hypophysectomy
	Adenohypophysectomy
—	Sham hypophysectomy
Bromocriptine (1 injection 5 mg/kg)	—

evidence implicating prolactin as the inhibitor of luteal function is very strong, there are also a number of puzzling inconsistencies and contradictions. These conflicting results may reflect a basic difference between the action of prolactin in marsupials as compared to eutherians and illustrate the dangers inherent in extrapolating knowledge gained in one species in an attempt to solve problems in another. There may also be many other, as yet unexplored endocrine factors involved in this complex problem.

V. Parturition

A. Overview

Marsupials give birth to minute young, which range in weight from less than 4 mg in the honey possum (Renfree, 1980a) to 750 mg in the largest kangaroos (Poole, 1975). Yet these offspring reach the pouch region unaided and become firmly attached each to one teat. Despite these differences from eutherian mammals, which deliver much larger offspring, there is growing evidence that parturition and the initiation of lactation are under similar endocrine controls in marsupials as those found in eutherians. In marsupials, the corpus luteum and both parts of the pituitary are critically involved and, in some species, the fetus or the placenta may determine the time of birth. The evidence for these endocrine controls will be considered first, in relation to the preparation of the genital tract and mammary gland for birth, second, in relation to the initiation of parturition, and finally in relation to the control of early lactation.

As described in detail in Section IV (Fig. 3), the Müllerian ducts of the female marsupial do not fuse posteriorly to form a single vagina and cervix, but instead two lateral vaginas surround the ureters and become secondarily fused anteriorly as a median vaginal cul-de-sac into which the two uteri open (Fig. 3). At parturition, the yolk sac membranes rupture, the fetus leaves the uterus, passes into the cul-de-sac, and then forsaking the lateral vaginas, continues directly through the connective tissue that joins the posterior wall of the cul-de-sac to the anterior wall of the urogenital sinus and thence to the exterior. In the honey possum and most kangaroos this pseudovaginal canal remains patent after the first parturition and becomes lined with epithelium. But in all other marsupials the rough tear is rapidly repaired so that, a few days after birth, no evidence of the canal remains (Hill, 1899). In the American opossum and in the brushtail possum the region where the pseudovaginal canal will form becomes loose-textured prior to parturition and the cervices become soft and edematous. These changes are not observed after ovariectomy, but exogenous progesterone will induce loosening in the pseudovaginal region (Risman, 1947; Tyndale-Biscoe, 1966).

There are also quite marked changes in the pouch region and in the mammary glands prior to parturition. The skin becomes granulomatous and exudes a moist, clear secretion and the teats become turgid and each one develops an apical button-like protuberance which the neonatus can grasp in its mouth. The apparent role of the corpus luteum in effecting these changes is discussed in Section V,E. Finally, in several species that have been observed throughout parturition, such as the red kangaroo (Sharman and Calaby, 1964) and the bandicoot (Lyne, 1974), the female undergoes a distinct sequence of postures and behavioral patterns which is not seen in nonpregnant females and so may have an underlying endocrine basis.

B. Role of the Corpus Luteum

Ovariectomy in late pregnancy of the polytocous opossum prevented parturition (Hartman, 1925b; Renfree, 1974) as did removal of the corpus luteum, or the ovary bearing it, in the monotocous brushtail possum (Sharman, 1965a) and quokka (Tyndale-Biscoe, 1963b). In most instances in all these species the fetuses had reached full term and were dead, either still inside the uterus, or, more commonly, in the vaginal cul-de-sac. The importance of the corpus luteum was further demonstrated in the tammar wallaby when gestation was induced with progesterone during seasonal quiescence (Renfree and Tyndale-Biscoe, 1973a). In this instance, the animals were intact, but their corpora lutea remained inactive during seasonal quiescence. Although the fetuses reached full term, all but one died in the uterus or cul-de-sac. These results all indicate that an active corpus luteum must be present late in pregnancy to prepare the genital tract and, especially the pseudovaginal region, for birth. In the tammar wallaby, Young and Renfree (1979) observed 4 of 10 pregnant animals to deliver young by day 27 after lutectomy on days 17 or 21, but none of the young lived for more than a day. By contrast, 3 of 10 pregnant animals lutectomized on days 23 or 25 had live young on day 27 which survived. The experimental design did not exclude the possibility that abortion occurred between surgery and day 27, but the low proportion of live deliveries in all the animals reinforces the conclusion that the corpus luteum is important for parturition. These results also suggest that the corpus luteum is necessary until at least day 23 for full development of the mammary gland and for adequate lactation to occur (see Section V,E). Clark (1968) observed similar results in the red kangaroo when development of the quiescent embryo was induced with exogenous progesterone 4–20 days before the resumption of development of the corpus luteum. Young born 10 days or more early failed to survive in the pouch for more than a day, presumably also because the mammary glands were not fully developed for lactation.

As noted above (Section IV,A), progesterone is the major steroid hormone of the luteal tissue of the opossum (Cook and Nalbandov, 1968), the brushtail possum (Shorey and Hughes, 1973a), and tammar wallaby (Renfree *et al.*, 1979). Progesterone concentrations in the peripheral circulation are highest in all these species, and also the quokka (Cake *et al.*, 1980) and bandicoot (Gemmell, 1981), just prior to parturition (Fig. 6). In all these species except the bandicoot, the progesterone concentration declines quite rapidly just before parturition. In the opossum the fall in progesterone coincides with a rise in estradiol, so that there is a marked but transient change in the ratio of the two hormones (Harder and Fleming, 1981). In the tammar wallaby the decline in progesterone is very rapid indeed and takes less than 8 hours (Hinds and Tyndale-Biscoe, 1982a; Tyndale-Biscoe *et al.*, 1982) and possibly more frequent sampling of the quokka will disclose similar rates. The progesterone profiles and effects of lutectomy indicate that, in these four species, parturition is corpus luteum-dependent as it is in the goat (Currie and Thorburn, 1977), the rat (Morishige *et al.*, 1973), and several other eutherian mammals. By analogy with the goat, prostaglandin might have been expected to be involved. In the tammar wallaby, a very brief peak of PGFM was detected within 1 hour of parturition (Tyndale-Biscoe *et al.*, 1982) (Fig. 6), but none has been detected in the brushtail possum (G. Jenkins, personal communication). Conversely, the decline in progesterone in the bandicoot does not begin until 10 days after parturition and does not reach basal levels until day 19, but there is a well defined peak of PGFM at parturition (Fig. 6) and detectable levels were measured in this species during the day preceding parturition and for 2 days thereafter (Gemmell *et al.*, 1980). It may therefore be unwise to assume that the same control of parturition operates in all marsupials.

Progesterone is not the only hormone in the corpus luteum of the brushtail possum or the tammar wallaby. In both species relaxin activity, as measured by the mouse pubic symphysis bioassay of Steinetz *et al.* (1969), can be detected in the corpus luteum from mid-pregnancy to parturition (Tyndale-Biscoe, 1969; 1981). However, this hormone could not be detected in other ovarian tissue nor in the corpora lutea 1–5 days postpartum. Relaxin was not detected in peripheral or ovarian vein plasma, but the pattern of concentration in the corpora lutea of both species was similar to that observed for progesterone. A conspicuous feature of the fine structure of luteal cells of all the species so far examined is small, electron-dense bodies about 200 nm in diameter. In the brushtail possum (Shorey and Hughes, 1973b) and in the tammar wallaby (Tyndale-Biscoe, 1981) the greatest abundance of these bodies coincides with the peak concentrations of relaxin and progesterone and, furthermore, these granules have disappeared 1 day postpartum when the levels of both hormones have declined. Similar granules have been

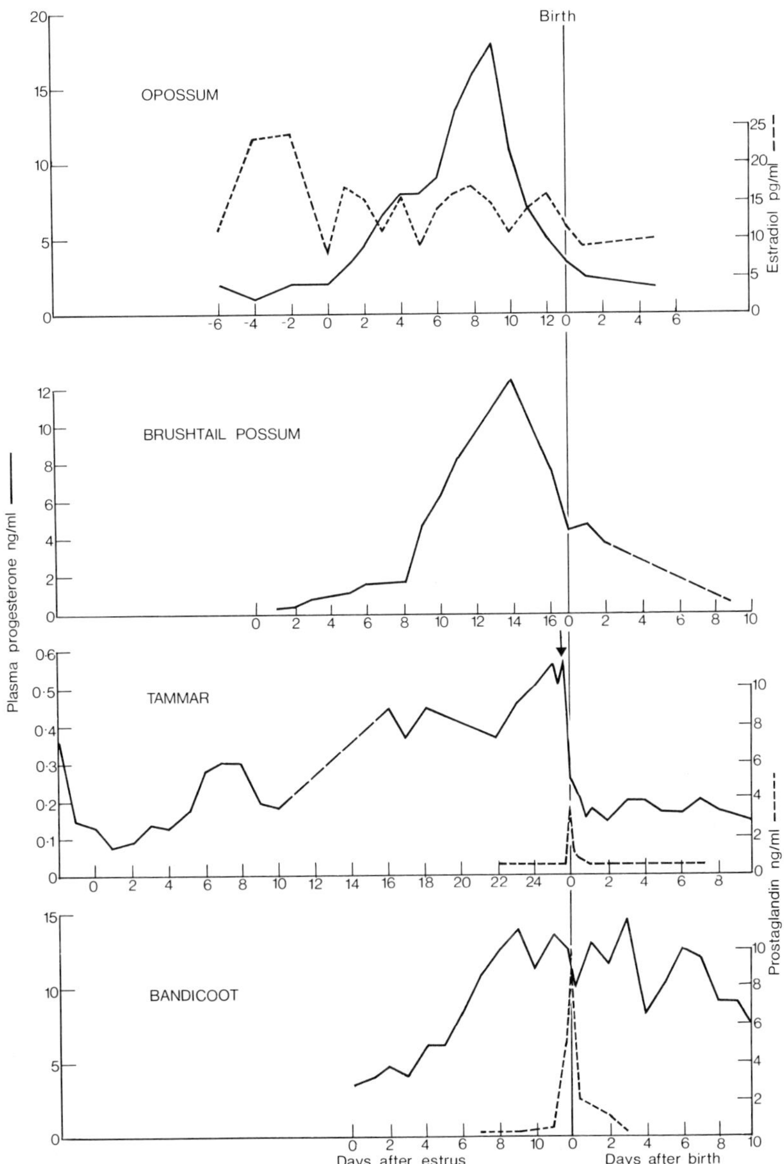

Fig. 6. Profiles of peripheral plasma progesterone (ng/ml) throughout pregnancy and the first 10 days after birth in four marsupials. The values are aligned on the day of birth in order to show the different patterns of pre- and postpartum decline in progesterone. For the opossum, profiles of estradiol (pg/ml) are also shown and for the tammar wallaby and the bandicoot values (ng/ml) for the metabolite of prostaglandin F2α (PGFM) are shown. In the tammar wallaby there is a very brief pulse of prolactin ↓ at about 4 hours before birth and coinciding with the steep decline in progesterone. (Data from Harder and Fleming, 1981; L. A. Hinds, unpublished; Tyndale-Biscoe *et al.*, 1982; Gemmell, 1981; Gemmell *et al.*, 1980.)

observed in the four-cycd opossum (Enders, 1973) and in the red-necked wallaby (Walker and Hughes, 1981), and in the pig similar structures have been inferred to be associated with the storage of relaxin (Belt *et al.*, 1971). However, an alternative view proposed by Gemmell *et al.* (1974) is that these structures are associated with progesterone secretion. Gemmell (1979) has correlated the presence of similar granules in bandicoot luteal cells with progesterone levels in plasma up to 11 days postpartum. The role of relaxin in parturition in marsupials is still unclear, as attempts to induce parturition or softening of the pseudovaginal region with procine relaxin have been unsuccessful (Tyndale-Biscoe, 1966; Renfree and Young, 1979), although a similar preparation did facilitate fetal survival and parturition in the quokka (Tyndale-Biscoe, 1963b).

C. *Role of the Pituitary*

Tammar wallabies hypophysectomized in mid-pregnancy carried to full term and their corpora lutea were fully grown, but the fetuses were found dead in the uterus 2 days after the expected time of birth (Hearn, 1973, 1974). In subsequent studies, the levels of progesterone in hypophysectomized tammar wallabies have been observed to be the same as that in intact animals (L. A. Hinds and C. H. Tyndale-Biscoe, unpublished data) and so the effect of hypophysectomy is unlikely to be mediated by a lack of luteotrophic support for the corpus luteum. In the animals in which the neurohypophysis was left intact, the uteri were empty but parturition did not occur (Hearn, 1973). This suggests that a lack of oxytocin may have been at least partially responsible for the failure of the fetus to leave the uterus in hypophysectomized animals.

In the brushtail possum, the results of adenohypophysectomy were similar to lutectomy and full-term fetuses were found dead in the uterus or cul-de-sac. However, if, in this species, the pituitary was removed before or on day 8 of the 17-day gestation period, the subsequent maximum level of plasma progesterone on day 14 was significantly lower than that observed in sham-operated or in intact females (C. H. Tyndale-Biscoe, C. A. Horn, and L. A. Hinds, unpublished data). Therefore, the anterior pituitary may act indirectly through its effect on the corpus luteum which has been already shown to be essential to parturition.

In pregnant tammar wallabies there is a transient but marked rise in plasma prolactin 4 hours before the rapid fall in progesterone and parturition (Tyndale-Biscoe *et al.*, 1982) (Fig. 6). An analogous pulse does not occur at the equivalent time in the nonpregnant cycle of the same females, so it is appropriate to consider whether this pulse may be part of the pituitary signal to initiate parturition. Its timing is also suggestive of a role in the sudden decline in progesterone secretion by the corpus luteum. If this is so, the effect of adenohypophysectomy on parturition may be caused by abolition of this surge.

Because postpartum estrus and ovulation follow very soon after parturition in the tammar wallaby (and also in most other macropodids), it was not surprising to discover that a LH preovulatory surge occurs 16 hours after the progesterone fall and onset of parturition (Tyndale-Biscoe *et al.,* 1982) and also that this surge and postpartum estrus and ovulation were abolished by hypophysectomy as late as day 23 (Hearn, 1973).

D. Role of the Fetus and/or Placenta

Harder and Fleming (1981) and Fleming and Harder (1981) concluded that there was no evidence for a fetal influence on steroid hormone profiles or endometria in the American opossum and, at present, the only evidence for such effects comes from species of the Macropodidae. In the experiments of Clark (1968) referred to above, the time of parturition and postpartum estrus was separated by up to 20 days in the red kangaroo and so clearly parturition in this species can occur independently of the stage of development reached by the corpus luteum. Similarly, when the two species (Eastern and Western) of grey kangaroo were cross-mated, the length of the gestation period of the hybrids was intermediate between that of the two parental species (Kirsch and Poole, 1972; Poole, 1975) reflecting the hybrid genotype of the fetus. More recently it has been shown for three species of wallaby that the interval between one estrus and the next is significantly shorter if the female is pregnant (Merchant, 1976, 1979; Merchant and Calaby, 1981). It has since been shown (Tyndale-Biscoe *et al.,* 1982) that the decline in plasma progesterone occurred 3 days earlier and more precipitately in females when they were undergoing a pregnant cycle compared to a nonpregnant one (see Fig. 1b). Estrus, the LH surge, and ovulation, which all follow the fall in progesterone sequentially (see Fig. 2), are also advanced in time in the pregnant cycle.

The inference drawn from these differences between pregnant and nonpregnant animals, especially with respect to the prolactin surge and the precocious demise of the corpus luteum, is that the fetus or the placenta provides a signal that initiates luteolysis. It seems unlikely that prostaglandin $F2\alpha$ is the agent because its metabolite was hardly detectable in the plasma. While there is a vascular route by which prostaglandin could be conveyed more directly from the gravid uterus to the ipsilateral corpus luteum (Lee and O'Shea, 1978), parturition has occurred in ovariectomized females bearing ovarian grafts where such a route would not exist (Tyndale-Biscoe and Hearn, 1981).

At present there is no more direct evidence for a fetal role in parturition, but, as in the fetuses of eutherian mammals, the adrenal cortex of the tammar wallaby has differentiated by day 22; 3β-hydroxysteroid dehydrogenase activity was detected in it at this stage (Call *et al.*, 1980) and cortisol and androgen were detected in the plasma of two fetuses on days 24 and 25 (Catling and Vinson, 1976). While the yolk sac placenta and endometrial tissue of the tammar wallaby have been shown to be capable of some of the steps of steroid biosynthesis and catabolism (Heap *et al.*, 1980), aromatase activity was not detected nor was any evidence for estrogen synthesis obtained. Indeed, the role of estrogen at parturition remains enigmatic; its presence is implicit in several of the steps from late pregnancy to postpartum estrus and in the preövulatory LH surge, and yet it has so far proved singularly difficult to detect even by sensitive radioimmunoassay methods (see Renfree and Heap, 1977; Evans *et al.*, 1980).

E. Mammary Gland Development

Since pregnancy in marsupials appears to exert so little endocrine influence on the mother, the question of the effect of pregnancy on the mammary gland arises, particulary whether pregnancy influences mammary gland development in marsupials in the way in which it is known to influence the mammary glands of eutherians (Linzell, 1959). Certainly the size and external appearance of the glands and teats in marsupials do not appear to be markedly influenced by gestation, although slight changes have been observed during the estrous cycle (O'Donoghue, 1911; Sharman, 1962).

O'Donoghue (1911) showed that the slight enlargement and subsequent regression of the mammary glands of the Eastern quoll (native cat) during successive estrous cycles showed a high degree of correlation with the development and regression of the corpora lutea. This was subsequently observed in other marsupials, including the American opossum (Hartman, 1923) and the brushtail possum (Sharman, 1962). Furthermore, the glands reached their maximum size and degree of lobuloalveolar growth at the stage of the estrous cycle at which parturition usually occurs and it was also observed that a small volume of clear fluid could be expressed from each teat at this time (Sharman, 1962; Sharman and Calaby, 1964).

An intriguing series of transfer experiments provided the ultimate confirmation that pregnancy was certainly not necessary for the establishment of normal lactation. In these experiments, the donor (pregnant) and recipient (nonpregnant) animals were synchronized so that newborn young could be transferred when the mammary glands of the donor and recipient animals were at a comparable stage of development. Provided the donor and recipient animals were synchronized to within a day or so, the transferred young developed just as successfully as those reared by their natural mothers (Sharman, 1962; Sharman and Calaby, 1964; Merchant and Sharman, 1966). Merchant and Sharman (1966) were also able to achieve the successful transfer of a pouch young to the pouch of a different species: tammar wallaby to red kangaroo, red kangaroo to grey kangaroo, and swamp wallaby to red kangaroo. The swamp wallaby reared on the red kangaroo teat became obese (presumably due to an oversupply of milk) but the other transfers developed essentially normally. Further confirmation of the lack of influence of pregnancy on mammary gland development comes from the observation that pregnancy has no effect on the weight of mammary glands or on the concentration of prolactin receptors in the glands (F. Stewart, unpublished).

Since, in the tammar wallaby, estrus coincides approximately with the expected time of parturition (and, therefore, mammary gland development) it was of interest to examine whether mammary growth was due to the endocrine influence of estrus, the preceding luteal phase, or both. Lutectomy experiments indicated that estrus alone has very little effect and the corpus luteum was necessary for the full increase in mammary gland weight and in prolactin receptor numbers normally seen at estrus in the tammar wallaby (F. Stewart, unpublished).

It is therefore reasonable to conclude that pregnancy has no discernible effect on mammary gland development in marsupials and is certainly not necessary for the establishment of successful lactation. However, the small degree of growth which occurs during the estrous cycle and which is apparently stimulated by secretions from the corpus luteum does appear to be necessary.

VI. Conclusions

The main conclusion to emerge from any review of marsupial reproduction is the pervasive and paramount importance of the corpus luteum to pregnancy, to parturition, and to mammogenesis.

While it is young and growing, the corpus luteum inhibits follicular development by some means not involving progesterone and, at the same time, progesterone from the corpus luteum stimulates the endometrial growth and secretion upon which the embryo depends. In macropodids a transient pulse of progesterone, arising from a briefly altered rate of secretion by the corpus luteum, occurs in the first week of pregnancy and may be necessary to stimulate blastocyst expansion and differentiation. The mature corpus luteum provides progesterone and relaxin which, together or separately, are necessary for the preparation of the pseudovaginal birth canal for parturition. The mature corpus luteum also stimulates lobulo-alveolar growth in the mammary gland and the development of prolactin-specific receptors in mammary tissue.

In some species the decline in progesterone from the corpus luteum is closely associated with the onset of parturition, postpartum estrus, and the preovulatory LH surge.

Despite its profound importance to reproduction, the marsupial corpus luteum is largely autonomous. The pituitary is essential for its formation, but thereafter it is not necessary for luteal function and there is no evidence that the uterus is luteolytic. Only in the Macropodidae has an external control of the corpus luteum developed, in which pituitary prolactin is luteostatic and at the end of gestation may be briefly luteolytic.

The paramountcy and autonomy of the corpus luteum in marsupials stand in marked contrast to the eutherian mammals in which the corpus luteum is usually subordinate to the pituitary, the placenta, or the uterus. This perhaps reflects the relative importance of pregnancy and lactation in these two groups of mammals.

References

Amoroso, E. C., Heap, R. B., and Renfree, M. B. (1980). *In* "Hormones and Evolution" (E. J. W. Barrington, ed.), Vol. II, pp. 925–989. Academic Press, New York.

Belt, W. D., Anderson, L. L., Cavazos, L. E., and Melampy, R. M. (1971). *Endocrinology* **89**, 1–10.

Berger, P. J. (1966). *Nature (London)* **211**, 435–436.

Bradshaw, S. D., McDonald, I. R., Hahnel, R., and Heller, H. (1975). *J. Endocrinol.* **65**, 451–452.

Cake, M. H., Owen, F. J., and Bradshaw, S. D. (1980). *J. Endocrinol.* **84**, 153–158.

Call, R. N., Catling, P. C., and Janssens, P. A. (1980). *Aust. J. Zool.* **28**, 249–259.

Catling, P. C., and Sutherland, R. L. (1980). *J. Endocrinol.* **86**, 25–33.

Catling, P. C., and Vinson, G. P. (1976). *J. Endocrinol.* **69**, 447–448.

Clark, M. J. (1967). *Aust. J. Zool.* **15**, 673–683.

Clark, M. J. (1968). *J. Reprod. Fertil.* **15**, 347–355.

Clark, M. J., and Sharman, G. B. (1965). *J. Reprod. Fertil.* **10**, 459–461.

Cook, B., and Nalbandov, A. V. (1968). *J. Reprod. Fertil.* **15**, 267–275.

Cook, B., Karsch, F. J., Graber, J. W., and Nalbandov, A. V. (1977). *J. Reprod. Fertil.* **49**, 399–400.

Currie, W. B., and Thorburn, G. D. (1977). *J. Endocrinol.* **73**, 263–278.

Enders, A. C. (1973). *Biol. Reprod. 8,* 158–182.

Evans, S. M., Tyndale-Biscoe, C. H., and Sutherland, R. L. (1980). *J. Endocrinol.* **86**, 13–24.

Farmer, S. W., and Papkoff, H. (1974). *Proc. Soc. Exp. Biol. Med.* **145**, 1031–1036.

Farmer, S. W., Licht, P., Gallo, A. B., Mercado-Simmen, R., Delisle, F. E., and Papkoff, H. (1981). *Gen. Comp. Endocrinol.* **43**, 336–345.

Fleming, M. W., and Harder, J. D. (1981). *J. Reprod. Fertil.* **63,** 21–24.
Flint, A. P. F., and Renfree, M. B. (1982). *J. Endocrinol.* **95.**
Gallo, A. B., Licht, P., Farmer, S. W., Papkoff, H., and Hawkins, J. (1978). *Biol. Reprod.* **19,** 680–687.
Gemmell, R. T. (1979). *Aust. J. Zool.* **27,** 501–510.
Gemmell, R. T. (1981). *Gen. Comp. Endocrinol.* **44,** 13–19.
Gemmell, R. T., Stacy, B. D., and Thorburn, G. D. (1974). *Biol. Reprod.* **11,** 447–462.
Gemmell, R. T., Jenkin, G., and Thorburn, G. D. (1980). *J. Reprod. Fertil.* **60,** 253–256.
Godfrey, G. K. (1975) *J. Zool.* **175,** 541–555.
Harder, J. D., and Fleming, M. W. (1981). *Science* **212,** 1400–1402.
Hartman, C. G. (1921. *Annu. Rep. Smithsonian Inst.* pp. 347–364.
Hartman, C. G. (1923). *Am. J. Anat.* **32,** 353–421.
Hartman, C. G. (1925a). *Am. J. Anat.* **35,** 25–29.
Hartman, C. G. (1925b). *Am. J. Physiol.* **71,** 436–454.
Heap, R. B., Renfree, M. B., and Burton, R. D. (1980). *J. Endocrinol.* **87,** 339–349.
Hearn, J. P. (1972). *J. Reprod. Fertil.* **28,** 132.
Hearn, J. P. (1973). *Nature (London)* **241,** 207–208.
Hearn, J. P. (1974). *J. Reprod. Fertil.* **39,** 235–241.
Hearn, J. P. (1975). *J. Endocrinol.* **64,** 403–416.
Hill, J. P. (1897). *Q. J. Microsc. Sci.* **40,** 385–446.
Hill, J. P. (1899). *Proc. Linn. Soc. N. S. W.* **24,** 42–82.
Hill, J. P. (1918). *Q. J. Microsc. Sci.* **63,** 91–139.
Hinds, L. A., and Tyndale-Biscoe, C. H. (1982a). *J. Endocrinol.* **93,** 99–107.
Hinds, L. A., and Tyndale-Biscoe, C. H. (1982b). *Biol. Reprod.* **29,** 391–398.
Hinds, L. A., Evans, S. M., and Tyndale-Biscoe, C. H. (1983). *J. Reprod. Fertil.* **67.**
Hughes, R. L. (1974). *J. Reprod. Fertil.* **39,** 173–186.
Hughes, R. L., and Shorey, C. D. (1973). *J. Reprod. Fertil.* **32,** 25–32.
Kennaway, D., and Seamark, R. F. (1976). *J. Reprod. Fertil.* **46,** 503–504.
Kirsch, J. A. W., and Poole, W. E. (1972). *Aust. J. Zool.* **20,** 315–339.
Lee, C. S., and O'Shea, J. D. (1978). *J. Morphol.* **154,** 95–114.
Lemon, M. (1972). *J. Endocrinol.* **55,** 63–71.
Linzell, J. L. (1959). *Physiol. Rev.* **39,** 534–576.
Lyne, A. G. (1974). *Aust. J. Zool.* **22,** 303–309.
Lyne, A. G. (1976). *Aust. J. Zool.* **24,** 513–521.
Lyne, A. G., and Hollis, D. E. (1977). *In* "Reproduction and Evolution" (J. H. Calaby and C. H. Tyndale-Biscoe, eds.), pp. 293–302. Australian Academy of Science, Canberra.
Lyne, A. G., and Hollis, D. E. (1979). *Aust. J. Zool.* **27,** 881–899.
McCrady, E. (1938). *Am. Anat. Mem.* **16,** 1–233.
McNeilly, A. S., and Friesen, H. G. (1978). *Endocrinology* **102,** 1539–1547.
McNeilly, A. S., and Land, R. B. (1979). *J. Reprod. Fertil.* **56,** 601–609.
Merchant, J. C. (1976). *Aust. Wildlife Res.* **3,** 93–103.
Merchant, J. C. (1979). *J. Reprod. Fertil.* **56,** 459–463.
Merchant, J. C., and Calaby, J. H. (1981). *J. Zool.* **194,** 203–217.
Merchant, J. C., and Sharman, G. B. (1966). *Aust. J. Zool.* **14,** 593–609.
Morishige, W. K., Pepe, G. J., and Rothchild, I. (1973). *Endocrinology* **92,** 1527–1530.
Niswender, G. D. (1974). *Endocrinology* **94,** 612–615.
Niswender, G. D., Reichert, L. E., Midgley, A. R., and Nalbandov, A. V. (1969). *Endocrinology* **84,** 1166–1173.
O'Donoghue, C. H. (1911). *Q. J. Microsc. Sci.* **57,** 187–234.
Padykula, H. A., and Taylor, J. M. (1976). *Anat. Rec.* **186,** 357–386.

Padykula, H. A., and Taylor, J. M. (1977). *In* "Reproduction and Evolution" (J. H. Calaby and C. H. Tyndale-Biscoe, eds.), pp. 303–323. Australian Academy of Science, Canberra.
Pilton, P. E., and Sharman, G. B. (1962). *J. Endocrinol.* **25,** 119–136.
Poole, W. E. (1975). *Aust. J. Zool.* **23,** 333–353.
Poole, W. E., and Catling, P. C. (1974). *Aust. J. Zool.* **22,** 277–302.
Renfree, M. B. (1972). *Nature (London)* **240,** 475–477.
Renfree, M. B. (1973a). *Dev. Biol.* **33,** 41–49.
Renfree, M. B. (1973b). *Dev. Biol.* **33,** 62–79.
Renfree, M. B. (1974). *J. Reprod. Fertil.* **39,** 127–130.
Renfree, M. B. (1975). *J. Reprod. Fertil.* **42,** 163–166.
Renfree, M. B. (1979). *Nature (London)* **278,** 549–551.
Renfree, M. B. (1980a). *Search* **11,** 81.
Renfree, M. B. (1980b). *In* "Comparative Physiology: Primitive Mammals" (K. Schmidt-Nielsen, L. Bolis, and C. R. Taylor, eds.), pp. 269–284. Cambridge Univ. Press, London and New York.
Renfree, M. B. (1981). *Nature (London)* **293,** 100–101.
Renfree, M. B., and Heap, R. B. (1977). *Theriogenology* **8,** 164.
Renfree, M. B., and Tyndale-Biscoe, C. H. (1973a). *Dev. Biol.* **32,** 28–40.
Renfree, M. B., and Tyndale-Biscoe, C. H. (1973b). *J. Reprod. Fertil.* **32,** 113–115.
Renfree, M. B., and Tyndale-Biscoe, C. H. (1978). *In* "Methods in Mammalian Reproduction" (J. C. Daniel, ed.), pp. 307–331. Academic Press, New York.
Renfree, M. B., and Young, I. R. (1979). *J. Steriod Biochem.* **11,** 515–522.
Renfree, M. B., Green, S. W., and Young, I. R. (1979). *J. Reprod. Fertil.* **57,** 131–136.
Renfree, M. B., Lincoln, D. W., Almeida, O. F. X., and Short, R. V. (1981). *Nature (London)* **293,** 138–139.
Reynolds, H. C. (1952). *Univ. Calif. Berkeley Publ. Zool.* **52,** 223–284.
Risman, G. C. (1947). *J. Morphol.* **81,** 343–397.
Sadleir, R. M. F. S., and Tyndale-Biscoe, C. H. (1977). *Biol. Reprod.* **16,** 605–608.
Selwood, L. (1980). *Aust. J. Zool.* **28,** 649–668.
Selwood, L. (1981). *J. Reprod. Fertil. Suppl.* **29,** 79–82.
Sernia, C., and Tyndale-Biscoe, C. H. (1979). *J. Endocrinol.* **83,** 79–89.
Sernia, C., Hinds, L. A., and Tyndale-Biscoe, C. H. (1980). *J. Reprod. Fertil.* **60,** 139–147.
Sharman, G. B. (1954). *Nature (London)* **173,** 302–303.
Sharman, G. B. (1955a). *Aust. J. Zool.* **3,** 56–70.
Sharman, G. B. (1955b). *Aust. J. Zool.* **3,** 156–161.
Sharman, G. B. (1959). *Monogr. Biol.* **8,** 332–368.
Sharman, G. B. (1962). *J. Endocrinol.* **25,** 375–385.
Sharman, G. B. (1965a). *Excerpta Med.* **83,** 669–674.
Sharman, G. B. (1965b). *Z. Saugetierk.* **30,** 10–20.
Sharman, G. B. (1965c). *Viewpoints Biol.* **4,** 1–28.
Sharman, G. B. (1970). *Science* **167,** 1221–1228.
Sharman, G. B., and Berger, P. J. (1969). *Adv. Reprod. Physiol.* **4,** 211–240.
Sharman, G. B., and Calaby, J. H. (1964). *CSIRO Wildlife Res.* **9,** 58–85.
Sharman, G. B., Calaby, J. H., and Poole, W. E. (1966). *Symp. Zool. Soc. London* **15,** 205–232.
Shorey, C. D., and Hughes, R. L. (1973a). *Aust. J. Zool.* **21,** 1–20.
Shorey, C. D., and Hughes, R. L. (1973b). *Aust. J. Zool.* **21,** 477–489.
Steinetz, B. G., Beach, V. L., and Kroc, R. L. (1969). *In* "Methods in Hormone Research" (R. I. Dorfman, ed.), Vol. II, pp. 481–513. Academic Press, New York.
Stewart, F., and Tyndale-Biscoe, C. H. (1982). *J. Endocrinol.* **92,** 63–72.

Stewart, F., Allen, W. R., and Moor, R. M. (1976). *J. Endocrinol.* **71**, 371–382.
Stewart, F., Sutherland, R. L., and Tyndale-Biscoe, C. H. (1981). *J. Endocrinol.* **89**, 213–223.
Sutherland, R. L., Evans, S. M., and Tyndale-Biscoe, C. H. (1980). *J. Endocrinol.* **86**, 1–12.
Thorburn, G. D., Cox, R. I., and Shorey, C. D. (1971). *J. Reprod. Fertil.* **24**, 139.
Tyndale-Biscoe, C. H. (1963a). *In* "Delayed Implantation" (A. C. Enders, ed.), pp. 15–32. Chicago Univ. Press, Chicago, Illinois.
Tyndale-Biscoe, C. H. (1963b). *J. Reprod. Fertil.* **6**, 25–40.
Tyndale-Biscoe, C. H. (1966). *Symp. Zool. Soc. London* **15**, 233–250.
Tyndale-Biscoe, C. H. (1968). *Aust. J. Zool.* **16**, 577–602.
Tyndale-Biscoe, C. H. (1969). *J. Reprod. Fertil.* **19**, 191–193.
Tyndale-Biscoe, C. H. (1970). *J. Reprod. Fertil.* **23**, 25–32.
Tyndale-Biscoe, C. H. (1973). "Life of Marsupials." Arnold, London.
Tyndale-Biscoe, C. H. (1979). *In* "Maternal Recognition of Pregnancy" (CIBA Symposium 64), pp. 173–190. Excerpta Medica, Amsterdam.
Tyndale-Biscoe, C. H. (1981). *In* "Relaxin" (F. Greenwood, H. Niall, and G. Bryant-Greenwood, eds.), pp. 225–232. Elsevier/North Holland, Amsterdam.
Tyndale-Biscoe, C. H. (1983). *In* "Marshalls Physiology of Reproduction" (G. E. Lamming, ed.), 4th Ed. Churchill, London. (In press).
Tyndale-Biscoe, C. H., and Hawkins, J. (1977). *In* "Reproduction and Evolution" (J. H. Calaby and C. H. Tyndale-Biscoe, eds.), pp. 245–252. Australian Academy of Science, Canberra.
Tyndale-Biscoe, C. H., and Hearn, J. P. (1981). *J. Reprod. Fertil.* **63**, 225–230.
Tyndale-Biscoe, C. H., and Hinds, L. A. (1981). *J. Reprod. Fertil. Suppl.* **29**, 111–117.
Tyndale-Biscoe, C. H., and Hinds, L. A. (1983). *Gen. Comp. Endocrinol.* (in press).
Tyndale-Biscoe, C. H., and Rodger, J. C. (1978). *J. Reprod. Fertil.* **52**, 37–43.
Tyndale-Biscoe, C. H., Hearn, J. P., and Renfree, M. B. (1974). *J. Endocrinol.* **63**, 589–614.
Tyndale-Biscoe, C. H., Hinds, L. A., Horn, C. A., and Jenkin, G. (1982). *J. Endocrinol.* **95.**
Walker, M. T., and Hughes, R. L. (1981). *J. Reprod. Fertil. Suppl.* **29**, 151–158.
Waring, H., Moir, R. J., and Tyndale-Biscoe, C. H. (1966). *Adv. Comp. Physiol. Biochem.* **2**, 237–376.
Welschen, R., Osman, P., Dullaart, J., de Greef, W. J., Uilenbroek, J. T. J., and de Jong, F. H. (1975). *J. Endocrinol.* **64**, 37–47.
Young, I. R., and Renfree, M. B. (1979). *J. Reprod. Fertil.* **56**, 249–254.,

THE ENDOCRINOLOGY OF THE PREIMPLANTATION PERIOD

J. K. Findlay

MEDICAL RESEARCH CENTRE
PRINCE HENRY'S HOSPITAL
MELBOURNE, VICTORIA, AUSTRALIA

I. Introduction 36
A. Time of Implantation 36
B. Morphological Aspects 37
C. Synchronous Development and Recognition of Pregnancy 37
D. Scope of the Review 38
II. Steroids 39
A. Steroid Hormones and Implantation 39
B. Steroid Receptors in the Uterus 42
III. Endometrial Proteins 46
IV. Prostaglandins 50
A. Tissue Levels and Production 50
B. Prostaglandins and Luteal Function 53
C. Prostaglandins, Endometrial Vascular Permeability, and Decidualization 56
V. Histamine 59
A. A Mediator of Estrogen Action? 59
B. Histamine and the Blastocyst 60
VI. Conclusions 60
References 61

Current Topics in
Experimental Endocrinology, Vol. 4

ISBN 0-12-153204-6

I. Introduction

A. Time of Implantation

The period between fertilization and implantation varies between species, especially those exhibiting embryonic diapause (Wimsatt, 1975; Renfree, 1981). Embryonic diapause gives rise to either facultative or obligatory delay in implantation for a period of days or months, depending on the season, lactation, or pregnancy. Implantation normally takes place during the life span of the corpus luteum (CL) (Table I) with the exception of some ungulates (Table II). Implantation can occur at various stages of development of the blastocyst (Tables I and II), and following diapause, may require (re)activation of the blastocyst and the quiescent CL.

Since this article will concentrate mainly on the interaction of the blastocyst and the maternal environment prior to implantation, it is important to define when implantation begins. The process of implantation involves a number of steps which have been described morphologically but not all these steps are understood biochemically.

Table I

A Comparison of the Stage of Pregnancy of Definitive Attachment and the Developmental Stage of the Embryo at Attachment[a]

Species	Implantation (days after fertilization)	Developmental stage of the embryo
Primates		
Human	5.5–6	
Chimpanzee	9–10	} Blastocyst
Baboon	8–9	
Rhesus	8–9	
Marmoset	After 8	Not known
Rodents		
Rabbit	7	Bilaminar blastocyst
Mouse	6	
Rat	5	} Blastocyst, some entoderm
Hamster	4.3	
Guinea pig	6	Unilaminar blastocyst
Carnivoers		
Dog	11–12	
Cat	13–14	} Bilaminar blastocyst
Ferret	12±	

[a]From Wimsatt (1975) and Hearn (1980).

Table II
A Comparison of the Times (Days Postcoitum) of Maternal Recognition of Pregnancy, Attachment, and Parturition in Ungulate Farm Animals Which Have an Elongated Chorionic Vesicle with Allantios at the Time of Attachment[a]

Species	Day by which the embryo must be present for luteal maintenance	Definitive attachment	Parturition
Ewe	12–13	16	145
Cow	16–17	18–22	282
Sow	12	18	114
Mare	14–16	36–38	340

[a]From Wimsatt (1975) and Findlay (1981).

B. Morphological Aspects

Implantation involves apposition (or association) of trophoblast and endometrium sometimes only at specialized areas of the endometrium, interdigitation of the respective cellular microvilli, and varying degrees of penetration of trophoblastic cells into the maternal and endometrial lining (Wimsatt, 1975; Enders and Schlafke, 1979). In most species, an increase in vascular permeability occurs in the endometrial implantation site(s) at or before apposition of the trophoblast and the endometrium. Since the increase in endometrial vascular permeability depends on a viable blastocyst and is followed by cell–cell interactions, it can be conveniently defined as the beginning of implantation. The process of interdigitation and penetration of endometrial cells by the trophoblast may take from 1 to 2 days for most species or up to 2–3 weeks as in the cow (King *et al.*, 1981).

C. Synchronous Development and Recognition of Pregnancy

During the preimplantation period, the embryo and the uterus develop in a coordinated synchronous manner, so that the uterus is receptive when the blastocyst is capable of implanting. Embryo transfer experiments have demonstrated that the blastocyst becomes increasingly dependent on the uterine environment for survival and growth (Heap *et al.*, 1979a). In turn, the uterine environment must undergo continual modification to cope with the needs of the embryo. Coordination of this synchrony of development rests mainly with the maternal steroids, probably acting on the endometrium to control glandular secretion. An influence of the embryo on this glandular secretion will be discussed in this article. The hormonal requirements for implantation are discussed in Section II,A,1.

Asynchronous transfer of embryos to "younger" or "older" uteri has established the limits of tolerance, as well as the time when an embryo must be present to prevent regression of the CL in those species in which implantation does not begin until after the expected time of regression of the CL. This has been described as the maternal recognition of pregnancy (Short, 1969) and is an endocrine form of recognition since it pertains to maintenance of the CL. There may be other forms of recognition not necessarily directly related to CL function (Findlay *et al.,* 1980). The recognition by the maternal system depends on the stage of development of the blastocyst and its capacity to produce the signals. This is demonstrated by the fact that "young" sheep blastocysts transferred to an older uterus have rapid but fatally modified growth because they fail to prevent luteolysis of the CL (Lawson and Findlay, 1977) even if they are transferred back to a synchronous uterus 3 days later (Wilmut and Sales, 1981). Thus, the sheep blastocyst depends on the support of the uterus to grow and develop so it can exert an antiluteolytic influence on the uterus. In rodents, the blastocyst may play a more passive role prior to and during the early stages of implantation (Martin, 1980).

D. Scope of the Review

The remainder of this article will be confined to the influence of the blastocyst on the maternal system prior to and during implantation. This idea was given substance by Deanesly (1967), who showed in guinea pigs that fertilized eggs have "a specific capacity to induce changes in the endometrium," a property appreciably greater than that of artificial traumatization. Signals to or influences on the maternal system have been easier to define than the maternal influences on growth and expansion of the blastocyst and the expression of the embryonic signals. Nevertheless, the absence of a signal may not mean the blastocyst is not producing it—it may mean that the maternal system is ignoring it. And it is likely that not all the signals are involved with implantation per se.

Some of the most interesting advances in recent years have been demonstrations of the capacity of the preimplantation trophoblast to secrete a number of hormones. The demonstration of the presence of a hormone or factor in the blastocyst or the capacity of the embryonic tissue to synthesize the hormone or factor does not imply a physiological role. At the very least, the following criteria should be satisfied for the physiological process under study.

1. Removal of the endogenous factor by tissue ablation or specific synthesis inhibitors, or preventing its action by the use of specific antagonists or antibodies, should prevent the process.

2. Replacement therapy with the factor should reverse the block imposed by the above-mentioned manipulations.

3. The factor should be produced and detected in the tissues of interest on the correct time scale related to the process.

4. A physiological stimulus/inhibitor for synthesis and release of the factor should be identified, and, if blocked, this in turn should modify the process being investigated.

These criteria are essential because they help to evaluate the physiological role of blastocyst factors such as estrogen, prostaglandin (PG), histamine, trophoblastin, chorionic gonadotrophin (CG) etc. on the endometrium during the preimplantation and implantation period. The local nature of the interaction between the blastocyst and the endometrium, the problems of accessibility of inhibitors to the uterine lumen, and of embryonic tissue ablation have made interpretation of the available data difficult.

II. Steroids

A. Steroid Hormones and Implantation

1. Ovarian Steroids

Although progesterone priming of the endometrium may be essential for successful implantation in most species (Amoroso and Perry, 1977), an absolute requirement for estradiol is not common (Marcus and Shelesnyak, 1970). Aitken (1979a) has provided an informative discussion of these hormonal requirements in relation to the occurrence or absence of delayed implantation. The experimental data are based on the exogenous steroid requirements for implantation in ovariectomized, and in some cases, adrenalectomized animals. An estrogen requirement has been demonstrated only in animals which show facultative delayed implantation, e.g., the rat and mouse. In these rodents, the following sequence of hormonal stimulation appears necessary: (1) priming of the uterus with estradiol during proestrus, (2) conditioning of the uterus with progesterone during the first 4 days of pregnancy, and (3) the induction of those endometrial changes required for implantation by "nidatory" estradiol.

In species which do not exhibit embryonic diapause, such as the sheep (Cumming *et al.*, 1974), hamster (Harper *et al.*, 1969), guinea pig (Deanesly, 1960), rabbit (Chàmbon, 1949), and ferret (Wu and Chang, 1972), progesterone alone will allow implantation to occur. In certain circumstances implantation can occur in ovariectomized guinea pigs in the absence of any exogenous steroids (see Martin, 1980). While exogenous estrogen is not obligatory in this group, it is facilitatory, because it improves the survival rate of embryos in the sheep (Miller and Moore, 1976) and rabbit (Chàmbon, 1949). Very little is known about the hormonal requirements for implantation in primates, although it is thought that progesterone only is required, with estradiol playing a facilitatory role (Hearn, 1980; Aitken, 1979a). Ovarian estrogen can be measured during the luteal phase at the time of implantation in these species. However, it is possible that the blastocysts are able to manufacture estrogens which may act locally to facilitate implantation.

2. Blastocyst Steroids

Rabbit blastocysts contain progestins (Seamark and Lutwak-Mann, 1972) and estradiol-17β (Dickman *et al.,* 1975; Bullock, 1977) and cow blastocysts contain progesterone and testosterone (Shemesh *et al.,* 1979) in picogram quantities. It is quite feasible for these steroids to have been taken up from the uterine lumen which contains measurable quantities of progestins (Fowler *et al.,* 1976) and estrogens (Eiler *et al.,* 1974). In the pig both estrone and estradiol concentrations are higher in uterine flushings from pregnant compared to nonpregnant sows from day 12 onward (Zavy *et al.,* 1980).

In an earlier review of this literature, Bullock (1977) drew attention to the importance of distinguishing between the presence of steroids in the blastocyst and its capacity to synthesize and metabolize steroids *de novo.* Biochemical criteria are needed to demonstrate synthesis. Histochemical methods of identifying enzymes associated with steroid synthesis lack specificity, and the results are difficult to interpret. The presence of an enzyme does not necessarily indicate its functional activity. While Dickmann and his colleagues (Dickmann and Sen Gupta, 1974; Dickmann *et al.,* 1976) have demonstrated histochemically Δ^5-3β- and 17β-hydroxysteroid dehydrogenase in preimplantation embryos of the rat, mouse, rabbit, and hamster, biochemical evidence for steroid synthesis in these species is available only for the rabbit (Huff and Eik-Nes, 1966; George and Wilson, 1978; Singh and Booth, 1978). Neither the mouse (Sherman *et al.,* 1977) nor the rat (Marcal *et al.,* 1975) embryo can synthesize or metabolize steroids prior to implantation. Implantation was not prevented in the hamster treated with progesterone and inhibitors of steroidogenesis (Brodie *et al.,* 1978; Evans and Kennedy, 1980) suggesting that neither maternal nor blastocyst estrogen production is essential for implantation in that species. These experiments and those using antiestrogens can be criticized on grounds that the drug may not have reached the embryo or that it had toxic effects on the embryo (Bullock, 1977) and so this approach cannot be used to resolve the requirements of blastocyst or maternal steroids for implantation.

In addition to the rabbit, definitive evidence for aromatase activity and estrogen synthesis by the preimplantation blastocyst has been obtained for the sow (Perry *et al.,* 1973; Gadsby *et al.,* 1980), mare (Zavy *et al.,* 1979a) and roe deer (but not before blastocyst activation) (Gadsby *et al.,* 1980). Aromatase activity in rabbit blastocysts is absent on day 6 but is present on day 6.5–7 (i.e., at implantation) and reaches a maximum on day 8 (George and Wilson, 1978; Gadsby *et al.,* 1980). In the pig, aromatase activity is not normally detected before day 12 when the blastocyst is still spherical; however, the activity increases dramatically thereafter coincident with elongation and formation of the tubular or filamentous blastocyst (Flint *et al.,* 1979a) and the appearance of increased quantities of estrogen in the uterine lumen (Zavy *et al.,* 1980). The conversion of androstenedione to estrogen is low or undetectable in embryonic tissues from the cow (Eley *et al.,* 1979; Gadsby *et al.,* 1980), sheep, ferret, plains viscacha (Gadsby *et al.,* 1980), and tammar wallaby (Heap *et al.,* 1980). The apparent absence of aromatase activity, however, does not mean that blastocysts or early embryonic tissues are devoid of steroid metabolizing activity. Androstenedione is metabolized extensively to other neutral steroids by trophoblast of the cow, sheep (Gadsby *et al.,* 1980; Chenault and Hruska, 1979), and wallaby (Heap *et al.,* 1980). By 2–5 days after attachment, ovine trophoblast has been demonstrated to have the capacity to synthesize (Marcus *et al.,* 1979a) and extensively metabolize progesterone (Marcus *et al.,* 1979b). Flood and Ghazi (1981) have demonstrated histochemically that ovine trophoblast acquires 3β-hydroxysteroid dehydrogenase at this time. Cow blastocysts obtained on days 13–16 postcoitum (pc) (Shemesh *et al.,* 1979) and yolk sac membranes from the quokka (Bradsaw *et al.,* 1975) can also synthesize progesterone; cow blastocysts can also synthesize testosterone (Shemesh *et al.,* 1979). An important gap in our knowledge is information on the steroidogenic potential of primate blastocysts.

The pronounced aromatase activity in trophoblast of the sow and mare, at the time when the signal for maintenance of the CL takes place, has been associated with the superficial form of implantation in these species (Gadsby *et al.,* 1980). Evidence is accumulating for a luteotrophic role of blastocyst estrogen in establishing pregnancy in these species, particularly in the pig (Bazer and Thatcher, 1977; Flint *et al.,* 1979a; Section IV,A,2).

The lack of aromatase activity in trophoblast of most species may reflect inadequacies of the techniques used. To date, the emphasis has been on conversion of radiolabeled precursors or on production form endogenous substrate *in vitro.* In view of the recent interest in high and low density lipoprotein as a percursor for steroidogenesis in human trophoblastic cells in culture (Winkel *et al.,* 1980), it would seem appropriate to study steroidogenic activity of the blastocyst using these substrates as steroid precursors.

B. Steroid Receptors in the Uterus

1. General Principles

The local production and action of steroids can be approached by a study of the steroid receptors and the effects of competitive inhibitors of those receptors on implantation. The literature on estrogen (ER) and progesterone receptor (PR) in the nonpregnant uterus is voluminous (see Muldoon, 1980) and is in stark contrast to data in the pregnant uterus. The main principles of ER and PR in the nonpregnant uterus can be summarized as follows:

1. The synthesis of both ER and PR is stimulated by estrogen and inhibited by progesterone.
2. The binding of steroid to its receptor in the cytosol is followed by translocation of the steroid-receptor complex to the nucleus where it associates with acceptor sites on the chromatin. This association leads to transcription of RNA species coding for the synthesis of steroid-dependent proteins in the target cells.
3. The ratio of cytoplasmic to nuclear receptor tends to vary with the circulating level or local concentration of the steroid. Thus, the levels of both ER and PR tend to be highest during the proliferative or follicular phase of the cycle when estrogen levels are high. The postovulatory rise in progesterone is associated with a decline in both ER and PR (Table III) which reach a nadir in the luteal phase.

Some caution should be exercised before accepting this as dogma. First,

Table III

The Concentration[a] and Subcellular Distribution of Estrogen and Progesterone Receptors in the Human Endometrium during the Normal Menstrual Cycle[b]

	Estrogen receptor				Progesterone receptor			
Phase	Total	Cytosol	Nuclei	Rc/RN	Total	Cytosol	Nuclei	Rc/RN
Early proliferative	1.5	1.1	0.4	2.7	1.5	1.2	0.2	6.0
Late proliferative	1.9	1.0	0.9	1.1	3.0	3.0	0.5	4.8
Early secretory	1.2	0.4	0.8	0.5	1.9	0.9	1.0	0.9
Late secretory	0.7	0.3	0.4	0.7	0.9	0.7	0.2	3.5

[a]Picomoles per milligram DNA.
[b]From Bayard *et al.* (1978).

the experimental data are based mainly on whole uteri or endometrium rather than specific cell types. There is evidence in the rat that ER may be present in stromal cells rather than epithelial cells (Talley *et al.,* 1977; McCormack and Glasser, 1980). Second, progesterone can increase ER synthesis in rat endometrium (Martel and Psychoyos, 1978), and despite inhibition of ER levels, progesterone is without effect on estradiol-induced protein synthesis, RNA–DNA ratios, and enzyme activities in the endometrium of the ovariectomized ewe (Stone *et al.,* 1979; Miller *et al.,* 1979; Findlay *et al.,* 1981). The need to retain some endometrial responsiveness to estradiol during the period of progesterone domination might be important for implantation. Recently, Zelinski *et al.* (1980) showed that high doses of estradiol can provoke significant increases in ovine endometrial ER and PR during the mid-luteal phase, but only 24 hours after treatment.

Third, the significance of the subcellular distribution of steroid receptor should be treated with caution (Baulieu *et al.,* 1980). Although steroid action is generally thought to occur by a transcriptional mechanism involving the nuclear receptor (but see Pietras and Szego, 1979), the presence of nuclear receptors does not necessarily prove that it is engaged in hormonal activity. "Translocation" should not be interpreted as "activation" and "acceptor" site is not necessarily synonymous with "effector" site (Baulieu *et al.,* 1980). It is for these reasons that one should measure both cytoplasmic and nuclear receptors in order to obtain the total concentration of intracellular receptors. A detailed critique on the physiology of steroid receptors has been written recently by Muldoon (1980).

With these principles and reservations in mind, let us now examine what happens to steroid receptors in the uterus prior to and during implantation. Most of the data pertains to ER.

2. Species by Species

In the rat, the amount of labeled estradiol measured in the sites of implantation was less than in the interimplantation sites on day 6 of normal pregnancy (Sartor, 1977) or by 14–16 hours after estrogen priming of "delayed-implanting" rats (Ward *et al.,* 1978). The decreased amount of radioactivity in the implantation sites was attributed to decreased uptake rather than differences in retention, suggesting decreased availability of ER. Subsequently, Martel and Psychoyos (1981) observed a 50–60% decrease in cytoplasmic ER concentration and no change in nuclear concentration in the endometrium surrounding the blastocyst 24 hours after injection of estradiol, compared with the concentration in interimplantation sites or in uteri from control delayed-implanting rats. This contrasts with the observations of Logeat *et al.* (1980) where the concentration of both ER and PR increased dramatically in the nuclear compartment of implantation sites on the morning of day 6 of normal pregnancy. Martel and Psychoyos (1981) attribute this discrepancy to the steroid binding capacity of Trypan blue, used by Longeat *et al.* (1980) to reveal implantation sites, in contrast to the relatively low steroid binding capacity of Evan's blue used by the former authors. In addition, there may be differences in steroid receptor concentrations between rats with natural pregnancy and estrogen-primed rats with delayed implantation. In two longitudinal studies, the concentration of nuclear ER either fluctuated with a circadian rhythm (Martel and Psychoyos, 1976), or increased up to day 5 (Myatt *et al.*, 1980) and then decreased at the time of implantation. The temporal pattern of cytoplasmic ER showed a continual increase up to day 6 (Mester *et al.*, 1974; Myatt *et al.*, 1980). The objectives of these studies did not include a comparison of steroid receptor levels in implantation and interimplantation sites in pregnant and nonpregnant horns with time after mating, and the studies differed in that some used whole uteri and others used endometrium. It is difficult to reconcile the results of the longitudinal studies with those of Martel and Psychoyos (1981) and Logeat *et al.* (1980), particularly in relation to the nuclear ER levels. If one excludes the data of Logeat *et al.* on the basis of binding of steroid to Trypan blue, then there would appear to be a decrease in total endometrial steroid receptor concentrations at about the time of implantation. Furthermore, the capacity of the rat blastocyst to synthesize estrogen is controversial (Section II,A,2), nevertheless, there is a rise in peripheral estrogen secreted by the ovary late on day 3, and continuing into day 4 (O'Grady and Bell, 1977).

In the preimplantation period of sheep, cytosol ER levels are lower in caruncular (attachment) endometrium of pregnant than nonpregnant ewes on days 9, 13, and 15 but not on day 11. In intercaruncular endometrium, the levels are lower on day 15 of pregnancy compared to nonpregnancy but not on other days tested (Findlay *et al.*, 1982). We have also observed that when the blastocyst was confined to one uterine horn of the ewe on day 2, there was a decrease in cytosolic and total ER and only in caruncular endometrium in the pregnant horn on day 15. Irrespective of pregnancy status, the levels of ER were approximately twofold higher in caruncular compared to intercaruncular endometrium (Findlay *et al.*, 1982), consistent with the steroid concentrations in these tissues (Challis *et al.*, 1976). We concluded that the changes in ER appeared to result from a local rather than systemic action of the blastocyst, and that the effects on ER were confined mainly to caruncular endometrium. Furthermore, the decrease in cytosolic ER was unlikely to have been due to translocation of receptor to the nucleus because the proportion of ER in the nucleus did not change in the experiment with the blastocyst confined to one horn. Similar studies on PR have not been published. In summary, the presence of a preimplantation blastocyst was associated with a decrease in cytosolic ER mainly in the caruncular endometrium well before the time of attachment in the ewe. In this species, there is no conclusive evidence of either a capacity of the blastocyst to synthesize estrogen or progesterone before implantation or of a specific perinidatory rise in estrogen. I am not aware of similar studies of steroid receptors in other ungulates during early pregnancy.

In the pig, pregnancy does not significantly alter the quantitative or qualitative pattern of cytoplasmic ER from day 10 to 20, during which time the receptor levels declined (Deaver and Guthrie, 1980). Of interest was the high concentrations of cytoplasmic ER in the endometrium of the mid-luteal phase relative to the follicular phase in contrast to most other species (Aitken, 1979b). Pack *et al.* (1979) observed that nuclear ER levels in the sow endometrium increased from the time of mating up to day 5 of pregnancy, but from day 10 onward, the nuclear ER were undetectable until a brief period around day 17. In the nonpregnant sow, a sharp increase in nuclear ER levels would be expected at around day 17 (Pack *et al.*, 1978). Thus, in the pregnant and nonpregnant pig, both nuclear and cytoplasmic ER are maximal in the early luteal phase and then decrease toward the time of implantation or next estrus, when there is a suppression of nuclear ER levels if the animal is pregnant. The nuclear and cytoplasmic levels of ER are inversely related to estrogen sulfotransferase activity in the endometrium (Pack *et al.*, 1978, 1979) and to the time when the blastocyst begins to produce significant quantities of estrogen (Section II,A,2). Pack *et al.* (1979) claim that progesterone-dependent sulfurylation of estrogen prevents ER complexes being formed, so allowing progesterone in association with its receptor to convert the endometrium from a proliferative to a secretory one. How this relates to the role of estrogen in the redistribution of PG, the production of lactoferrin etc. in early pregnancy in the pig (Bazer and Thatcher, 1977) is not clear.

A comparison of ER and PR in decidual tissue of humans prior to and during implantation has not been reported. The only data available are from human decidual tissue collected at 8–10 weeks of gestation. Levy *et al.* (1980) were unable to detect cytoplasmic ER or PR, whereas nuclear concentrations of these receptors were higher than the levels observed in the early follicular phase. Kreitman and Bayard (1979) noted a similar distribution of ER and PR in favor of the nucleus, with levels comparable to those in the menstrual cycle.

In Rhesus monkeys, the late luteal phase during the fertile cycle was associated with a relative increase in nuclear receptors for estrone compared to estradiol-17β (Kreitmann-Gimbal *et al.*, 1981). These authors concluded from experiments in which nonpregnant monkeys were treated with hCG and progesterone that this rise in nuclear estrone receptors was probably due to progesterone rather than the preimplantation blastocyst. A similar change in estrogen binding was noted in cytosol of decidualized human endometrium from an infertile cycle (B. Kreitmann *et al.*, 1979), and, in both species, might be related to the progesterone-dependent 17β-hydroxysteroid dehydrogenase present in the endometrium (Tseng and Gurpide, 1974; O. Kreitmann *et al.*, 1979).

The overall impression on the limited data available is that total ER and PR levels are suppressed in the presence of a blastocyst in the periimplantation period as they are during the luteal phase. This does not accord well with an obligatory requirement for progesterone and a facilitatory or obligatory need for estrogen, but it does agree with the suppressive action of progesterone on ER and PR. The possibilities are that the number of steroid receptors remaining in specific cell types is sufficient to account for the endometrial responses, that the blastocyst can in some way modulate the tissue response to the steroid, despite the low levels of receptor, or that the steroids might not act via the "classical" receptor system. The next section will consider modulation by the blastocyst of the endometrial biosynthetic and secretory activity, some of which is steroid dependent.

III. Endometrial Proteins

It is well established in most species that the endometrium is under the control of ovarian steroids, although there may be differentiation between areas and cell types with respect to steroid action and cellular response. The activation of many enzymes associated with intermediary metabolism, the synthesis of the steroid receptor proteins and some of the secreted proteins are steroid dependent, showing changes related to estrogen and progesterone concentration in the circulation (Aitken, 1979b; Bazer, 1975; Findlay *et al.*, 1980; Finn and Porter, 1975; O'Grady and Bell, 1977). For example, in the sheep (Findlay *et al.*, 1980, 1981), lysosomal enzymes such as acid and alkaline phosphatase and β-glucuronidase have a greater activity in caruncular than in intercaruncular endometrium and reach their highest activity during the luteal phase of the normal cycle. In some species, specific proteins, known to be under the influence of steroids, are secreted into the uterine lumen. Examples are lactoferrin or "purple protein" in the pig (Bazer, 1975) and uteroglobin or blastokinin in the rabbit (Beier and Mootz, 1979). The estrogen-dependent, induced-protein synthesized by rat uterus now appears to consist of several components (Manak *et al.*, 1980). In addition to regulation by ovarian steroids, there may also be a local action of the early embryo on endometrial protein synthesis and secretion.

The proteins secreted into the uterine lumen may serve several functions including the protection and nurturing of the blastocyst and facilitation of implantation. The degree of secretory activity exhibited by the uterus varies considerably between species and has been related to the degree of embryonic expansion and growth preceding implantation (Boyd and Hamilton, 1952) and to the mode of implantation (Martin, 1980). Thus in ruminants and pigs, there is substantial growth of the preimplantation blastocyst, associated with a copious secretion from the endometrial glands (Amoroso, 1952). The protein content of the luminal fluid increases dramatically in the few days prior to implantation in the sheep (Roberts *et al.*, 1976; Ellinwood *et al.*, 1979a), pig (Zavy *et al.*, 1980), and horse (Zavy *et al.*, 1979b). The quantitative but not the qualitative pattern of luminal proteins is changed in the pig and horse, with both species apparently possessing similar types of protein. This has been related to the diffuse epitheliochorion type of placentation in these species (Zavy *et al.*, 1979b). The analogy might now be extended following the recent discovery by Flint (1981) of a CG in the pig with LH-like bioactivity (Section IV,B,5). *In vitro* studies on pig endometrium confirm that tissue underlying a conceptus is quantitatively more active in the synthesis of secretory (Basha *et al.*, 1980) but not membrane protein (Mullins *et al.*, 1980). The contribution to the luminal protein by pig blastocyst is not known, since there are only preliminary studies on the pattern of soluble proteins synthesized *in vitro* (Jones *et al.*, 1976; Heap *et al.*, 1979a). Of particular interest was the capacity of synchronous but not asynchronous endometrium to stimulate protein synthesis by the blastocyst *in vitro* (Heap *et al.*, 1979a).

In sheep and cows, there is also evidence of an embryonic influence on the patterns of protein. Although many of the proteins in luminal fluid are of serum origin, electrophoretic analysis has revealed up to five bands which appear to be nonserum "pregnancy-specific" proteins in the uterine lumen (Roberts and Parker, 1974a; Roberts *et al.*, 1976; Gibbons *et al.*, 1977) coincident with blastocyst expansion. Numerous glycosidases also appear in uterine fluids of the sheep and cow at this stage (Roberts and Parker, 1974b; Roberts *et al.*, 1976).Although the origin of these enzymes is unknown, they may be important for modifying glycoprotein in the lumen and on the cell surfaces to facilitate implantation. Laster (1977) described increased RNA concentration in bovine endometrium in the presence of a blastocyst, and a pregnancy-specific protein. However, Wathes (1980) was not able to demonstrate either a qualitative or quantitative alteration in protein synthesis *in vitro* by bovine endometrium cocultured with chorion.

Pregnancy-associated protein(s) are present in the trophoblast, uterine lumen, and endometrium of pregnant ewes and in endometrium of some nonpregnant ewes (Findlay *et al.*, 1979; Staples *et al.*, 1978; Staples, 1980).

This and the presence of a quantitative but not a qualitative change in endometrial protein synthesis *in vitro* (Findlay *et al.*, 1981, 1982) suggest that the influence of the ovine blastocyst on endometrial protein synthesis is probably quantitative rather than qualitative and that the pregnancy proteins in the lumen might originate from the blastocyst. The nature of proteins synthesized by the sheep blastocyst remains largely unknown with the exception of trophoblastin (Section IV,B,3).

In rabbits, carnivores, and macropod marsupials, all of which have central implantation and some degree of blastocyst expansion before attachment (Wimsatt, 1975), there is considerable uterine secretion which is probably important in regulating implantation (Martin, 1980; Renfree, 1980) [the exception is the roe deer, see Aitken (1979a)]. Evidence for local induction of enhanced uterine secretory activity by the blastocyst has been described for the rabbit (Daniel, 1972) and the tammar wallaby (Renfree, 1972). Distinct proteins have been identified in the uterine secretions of the tammar (Renfree, 1973), whereas in the rabbit, the change is quantitative rather than qualitative. Uteroglobin, the major progesterone-dependent protein in rabbit uterus, is synthesized in the pregnant and nonpregnant endometrium and is present in the uterine lumen and blastocoele fluid. Uteroglobin is well characterized biochemically; it can bind progesterone, and it has antiprotease activity, yet we do not understand its biological role (see Aitken, 1979b). Beier and Mootz (1979) have suggested a role of uteroglobin together with other luminal proteins in synchronous development of the blastocyst and endometrium in preparation for implantation.

The rat, mouse, hamster, guinea pig, and human have eccentric or interstitial implantation and virtually no expansion of the blastocyst before implantation (Wimsatt, 1975). Martin (1980) considers that in the rodent species, progesterone stimulates epithelial proliferation and suppresses estrogen-induced secretion, which together with pinocytosis by epithelial cells of the endometrium has the net result of decreasing uterine luminal volume. This eventually closes the lumen allowing the microvilli of the apposing surfaces to interdigitate and begin implantation when the nidatory estrogen stimulus is received. Because one can induce in pseudopregnant mice the formation of implantation chambers indistinguishable from those formed in the presence of an "invasive" trophoblast, Martin (1980) argues that the blastocyst is largely passive in the early stages of implantation. Some of the biochemical evidence supports this suggestion. The uterine protein profiles observed during the early implantation phase of normal pregnancy closely resemble the pattern observed during the early phase of estrogen action in both the rat (Surani, 1977) and mouse (Aitken, 1977). However, Aitken (1977) noted an enhanced protein secretion in response to estrogen in the presence of the mouse blastocyst, and Given and Enders (1980) provided morphological and cytochemical evidence of increased secretory activity of the uterine glands during normal implantation. Decidualization in the rat is associated with a number of biochemical changes, e.g., increased alkaline phosphatase and ornithine decarboxylase activities and protein RNA and DNA content (O'Grady and Bell, 1977) and a posttransferrin protein (Bell *et al.,* 1977). But there is no compelling evidence that the rat or mouse blastocyst is better (or worse) than a nonspecific stimulus at stimulating these activities in the endometrium. In fact, in these rodents as in other species exhibiting embryonic diapause, most of the preimplantation signals are probably from uterus to blastocyst to first inhibit (or fail to stimulate) the blastocyst and, then following the nidatory estrogen stimulus, to activate the blastocyst (Weitlauf, 1978) in preparation for the sensitive phase of the uterus. Tzartos and Surani (1979) noted that luminal proteins on day 5 of pregnancy in the rat had a greater binding affinity for the rat blastocyst than did proteins from uterine fluid at proestrus. As the steroid requirements for nidation become less stringent, the blastocyst may assume a more positive role in decidualization (Martin, 1980). Thus implantation will proceed in ovariectomized, adrenalectomized hamsters with progesterone alone and in ovariectomized guinea pigs without exogenous progesterone (Section II,A,1). These steroid requirements do not appear to have been satisfied by a steroidogenic capacity of the blastocysts (Section II,A,2).

By analogy with the rodents, Martin (1980) has predicted that luminal closure rather than uterine secretion might be important in the human in which the blastocyst remains small and implantation is interstitial. Clemetson *et al.* (1973) found evidence of increased luminal absorption of water and sodium and a decrease in luminal volume during the human luteal phase. The luminal protein content falls following ovulation and reaches a nadir in the luteal phase in the baboon (Peplow *et al.,* 1973) and human (Maathuis and Aitken, 1978) at the expected time of implantation. A qualitative analysis of the proteins from the lumen of the human endometrium revealed a number of nonserum proteins including a posttransferrin (Aitken, 1979b) and a glycoprotein which might be progesterone-dependent (Sylvan *et al.,* 1981). There is a paucity of information on the qualitative and quantitative patterns of uterine proteins during early pregnancy in primates. Chorionic gonadotrophin (Hearn, 1980) and a prolactin of decidual origin (Maslar and Riddick, 1979) might be two proteins present.

The failure to detect changes in protein synthesis or secretion in some species may reflect inadequacies of the techniques. Despite this deficiency, the available data suggests a strong correlation between quantitative protein production and secretion into the uterine lumen and the degree of growth and expansion of the blastocyst in the preimplantation period. Mechanism(s) by which the blastocyst exerts this effect on protein synthesis are not known. Although it can be mimicked to some extent by estradiol there is no compelling evidence yet that blastocyst estrogen is the universal stimulant, with the exception of the pig (Section II,A,2). Furthermore, the levels of ER in the sheep and pig appear to be low at the time when luminal protein content is increasing (Section II,B,2). Surprisingly little is known about the contribution of the blastocyst to this pool of luminal protein in any of the species studied.

IV. Prostaglandins

A. Tissue Levels and Production

The precursors of the PG family are essential polyunsaturated fatty acids which occur partly membrane-bound in cells esterified to phospholipids. Of particular importance is 5,8,11,14-eicosatetraenoic acid, or arachidonic acid, the precursor of the biologically active 2-series PGs (Hagenfeldt, 1980; Fig. 1). Most cell types in the mammalian body possess the enzyme systems to convert arachidonic acid to PG, but the relative proportion of the products formed varies between different tissues and within the same tissue under different conditions. Very little is known about the factors that regulate the ratio between the different PGs, although in reproductive tissues the overall rates of synthesis are influenced by steroids and oxytocin (Section IV,A,2). The rate-limiting steps appear to be the activation of phospholipase-A_2 and the amount of prostaglandin synthetase. A further complication arises because newly synthesized PGs are generally not stored in tissues but are released to act locally and are metabolized very rapidly (Bito, 1975). Unless special precautions are taken, tissue concentrations probably reflect synthesis between the time of collection and storage and can be artificially increased because of tissue injury.

1. Prostaglandins in the Blastocyst

Notwithstanding these limitations, PGE_2 and $PGF_{2\alpha}$ have been measured in rabbit (Dickmann and Spilman, 1975), cow (Shemesh *et al.*, 1979), and sheep blastocysts (Hyland *et al.*, 1982), but not in rat blastocysts (Kennedy and Armstrong, 1981). Likewise, rabbit (Dey *et al.*, 1980), pig (Watson and Patek, 1979), cow (Shemesh *et al.*, 1979; Thatcher *et al.*, 1980), and sheep (Hyland *et al.*, 1982), but not rat blastocysts (Kennedy and Armstrong, 1981) can synthesize PGs *in vitro*. Kennedy and Armstrong (1981) speculate that this may reflect the differences in development of the embryo, where rabbit and particulary sheep and cow blastocysts are at a relatively more ad-

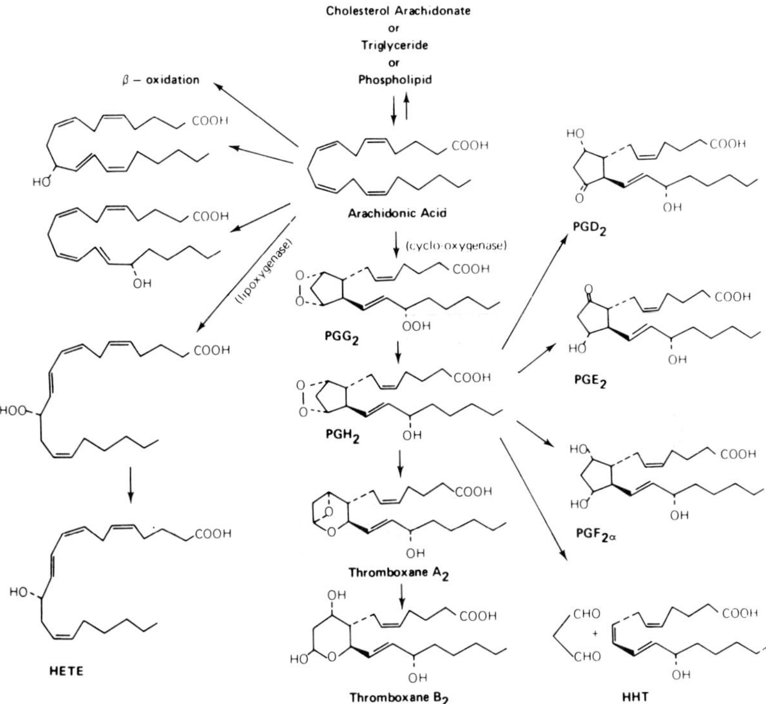

Fig. 1. The major metabolic pathways in the conversion of arachidonic acid. (From Ramwell *et al.*, 1977, reprinted with permission from the publishers.)

vanced stage when PG production has been demonstrated, compared to the rat blastocyst.

Little is known about metabolism of PGs by the blastocyst. Maule Walker *et al.* (1977) demonstrated the capacity of pig blastocysts to metabolize over 50% of labeled PGE_2 and $PGF_{2\alpha}$ to the 13,14-dihydro-15-keto prostaglandins, although the metabolites were not identified in a definitive manner. Guinea pig conceptuses metabolized up to 22% of the respective substrate, but at a very low rate (Maule Walker and Poyser, 1978).

2. Prostaglandins in the Endometrium and Uterine Lumen

Since Pickles (1957) demonstrated PG bioactivity in human menstrual fluid, the capacity of the uterus to synthesize and release PGs into the uterine vein and lumen has been described in most species studied (see reviews by Goding, 1974; Horton and Poyser, 1976; Bazer and Thatcher, 1977; Baird, 1978; Flint *et al.*, 1979a; Inskeep *et al.*, 1980; Inskeep and Murdoch, 1980; Findlay, 1981). Both the myometrium and the endometrium can synthesize PG, although recent evidence suggests that prostacyclins may be the major products in the myometrium, whereas PGE_2 and $PGF_{2\alpha}$ predominate in the endometrium, with endometrial endoperoxides also acting as substrates for myometrial synthesis of PGI_2 (Abel and Kelly, 1979). The cell types responsible for synthesis of the PG in the uterus have not been studied in depth. In sheep, both the caruncular (attachment sites) and intercaruncular portions of the endometrium can synthesize PGF (Findlay *et al.*, 1981). The increase in PGF content of the endometrium during the luteal phase has been attributed to an increase in cyclooxygenase activity in microsomes from stromal cells in caruncular endometrium (Huslig *et al.*, 1979) rather than increased availability of substrate (Horton and Poyser, 1976).

Control of PG synthesis by the uterus rests with the ovarian steroids, estradiol-17β and progesterone (Baird, 1978; Inskeep and Murdoch, 1980), and oxytocin (McCracken, 1980). For maximal release of PGs *in vivo,* the sheep requires a period of about 7 days of progesterone priming, then progesterone withdrawal and stimulation with estradiol. Oxytocin requires priming with both steroids for maximum response. The mechanism of action of steroids and oxytocin on PG synthesis and release remains speculative.

Considering that the tissue level of PG will depend on the rates of synthesis, release, and metabolism, it is surprising that relatively little attention has been paid to PG metabolism in the uterus. The 13,14-dihydro-15-keto metabolites are present in uterine tissues of ruminants (Inskeep and Murdoch, 1980) and women (Lundstrom and Green, 1978) and 15-keto dehydrogenase activity increases markedly in human endometrium during the luteal phase (Casey *et al.*, 1980). Neither the pregnant nor the nonpregnant uterus of the pig (Maule Walker *et al.*, 1977) and guinea pig (Maule Walker and Poyser, 1978) extensively metabolize $PGF_{2\alpha}$ and PGE_2.

In pregnancy, uterine production and content of PGs appear to either remain the same or increase above that observed in nonpregnant endometrium of the sheep, cow, pig, and horse (Inskeep *et al.*, 1980). In contrast, the production of PG in endometrial tissue of the human (Maathuis and Kelly, 1978; Abel *et al.*, 1980) and guinea pig (Poyser and Maule Walker, 1979) appears to be reduced. However, it should be pointed out that while the capacity of the endometrium to synthesize PG may not change, the relative abundance of PGE_2 and $PGF_{2\alpha}$ can change, as for example in the sheep (Ellinwood *et al.*, 1979a). Pregnancy in ungulates is associated with a dramatic increase in the content of PG in the uterine lumen just prior to implantation (sheep, Ellinwood *et al.*, 1979a; pig, Zavy *et al.*, 1980; cow, Thatcher *et al.*, 1979), raising the question of the relative contribution of the endometrium and blastocyst to this pool of PG.

B. Prostaglandins and Luteal Function

1. Maintenance of Luteal Function

A requirement for luteal progesterone for implantation and normal pregnancy is a widespread phenomenon (Amoroso and Perry, 1977; Section II,A,1). In those species in which the period of dependence on progesterone exceeds the length of the normal luteal phase, it becomes necessary to have an extension of the lifespan of the CL, with the option of placental production of progesterone at a later time. In some cases, the signal to extend the lifespan of the CL is given before implantation (Table II). Species such as the goat, sheep, cow, pig, and guinea pig, in which hysterectomy prevents regression of the CL in the nonpregnant state, the blastocyst is said to be antiluteolytic. The blastocyst signal in the ewe has been called trophoblastin (Martal *et al.,* 1979) and, in the pig, it is suggested that blastocyst estrogen is the luteotrophin (Bazer and Thatcher, 1977). In those species, e.g., the primates, in which hysterectomy does not influence luteal function, the blastocyst is said to be luteotrophic, the signal being a chorionic gonadotrophin. Recent evidence suggests that even in ruminants, the blastocyst, although predominantly antiluteolytic at the uterine level, may also have a luteotrophic influence at the ovarian level (Inskeep and Murdoch, 1980). In the pig it has been suggested that estrogen subserves both actions (Flint *et al.,* 1979a). There is now good evidence that the uterine luteolysin in ruminants, rodents, pigs, and guinea pigs is $PGF_{2\alpha}$ (Anderson *et al.,* 1969; Goding, 1974; Horton and Poyser, 1976), whereas the nature of the luteolysin in primates is not known. The remainder of this section will discuss blastocyst antiluteolysins and luteotrophins.

2. Estrogen

Evidence for an antiluteolytic and luteotrophic role of blastocyst estrogen in the pig is particularly strong (Flint *et al.,* 1979a); Bazer and Thatcher (1977) proposed a theory of maternal recognition of pregnancy in the pig in which blastocyst estrogen (Section II,A,2) acts on the endometrium to prevent $PGF_{2\alpha}$ release into the uterine vein (and so being luteolytic), at the same time facilitating exocrine release of PG (and protein) into the uterine lumen at the time when luteal sensitivity to $PGF_{2\alpha}$ is increasing. In addition to an action at the uterine level, estrogens may subsequently act on the CL to augment the luteotrophic action of LH. Robertson *et al.* (1980) argue, on the basis of studies with estrogen antisera and measurement of circulating estrogens, that the conjugated rather than the unconjugated estrogens are luteotrophic on the CL. These authors concede that it is possible that free estrogen may act locally on the endometrium to facilitate attachment and redirect PG release. However, estrone sulfate has not been shown to be luteotrophic in the normal cycle (Flint *et al.,* 1979a). Furthermore, the mechanism by which estrogen changes the direction of PG release by the porcine uterus remains obscure.

This theory obviously can apply only to species such as the pig and horse with demonstrable estrogen production by the blastocyst. Estrogens are essential for CL maintenance in the rabbit (Browning *et al.,* 1980) and are produced by the rabbit blastocyst at implantation (Section II,A,2). However, there is no evidence of a difference in circulating estradiol levels in pregnant and pseudopregnant rabbits with the exception of a rise in levels in pseudopregnant does during luteal regression (Browning *et al.,* 1980). This suggests that the estrogen requirement in the rabbit is probably fulfilled by the ovary rather than the blastocyst.

3. Trophoblastin

Moor (1968) described the antiluteolysin in sheep as a watersoluble, heat-labile, species-specific substance, present in trophoblast on days 14–15. The capacity of embryo extracts to extend the lifespan of the CL when infused into the uterine lumen (but not when infused systemically) has been confirmed in sheep (Lawson and Findlay, 1977; Martal *et al.,* 1979; Ellinwood *et al.,* 1979b) and cows (Northey and French, 1980) but not in guinea pigs (Poyser and Maule Walker, 1979). The ovine antiluteolysin, trophoblastin, is a protein which can be extracted at pH 9.6 from trophoblast from day 12 to day 25 (Martal *et al.,* 1979; Martal, 1981). The mechanism by which trophoblastin acts is not known, but in view of the luteolytic and luteotrophic actions of prostaglandin $F_{2\alpha}$ and E_2, respectively (Inskeep and Murdoch, 1980), trophoblastin may prevent the action of $PGF_{2\alpha}$ and promote the production of PGE_2 at the uterine level (Findlay, 1981). This could be achieved by a redistribution of PG away from the uterine venous drainage toward the uterine lumen as in the pig (Bazer and Thatcher, 1977) and observed in the sheep (Ellinwood *et al.,* 1979a), and by an alteration in the relative abundance of PGE_2 over $PGF_{2\alpha}$ due to changes in endometrial synthesis and metabolism and production of PGs by the blastocyst. Alternatively, trophoblastin may influence the receptors for estrogen (Findlay *et al.,* 1982) and oxytocin (McCracken, 1980) which are suppressed in pregnancy and are important for the secretion of PG.

4. Placental Lactogen (PL)

PL or chorionic somatomammotrophin has been found in human and nonhuman primates, ruminants, and rodents (Forsyth and Hayden, 1977; Martal and Djiane, 1977) but generally it is not present before implantation, except in ruminants. In sheep, PL is first detected in trophectoderm on day 16, when attachment is initiated, but it is not detected in blood until around days 40–50 (Martal and Djiane, 1977). PL is believed to originate from the binucleate cells (Martal *et al.,* 1977) which are of fetal origin and migrate through the microvillar junction of the endometrium to form the syncytium (Wooding *et al.,* 1980). A similar migration occurs in the bovine placentome (Wooding and Wathes, 1980). PL has been detected in bovine conceptuses collected between 17 and 25 days pc, at or shortly after the time of appearance of binucleate cells in the trophectoderm, but before the time of attachment (Flint *et al.,* 1979b). Since PL is not luteotrophic in sheep (Martal and Djiane, 1977), its role in implantation and early pregnancy in that species remains obscure (Martal, 1981). In rodents PL may be luteotrophic by stimulation of receptors for estrogen (Gibori *et al.,* 1979) and maintenance of receptors for LH (Chan *et al.,* 1980) in the CL.

5. Chorionic Gonadotrophins

All primates examined so far produce a CG at or after the time of vascularization of the implantation site and implantation of the blastocyst (Hearn, 1980; Findlay, 1980). Evidence to date suggests that CGs in nonhuman primates have a similar chemical structure, site of origin, and role to maintain the CL as hCG in the human. Pregnancy in equids is also associated with production of a CG, but not until after the time of implantation (Allen, 1979).

Claims that substances with similar radioreceptor and radioimmunoassay characteristics as a CG are present in preimplantation blastocysts of the rat (Haour *et al.,* 1976), mouse and hamster (Wiley, 1974; Wide and Hobson, 1978; Wide and Wide, 1979), rabbit (Haour and Saxena, 1974), sheep (Lacroix and Martal, 1979; Martal, 1981), and pig (Saunders *et al.,* 1980) should be treated with caution. The assays used are open to nonspecific interference by a variety of substances, and many of the extracts have not been tested in proper bioassays for luteotrophic activity.

Controversy exists about the presence of biologically active luteotrophic material in rabbit and ruminant blastocysts. Keyes and his colleagues did not find evidence from *in vitro* bioassays or from measurement of peripheral progesterone levels for a pregnancy luteotrophin in the rabbit until after the end of the first third of gestation (Holt *et al.,* 1976; Browning *et al.,* 1980; Browning and Wolf, 1981). Their observations are supported by Sundaram *et al.* (1975) and Ellinwood *et al.* (1979c). In contrast, Channing *et al.* (1978) describe a stimulating effect of rabbit blastocyst fluid on progesterone secretion by monkey granulosa cells *in vitro,* but a proper dose–response study with bioassay statistics was not performed. In the cow, increased secretion of progesterone by the CL is observed from day 10 of pregnancy (Lukaszewska and Hansel, 1980) and could be related to the capacity of preattachment bovine embryos to stimulate progesterone secretion by luteal tissue *in vitro*

(Hansel *et al.,* 1978) and to the presence of placental lactogen (Flint *et al.,* 1979b). Despite claims of luteotrophic activity in sheep blastocyst by radioreceptor assay (Lacroix and Martal, 1979) and *in vitro* assay (Godkin *et al.,* 1978), there is no evidence of a pregnancy associated increase in peripheral progesterone levels before implantation (Bindon, 1971). Using specific bio- and radioreceptor assays, Ellinwood *et al.* (1979b) were unable to find any evidence of LH or prolactin-like activity in 14- to 15-day-old sheep blastocysts. Preliminary data suggest that porcine blastocysts do have luteotrophic activity (Flint, 1981). If these substances are important for maintenance of CL function in early pregnancy the activity should be present in the circulation, but no evidence yet exists. It is possible that hCG and the other CG-like substances might be involved in the immunological protection of the conceptus (Amoroso and Perry, 1975).

C. *Prostaglandins, Endometrial Vascular Permeability, and Decidualization*

An increase in endometrial vascular permeability (EVP) is one of the earliest responses of the receptive endometrium of rodents to natural (blastocyst) or artificial deciduogenic stimuli (Psychoyos, 1973). Originally it was thought that estrogen was responsible for the EVP (Marcus and Shelesnyak, 1970). There is now evidence that PGs mediate the changes in EVP and may also influence decidualization in the rat, mouse, and hamster (see Lindner *et al.,* 1974; Kennedy, 1980; Kennedy and Armstrong, 1981 for references).

1. Endometrial Vascular Permeability

Indomethacin, an inhibitor of PG synthesis, will delay or inhibit the localized increase in EVP and implantation in pregnant animals, an effect partially reversed by exogenous PG. The "dye sites" or areas of EVP contain increased concentrations of PGs (PGE in particular) at the time of EVP. Studies in nonpregnant animals with artificially induced deciduomata also support a role for PGs in these processes. Since EVP is thought to be an essential prerequisite for the decidual cell reaction (Psychoyos, 1973), the effect of PG on implantation might be mediated by the increase in EVP. However, indomethacin still blocked the decidual reaction when administered into the uterine lumen 8 hours after the deciduogenic stimulus, by which time the increase in permeability had presumably occurred. This suggests that PGs are involved not only in EVP but also in the later stages of the decidual cell reaction.

While the timing of uterine sensitivity to the decidual cell reaction was not related to the ability of the uterus to produce PG, it may be related to its ability to respond to PG or to the presence of other mediators of EVP (Kennedy, 1980). Current evidence suggests that PGE_2 rather than $PGF_{2\alpha}$ and PGI_2 is responsible for the change in vascular permeability, although because of its instability in the experiments performed, a role for PGI_2 cannot be eliminated (Kennedy *et al.,* 1980). The mechanisms by which PGE_2 (PGI_2) cause EVP are not understood. Vasodilation accompanies EVP induced by artificial stimulus (Bitton *et al.,* 1965) and might be due to a PG of the E or I series. Kennedy and Armstrong (1981) have suggested that EVP may represent two components, vasodilation and vascular permeability, a situation analogous to the inflammatory response (Espey, 1980).

2. Decidualization

The decidualization of stromal cells requires prior exposure to the correct sequence of estrogen and progesterone, making the cells responsive to the stimulus (Marcus and Shelesnyak, 1970). An action of PGs in this process may depend on the stage of decidualization. In pseudopregnant rats, decidual cells proliferate vigorously and then stop dividing after about 4 days (Glasser and Clark, 1975) when PGE content is markedly increased in the deciduomata (Anteby *et al.,* 1975). Evidence for a positive action of PG during the early, proliferative phase of decidualization comes from studies in which indomethacin, instilled in the uterine lumen 8 hours after the stimulus, prevented decidualization (Sananes *et al.,* 1976; Tobert, 1976) or reduced decidual size but not number (Evans and Kennedy, 1978).

Not all the evidence favors a positive action of PG in decidualization. Peleg and Lindner (1980) explanted rat decidual cells during the proliferative phase, and found that estrogen and progesterone inhibited accumulation of PGE *in vitro* and inhibitors of PG synthesis had a stimulating effect on DNA synthesis. PGE, known to inhibit cell division in various culture systems (Pastan *et al.,* 1975), inhibited DNA synthesis by decidual cells in culture. Peleg and Lindner (1980) suggest that progesterone-induced stimulation of DNA synthesis may be due in part to its inhibitory effect on PGE accumulations by decidual cells, inferring that the rate of DNA synthesis may be influenced by steroid-induced changes in PGE tissue content. Subsequently, Peleg and Lindner (1981) demonstrated that indomethacin given ip before the deciduogenic stimulus reduced the number of polyploid cells (a measure of decidualization) in 4-day-old cultures. Indomethacin added to the cultures had no effect. They concluded that once triggered, the differentiation of endometrial cells into polyploid decidual cells *in vitro* is independent of PG. The inhibitory effect of indomethacin *in vivo* may have involved progesterone action since nuclear binding of the progesterone analog, R5020, was reduced by 50% in the uteri of indomethacin-treated, pseudopregnant rats (Peleg and Lindner, 1981). It remains to be determined if this effect of PG is independent of the changes in vascular permeability. If PGs are involved in EVP and decidualization in the rat, it is unlikely that they originate from the blastocyst because to date there is no evidence that rat blastocysts can make PG (Kennedy and Armstrong, 1981). Thus the PG is likely to be of uterine origin probably from the luminal epithelium (Lejeune *et al.,* 1981). The embryonic signal responsible for eliciting this response is not known, that is, if a signal is needed at all, since adequate uterine sensitivity and uterine closure may suffice (Martin, 1980).

The decidual cell reaction is by no means universal among mammals. It is especially marked in rodents, in members of the orders Insectivora and Arthropoidea (Finn and Porter, 1975), including the human (Noyes *et al.,* 1950). True decidual cells do not occur in most carnivores, artiodactyls (Finn and Porter, 1975), or marsupials (Renfree, 1980). However, some artiodactyls have been observed to have changes in uterine blood flow and EVP prior to implantation. Transient increases in blood flow to the gravid uterine horns of the ewe (Greiss and Anderson, 1970), cow (Ford *et al.,* 1979), and sow (Ford and Christenson, 1979) have been observed prior to implantation, during the period when the embryo must be present to ensure maintenance of the CL. In sheep, the blastocyst induces EVP within the caruncular (attachment areas) endometrium immediately prior to attachment (Boshier, 1970); a similar reaction has not been observed in the pig (Heap *et al.,* 1979b).

It has been suggested that the increased uterine blood flow results from a local influence of the blastocyst on the uterine vascular bed, whereby neurotransmitter effects on arterial smooth muscle cells are reduced resulting in vasodilation (Ford *et al.,* 1976, 1977; Pope and Stormshak, 1979). The nature of the substance(s) produced by the conceptus or gravid uterus is not known, however, estrogens and progesterone have been implicated. Although estrogen administration will increase uterine blood flow in the ewe (Huckabee *et al.,* 1970), cow (Roman-Ponce *et al.,* 1978), and sow (Dickson *et al.,* 1969), not all the evidence supports a role for estrogen as the vasodilatory agent. First, the pig is the only species in which there is sufficient evidence for a local increase in estrogen production by the blastocyst at the critical time (Section II,A,2). Second, the estrogen-induced flow response in the ewe begins 30 minutes after intraarterial injection and is inhibited by cyclohexamide (Killam *et al.,* 1973) suggesting that other local vasoactive agents may act as mediators in the action of estrogen (Resnik *et al.,* 1976). Resnik and Brink (1978, 1980) have shown that PGE_1, PGE_2, and PGI_2 increase uterine blood flow in sheep in contrast to $PGF_{2\alpha}$, which is vasoconstrictive. These authors suggest that the action of estrogen may be mediated via PGE_2 or PGI_2. The increased quantities of PGE_2 in the endometrium, uterine lumen, and blastocyst prior to implantation in sheep

(Sections II,A,1 and 2) suggest PGE_2 as the vasodilatory agent. However, perfusion of uterine arteries of pregnant and nonpregnant ewes with PGE_2 *in vitro* failed to alter the response of those arteries to nerve stimulation, compared to saline (Pope and Stormshak, 1979). The effects of PGI_2 should be investigated in this system, since PGI_2 is probably a major product in the sheep uterus (Jones *et al.*, 1977).

In the endometrium of women, there are generally lower concentrations of PGF and PGE during the proliferative phase compared with the late secretory phase (see Hagenfeldt, 1980). This is most likely related to the circulating levels of progesterone and estradiol-17β which control the production of PG by the endometrium (Abel and Baird, 1980) and are also important for the formation of the decidua (Long and Bradbury, 1951). PGE_2 and $PGF_{2\alpha}$ are the primary products in human endometrium, in contrast to the myometrium where the presence of 6-keto-$PGF_{2\alpha}$ indicates that a prostacyclin is the major product (Abel and Kelly, 1979). The concentrations of PGE and PGF were much lower in decidua of women with either an intrauterine device or ectopic and normal pregnancy than in proliferative or secretory endometrium (Maathius and Kelly, 1978; Abel *et al.*, 1980). Decreased conversion of arichadonic acid to PG *in vitro* was also noted in decidua of pregnancy (Abel and Kelly, 1979). The importance of these changes in PG levels to implantation in the human is not known. It is tempting to speculate that the PGs have a local vasodilatory rather than a vasopressive action to maintain blood flow to the decidua. Thus a predominance of prostacyclin and PGE over PGF would be preferable. PGs have also been implicated in menstrual blood flow with a balance between platelet prostaglandin and thromboxane synthesis being important for hemostasis (Hagenfeldt, 1980). An action of the implanting blastocyst on this balance could be important for maintaining the integrity of endometrial blood flow and the viability of the endometrial cells.

V. Histamine

A. A Mediator of Estrogen Action?

The fact that uterine vascular responses to estrogen administration closely resemble the tissue responses to local application of histamine led Holden (1939) to suggest that the actions of estrogen on the uterus are mediated by a dilator substance released from uterine cells under the influence of estrogen. Attempts to substantiate the hypothesis that histamine was the vasodilator intermediary in decidualization in rodents have not been successful (De Feo, 1967; Marcus and Shelesnyak, 1970). Cause and effect relationships cannot be inferred from the fact that the prenidatory rise in estrogen is followed by histamine release, and that implantation can be blocked by antiestrogens, by antihistamines, or by chronic histamine depletion. Under certain experimental conditons, it is possible to separate the effects of estrogen and histamine, suggesting that histamine release is not a necessary adjunct of estrogen action (Marcus and Shelesnyak, 1970).

B. Histamine and the Blastocyst

Nevertheless, the fact that antihistamines can interrupt implantation in rats (Shelesnyak, 1957), provided the antagonists interact with both the H1 and H2 receptors for histamine (Brandon and Wallis, 1977), indicates a role for histamine. Implantation can be induced in rats with delayed implantation by administration of histamine in combination with suboptimal amounts of estrogen (Brandon and Raval, 1979; Johnson and Dey, 1980). Day *et al.* (1979a) interrupted implantation in rabbits by intraluminal injection on day 5 of pregnancy of DL-α-methylhistidine, a specific inhibitor of histidine decarboxylase (HDC) which converts histidine to histamine. Because rabbit blastocysts and not endometrial tissue exhibited HDC activity, these authors suggested that implantation was interrupted by interference with embryonic HDC activity.

Once formed, histamine could act on the embryo via H2 receptors or on the endometrium via H1 receptors (Dey *et al.*, 1976b). In the embryo and uterus, histamine may exert its influence via synthesis of prostaglandins since histamine is known to influence phospholipase-A_2 activity (Blackwell *et al.*, 1978). Alternatively, histamine may promote embryonic growth (Kahlson, 1962). There is evidence that including an HDC inhibitor in the culture medium retarded the development of mouse embryos *in vitro* (Dey and Johnson, 1980). Because the action of histamine is probably mediated by activation of adenylate cyclase (Study and Greenguard, 1978) alterations in cyclic AMP and GMP in embryonic and uterine tissue should be examined following exposure to histamine.

VI. Conclusions

This brief survey of the literature has shown that the blastocysts of quite a number of species can produce a variety of agents capable of influencing endometrial and ovarian function in the preimplantation period. Definitive involvement of these agents in the endometrial processes prior to and during implantation remains conjectural, however. Indeed, it is paradoxical that in the rat, there is good evidence for an influence of prostaglandins and estradiol on the endometrium, yet the blastocysts of this species apparently lack the capacity to produce these agents. A relatively passive role of the blastocyst is suggested in the rat. By contrast, in ungulates where there is considerable growth and expansion of the blastocyst prior to attachment, there is good evidence for an influence of the blastocyst on endometrial metabolism and secretion but the nature of the agents responsible is not known. Of the blastocyst factors discussed, the luteotrophic properties of estradiol in pigs and CG in primates and the antiluteolysin, trophoblastin, in sheep seem best established. More work is needed on the relationship of the blastocyst and endometrium in primates. While sheep (Findlay, 1980) and guinea pigs (Aitken, 1980) can be used as models for the human, I support John Hearn's (1980) view that nonhuman primates are probably best if they can be used. Much of the work done so far has not unravelled the effects of a blastocyst on specific cell types within the endometrium. There is a varying degree of functional differentiation of the endometrium and efforts should be made to understand the function of epithelial and stromal cells from those regions now that techniques of cell separation are available (e.g., McCormack and Glasser, 1980).

Time and space did not permit me to review the increasing evidence of an effect of the endometrium on blastocyst growth. By exploiting the situations of delayed implantation in rodents (Weitlauf, 1978; Weitlauf and Kiessling, 1981), macropodids (Wallace, 1981), and roe deer (Aitken, 1979a) and trophoblast expansion in pigs (Flint, 1981), it should be possible to describe this influence in more detail. This aspect of blastocyst–endometrial interactions should not be divorced from influences of the blastocyst on the endometrium, because, as embryo transfer studies in sheep have shown (Lawson and Findlay, 1977; Wilmut and Sales, 1981), the signaling capacity of the blastocyst may be determined by its uterine environment.

Acknowledgments

I am indebted to Noelene Colvin, Caroline Donkin, and Elaine Griffiths for their editorial assistance and typing and to the Australian Wool Research Trust Fund and the National Health and Medical Research Council of Australia for financial support.

References

Abel, M. H., and Baird, D. T. (1980). *Endocrinology* **106,** 1599–1606.

Abel, M. H., and Kelly, R. W. (1979). *Prostaglandins* **18,** 821–828.

Abel, M. H., Smith, S. K., and Baird, D. T. (1980). *J. Endocrinol.* **85,** 379–386.

Aitken, R. J. (1977). *J. Reprod. Fertil.* **50,** 29–36.

Aitken, R. J. (1979a). *Ciba Found. Symp.* **64,** 53–83.

Aitken, R. J. (1979b). *In* "Oxford Review of Reproductive Biology" (C. A. Finn, ed.), Vol. I, pp. 351–382. Clarendon, Oxford.

Aitken, R. J. (1980). *In* "Animal Models in Human Reproduction" (M. Serio and L. Martini, eds.), pp. 299–317. Raven, New York.

Allen, W. R. (1979). *Ciba Found. Symp.* **64,** 323–352.

Amoroso, E. C. (1952). *In* "Marshalls Physiology of Reproduction" (A. S. Parkes, ed.), Vol. II, pp. 127–311. Longmans, London.

Amoroso, E. C., and Perry, J. S. (1975). *Philos. Trans. R. Soc., London Ser. B* **271,** 343–361.

Amoroso, E. C., and Perry, J. S. (1977). *In* "The Ovary" (S. Zuckerman and B. J. Weir, eds.), 2 Ed., Vol. II, Physiology, pp. 315–398. Academic Press, New York.

Anderson, L. L., Bland, K. P., and Melampy, R. M. (1969). *Recent Prog. Horm. Res.* **25,** 57–104.

Anteby, S. O., Bauminger, S., Zor, U., and Lindner, H. R. (1975). *Prostaglandins,* **10,** 991–999.

Baird, D. T. (1978). *In* "Control of Ovulation" (D. B. Crichton, N. B. Haynes, G. R. Foxcroft, and G. E. Lamming, eds.), pp. 217–233. Butterworths, London.

Basha, S. M. M., Bazer, F. W., and Roberts, R. M. (1980). *J. Reprod. Fertil.* **60,** 41–48.

Baulieu, E. -E., Mortel, R., and Robel, P. (1980). *WHO Symp., Geneva* pp. 266–290.

Bayard, F., Damilano, S., Robel, P., and Baulieu, E. -E. (1978). *J. Clin. Endocrinol. Metab.* **46,** 635–648.

Bazer, F. W. (1975). *J. Anim. Sci.* **41,** 1376–1382.

Bazer, F. W., and Thatcher, W. W. (1977). *Prostaglandins* **14,** 397–401.

Beier, H., and Mootz, V. (1979). *Ciba Found. Symp.* **64,** 111–140.

Bell, S. C., Reynolds, S., and Heald, P. J. (1977). *J. Reprod. Fertil.* **49,** 177–181.

Bindon, B. M. (1971). *J. Reprod. Fertil.* **24,** 146.

Bito, L. Z. (1975). *Prostaglandins* **9,** 851–855.

Bitton, V., Vassent, G., and Psychoyos, A. (1965). *C. R. Hebd. Seance Acad. Sci. Paris* **261,** 3474–3477.

Blackwell, G. J., Flower, R. J., Nijkamp, F. P., and Vane, J. R. (1978). *Br. J. Pharmacol.* **62,** 79–89.

Boshier, D. P. (1970). *J. Reprod. Fertil.* **19,** 51–61.

Boyd, J. D., and Hamilton, W. J. (1952). *In* "Marshalls Physiology of Reproduction" (A. S. Parkes, ed.), Vol. II, pp. 1–126. Longmans, London.

Bradshaw, S. D., McDonald, I. R., Hahnel, R., and Heller, H. (1975). *J. Endocrinol.* **65,** 451–452.

Brandon, J. M., and Raval, P. J. (1979). *Eur. J. Pharmacol.* **57,** 171–177.

Brandon, J. M., and Wallis, R. M. (1977). *J. Reprod. Fertil.* **50,** 251–254.

Brodie, A. M. H., Wu, J. -T., Marsh, D. A., and Brodie, H. J. (1978). *Biol. Reprod.* **18,** 365–370.

Browning, J. Y., and Wolf, R. C. (1981). *Biol. Reprod.* **24,** 293–297.

Browning, J. Y., Keyes, P. L., and Wolf, R. C. (1980). *Biol. Reprod.* **23,** 1014–1019.

Bullock, D. W. (1977). *In* "Development in Mammals" (M. H. Johnson, ed.), Vol. 2 pp. 199–208. Elsevier, Amsterdam.

Casey, M. L., Hamsell, D. L., MacDonald, P. C., and Johnson, J. M. (1980). *Prostaglandins* **19,** 115–122.

Challis, J. R. G., Louis, T. M., Robinson, J. S., and Thorburn, G. D. (1976). *J. Endocrinol.* **69,** 451–452.

Chàmbon, Y. (1949). *C. R. Seances Soc. Biol. Fil.* **143,** 1172.

Chan, J. S. D., Grinwich, D. L., Robertson, H. A., and Friesen, H. G. (1980). *Biol. Reprod.* **23,** 60–63.

Channing, C. P., Stone, S. L., Sakai, C. N., Haour, F., and Saxena, B. B. (1978). *J. Reprod. Fertil.* **54,** 215–220.

Chenault, J. R., and Hruska, R. L. (1979). *J. Anim. Sci.* **49,** (Suppl. 1), Abstr. 355.

Clemetson, C. A. B., Kim, J. K., De Jesus, T. P. S., Mallikarjuneswara, V. R., and Wilds, J. H. (1973). *J. Obstet. Gynaecol. Br. Commonw.* **80,** 553–561.
Cumming, I. A., Baxter, R. B., and Lawson, R. A. S. (1974). *J. Reprod. Fertil.* **40,** 443–446.
Daniel, J. C., Jr. (1972). *J. Reprod. Fertil.* **31,** 303–306.
Deanesly, R. (1960). *J. Reprod. Fertil.* **1,** 242–248.
Deanesly, R. (1967). *J. Reprod. Fertil.* **14,** 243–248.
Deaver, D. R., and Guthrie, H. D. (1980). *Biol. Reprod.* **23,** 72–77.
De Feo, V. J. (1967). *In* "Cellular Biology of the Uterus" (R. M. Wynn, ed.), pp. 191–290. Appleton, New York.
Dey, S. K., and Johnson, D. C. (1980). *J. Reprod. Fertil.* **60,** 457–460.
Dey, S. K., Johnson, D. C., and Santos, J. G. (1979a). *Biol. Reprod.* **21,** 1169–1173.
Dey, S. K., Villanueva, C., Chien, S. M., and Crist, R. D. (1979b). *Nature (London)* **278,** 648–649.
Dey, S. K., Chien, S. M., Cox, C. L., and Crist, R. D. (1980). *Prostaglandins* **19,** 449–453.
Dickmann, Z., and Sen Gupta, J. (1974). *Dev. Biol.* **40,** 196–198.
Dickmann, Z., and Spilman, C. H. (1975). *Science* **190,** 997–998.
Dickmann, Z., Dey, S. K., and Sen Gupta, J. (1975). *Proc. Natl. Acad. Sci. U.S.A.* **72,** 298–300.
Dickmann, Z., Dey, S. K., and Sen Gupta, J. (1976). *Vitam. Horm.* **34,** 215–242.
Dickson, W. M., Bosc, M. J., and Locatelli, A. (1969). *Am. J. Physiol.* **217,** 1431–1434.
Eiler, H., Bahr, J., and Nalbandov, A. (1974). *Proc. Annu. Meet. Soc. Study Reprod., 7th, Ottawa* Abstr. 97.
Eley, R. M., Thatcher, W. W., Bazer, F. W., and Fields, M. J. (1979). *J. Anim. Sci.* **149,** 294A.
Ellinwood, W. E., Nett, T. M., and Niswender, G. D. (1979a). *Biol. Reprod.* **21,** 845–856.
Ellinwood, W. E., Nett, T. M., and Niswender, G. D. (1979b). *Biol. Reprod.* **21,** 281–288.
Ellinwood, W. E., Seidel, G. E., and Niswender, G. D. (1979c). *Proc. Soc. Exp. Biol. Med.* **161,** 136–141.
Enders, A. C., and Schlafke, S. (1979). *Ciba Found. Symp.* **64,** 3–32.
Espey, L. L. (1980). *Biol. Reprod.* **22,** 73–106.
Evans, C. A., and Kennedy, T. G. (1978). *J. Reprod. Fertil.* **54,** 255–261.
Evans, C. A., and Kennedy, T. G. (1980). *Steroids* **36,** 41–52.
Findlay, J. K. (1980). *In* "Immunological Aspects of Reproduction and Fertility Control" (J. P. Hearn, ed.), pp. 63–81. MTP Press, Lancaster.
Findlay, J. K. (1981). *J. Reprod. Fertil. Suppl.* **30,** 171–182.
Findlay, J. K., Cerini, M., Sheers, M., Staples, L. D., and Cumming, I. A. (1979). *Ciba Found. Symp.* **64,** 239–259.
Findlay, J. K., Maule Walker, F. M., and Heap, R. B. (1980). *In* "Animal Models in Human Reproduction" (M. Serio and L. Martini, eds.), pp. 283–297. Raven, New York.
Findlay, J. K., Ackland, N., Burton, R. D., Davis, A. J., Maule Walker, F. M., Walters, D. E., and Heap, R. B. (1981). *J. Reprod. Fertil.* **62,** 361–377.
Findlay, J. K., Clarke, I. J., Swaney, J., Colvin, N., and Doughton, B. (1982). *J. Reprod. Fertil.* **64,** 329–339.
Finn, C. A., and Porter, D. G. (1975). *In* "Handbooks in Reproductive Physiology," Vol. 1. Elek Science, London.
Flint, A. P. F. (1981). *J. Reprod. Fertil. Suppl.* **29,** 215–227.
Flint, A. P. F., Burton, R. D., Gadsby, J. E., Saunders, P. T. K., and Heap, R. B. (1979a). *Ciba Found. Symp.* **64,** 209–238.
Flint, A. P. F., Henville, A., and Christie, W. G. (1979b). *J. Reprod. Fertil.* **56,** 305–308.
Flood, P. F., and Ghazi, R. (1981). *J. Reprod. Fertil.* **61,** 47–52.
Ford, S. P., and Christenson, R. K. (1979). *Biol. Reprod.* **21,** 617–624.

Ford, S. P., Weber, L. J., and Stormshak, F. (1976). *Biol. Reprod.* **15,** 58–65.
Ford, S. P., Weber, L. J., and Stormshak, F. (1977). *Biol. Reprod.* **17,** 480–483.
Ford, S. P.,Chenault, J. R., and Echternkamp, S. E. (1979). *J. Reprod. Fertil* **56,** 53–62.
Forsyth, I. A., and Hayden, T. J. (1977). *Symp. Zool. Soc. London* **41,** 135–163.
Fowler, R. E., Johnson, M. H., Walters, D. E., and Pratt, H. P. M. (1976). *J. Reprod. Fertil.* **46,** 427–430.
Gadsby, J. E., Heap, R. B., and Burton, R. D. (1980). *J. Reprod. Fertil.* **60,** 409–417.
George, F. W., and Wilson, J. D. (1978). *Science* **199,** 200–201.
Gibbons, R. A., Dixon, S. N., and Roberts, G. P. (1977). *Biochem. Soc. Trans.* **5,** 452–454.
Gibori, G., Richards, J. S., and Keyes, P. L. (1979). *Biol. Reprod.* **21,** 419–423.
Given, R. L., and Enders, A. C. (1980). *Am. J. Anat.* **157,** 169–179.
Glasser, S. R., and Clark, J. H. (1975). *In* "The Developmental Biology of Reproduction" (C. L. Makert and J. Papaconstantinov, eds.), pp. 311–345. Academic Press, New York.
Goding, J. R. (1974). *J. Reprod. Fertil.* **38,** 261–271.
Godkin, J. D., Cote, C., and Duby, R. T. (1978). *J. Reprod. Fertil.* **54,** 375–378.
Greiss, F. C., Jr., and Anderson, S. G. (1970). *Am. J. Obstet. Gynecol.* **106,** 30–38.
Hagenfeldt, K. (1980). *WHO Symp. Geneva* pp. 222–245.
Hansel, W., Lukaszewska, J., and Beal, W. (1978). *Proc. Annu. Meet. Soc. Study Reprod., 11th* p. 37.
Haour, F., and Saxena, B. B. (1974). *Science* **185,** 444–445.
Haour, F., Tell, G., and Sanchez, P. (1976). *C.R. Hebd. Seance Acad. Sci. Paris Ser. D* **82,** 1183–1186.
Harper, M. J. K., Dowd, D., and Elliot, A. (1969). *Biol. Reprod.* **1,** 253–257.
Heap, R. B., Flint, A. P. F., Gadsby, J. E., and Rice, C. (1979a). *J. Reprod. Fertil* **55,** 267–275.
Heap, R. B., Flint, A. P. F., and Gadsby, J. E. (1979b). *Br. Med. Bull.* **35,** 129–135.
Heap, R. B., Renfree, M. B., and Burton, R. D. (1980). *J. Endocrinol.* **87,** 339–349.
Hearn, J. P. (1980). *In* "Animal Models in Human Reproduction" (M. Serio and L. Martini, eds.), pp. 319–332. Raven, New York.
Holden, R. B. (1939). *Endocrinology* **25,** 593–596.
Holt, J. A., Heise, W. F., Wilson, W. M., and Keyes, P. L. (1976). *Endocrinology* **98,** 904–909.
Horton, E. W., and Poyser, N. L. (1976). *Physiol. Rev.* **56,** 595–651.
Huckabee, W. E., Crenshaw, C., Curet, L. B., Mann, L., and Barrow, D. H. (1970). *Q. J. Exp. Physiol.* **55,** 16–24.
Huff, R. L., and Eik-Nes, K. B. (1966). *J. Reprod. Fertil.* **11,** 57–63.
Huslig, R. L., Fogwell, R. L., and Smith, W. L. (1979). *Biol. Reprod.* **21,** 589–600.
Hyland, J. H., Manns, J. G., and Humphrey, W. D. (1982). *J. Reprod. Fertil.* **65,** 299–304.
Inskeep, E. K., and Murdoch, W. J. (1980). *Int. Rev. Physiol.* **22,** 325–356.
Inskeep, E. K., Wilson, L., Jr., Butler, W. R., Dierschke, D. J., Fritz, G. R., and Knobil, E. (1980). *In* "The Endometrium" (F. A. Kimball, ed.), pp. 287–309. Spectrum, New York.
Johnson, D. C., and Dey, S. K. (1980). *Biol. Reprod.* **22,** 1136–1141.
Jones, L. T., Heap, R. B., and Perry, J. S. (1976). *J. Reprod. Fertil.* **47,** 129–131.
Jones, R. L., Poyser, N. L., and Wilson, N. H. (1977). *Br. J. Pharmacol.* **59,** 436–437.
Kahlson, G. (1962). *Perspect. Biol. Med.* **5,** 179–197.
Kennedy, T. G. (1980). *Prog. Reprod. Biol.* **7,** 234–243.
Kennedy, T. G., and Armstrong, D. T. (1981). *In* "Cellular and Molecular Aspects of Implantation" (S. R. Glasser and D. W. Bullock, eds.), pp. 349–363. Plenum, New York.
Kennedy, T. G., Barbe, G. J., and Evans, C. A. (1980). *In* "The Endometrium" (F. A. Kimball, ed.), pp. 331–344. Spectrum Publications, New York.
Killam, A. P., Rosenfeld, C. R., Battaglia, F. C., Makowski, E. R., and Meschia, G. (1973). *Am. J. Obstet. Gynecol.* **115,** 1045–1052.
King, G. J., Atkinson, B. A., and Robertson, H. A. (1981). *J. Reprod. Fertil.* **61,** 469–474.

Kreitmann, B., and Bayard, F. (1979). *Acta Endocrinol. Copenhagen* **92**, 547–552.
Kreitmann, B., Faye, J. C., Derache, B., and Bayard, F. (1979). *J. Steroid Biochem.* **11**, 1253–1258.
Kreitmann-Gimbal, B., Bayard, F., and Hodgen, G. J. (1981). *J. Clin. Endocrinol. Metab.* **52**, 133–137.
Kreitmann, O., Kreitmann-Gimbal, B., Bayard, F., and Hodgen, G. J. (1979). *Steroids* **34**, 693–703.
Lacroix, M. C., and Martal, J. (1979). *C.R. Hebd. Séance. Acad. Sci. Paris Ser. D* **288**, 771–774.
Laster, D. B. (1977). *Biol. Reprod.* **16**, 682–690.
Lawson, R. A. S., and Findlay, J. K. (1977). *In* "Reproduction and Evolution" (J. H. Calaby and C. H. Tyndale-Biscoe, eds.), pp. 349–357. Australian Academy of Science, Canberra.
Lejeune, B., Van Hoeck, J., and Leroy, F. (1981). *J. Reprod. Fertil.* **61**, 235–240.
Levy, C., Robel, P., Gantray, J. P., De Brux, J., Verma, U., Descomps, B., Baulieu, E.-E., and Eychene, B. (1980). *Am. J. Obstet. Gynecol.* **136**, 646–651.
Lindner, H. R., Zor, U., Bauminger, S., Tsafriri, A., Lamprecht, S. A., Koch, Y., Anteby, S. O., and Schwartz, A. (1974). *In* "Prostaglandin Synthetase Inhibitors" (J. H. Robinson and J. R. Vane, eds.), pp. 271–287. Raven, New York.
Logeat, F., Santor, P., Vu Hai, M. T., and Milgrom, E. (1980). *Science* **207**, 1083–1085.
Long, R. C., and Bradbury, J. T. (1951). *J. Clin. Endocrinol. Metab.* **11**, 134–145.
Lukaszewska, J., and Hansel, W. (1980). *J. Reprod. Fertil.* **59**, 485–493.
Lundstrom, V., and Gréen, K. (1978). *Am. J. Obstet. Gynecol.* **130**, 640–646.
Maathuis, J. B., and Aitken, R. J. (1978). *J. Reprod. Fertil.* **52**, 289–295,
Maathuis, J. B., and Kelly, R. W. (1978). *J. Endocrinol.* **77**, 361–371.
McCormack, S. A., and Glasser, S. R. (1980). *Endocrinology* **106**, 1634–1649.
McCracken, J. A. (1980). *In* "Advances in Prostaglandin and Thromboxane Research" (B. Samuelsson, P. W. Ramwell, and R. Paoletti, eds.), Vol. 8, pp. 1329–1344. Raven, New York.
Manak, R. C., Wertz, N. C., Slabaughm, Denari, H., Wang, J.-T., and Gorski, J. (1980). *In* "Steroid Induced Uterine Proteins" (M. Beato, ed.), pp. 21–34. Elsevier, Amsterdam.
Marcal, J., Chew, M. J., Salomon, D. S., and Sherman, M. I. (1975). *Endocrinology* **96**, 1270–1279.
Marcus, G. J., and Shelesnyak, M. C. (1970). *In* "Advances in Steroid Biochemistry and Pharmacology" (M. H. Briggs, ed.), Vol. 2, pp. 373–438. Academic Press, New York.
Marcus, G. J., Ainsworth, L., and Lucis, R. (1979a). *Steroids* **34**, 295–303.
Marcus, G. J., Lucis, R., and Ainsworth, L. (1979b). *Steroids* **34**, 807–815.
Martal, J. (1981). *J. Reprod. Fertil. Suppl.* **30**, 201–210.
Martal, J., and Djiane, J. (1977). *J. Reprod. Fertil.* **49**, 285–289.
Martal, J., Djiane, J., and Dubois, M. (1977). *Cell Tissue Res.* **184**, 427–433.
Martal, J., Lacroix, M. C., Loudes, C., Saunier, M., and Wintenberger-Torres, S. (1979). *J. Reprod. Fertil.* **56**, 63–73.
Martel, D., and Psychoyos, A. (1976). *Endocrinology* **99**, 470–475.
Martel, D., and Psychoyos, A. (1978). *J. Endocrinol.* **76**, 145–154.
Martel, D., and Psychoyos, A. (1981). *Science* **211**, 1454–1455.
Martin, L. (1980). *Prog. Reprod. Biol.* **7**, 54–69.
Maslar, I. A., and Riddick, D. H. (1979). *Am. J. Obstet. Gynecol.* **135**, 751–754.
Maule Walker, F. M., and Poyser, N. L. (1978). *Br. J. Pharmacol.* **62**, 177–183.
Maule Walker, F. M., Patik, C. E., Leaf, C. F., and Watson, J. (1977). *Prostaglandins* **14**, 557–562.
Mester, I., Martel, D., Psychoyos, A., and Baulieu, E.-E. (1974). *Nature (London)* **250**, 776–778.
Miller, B. G., and Moore, N. W. (1976). *Aust. J. Biol. Sci.* **29**, 565–573.

Miller, B. G., Wild, J., and Stone, G. M. (1979). *Aust. J. Biol. Sci.* **32,** 549-560.
Moor, R. M. (1968). *J. Anim. Sci.* **27,** (Suppl. 1), 97-118.
Muldoon, T. G. (1980). *Endocrinol. Rev.* **1,** 339-364.
Mullins, D. E., Horst, M. N., Bazer, F. W., and Roberts, M. R. (1980). *Biol. Reprod.* **22,** 1181-1192.
Myatt, L., Chaudhuri, G., Elder, M. G., and Lim, L. (1980). *J. Endocrinol.* **87,** 357-364.
Northey, D. L., and French, D. R. (1980). *J. Anim. Sci.* **50,** 298-302.
Noyes, R. W., Hertig, A. T., and Rock, J. (1950). *Fertil. Steril.* **1,** 3-25.
O'Grady, J. E., and Bell, S. C. (1977). *In* "Development in Mammals" (M. H. Johnson, ed.), Vol. 1, pp. 165-243. North-Holland Publ., Amsterdam.
Pack, B. A., Christensen, C., Douraghy, M., and Brooks, S. C. (1978). *Endocrinology* **103,** 2129-2136.
Pack, B. A., Brooks, C. L., Dukelow, W. R., and Brooks, S. C. (1979). *Biol. Reprod.* **20,** 545-551.
Pastan, I. H., Johnson, G. S., and Anderson, W. B. (1975). *Annu. Rev. Biochem.* **44,** 491-522.
Peleg, S., and Lindner, H. R. (1980). *Mol. Cell. Endocrinol.* **20,** 209-218.
Peleg, S., and Lindner, H. R. (1981). *In* "Cellular and Molecular Aspects of Implantation" (S. Glasser and D. Bullock, eds.), pp. 431-433. Plenum, New York.
Peplow, V., Breed, W. G., and Eckstein, P. (1973). *Am. J. Obstet. Gynecol.* **116,** 780-784.
Perry, J. S., Heap, R. B., and Amoroso, E. C. (1973). *Nature (London)* **245,** 45-47.
Pickles, V. R. (1957). *Nature (London)* **180,** 1198-1199.
Pietras, R. J., and Szego, C. M. (1979). *J. Steroid Biochem.* **11,** 1471-1483.
Pope, W. F., and Stormshak, F. (1979). *Biol. Reprod.* **20,** 847-851.
Poyser, N. L., and Maule Walker, F. M. (1979). *Ciba Found. Symp.* **64,** 261-292.
Psychoyos, A. (1973). *In* "Handbook of Physiology" (R. O. Greep, E. B. Astwood, and S. R. Geiger, eds.), Sect. 7, Vol. II, Part 2, pp. 187-215. American Physiol. Soc., Washington, D. C.
Ramwell, P. W., Leovey, E. M. K., and Sintetos, A. L. (1977). *Biol. Reprod.* **16,** 70-87.
Renfree, M. B. (1972). *Nature (London)* **240,** 475-477.
Renfree, M. B. (1973). *Dev. Biol.* **32,** 41-49.
Renfree, M. B. (1980). *Prog. Reprod. Biol.* **7,** 1-13.
Renfree, M. B. (1981). *J. Reprod. Fertil. Suppl.* **29,** 67-78.
Resnik, R., and Brink, G. W. (1978). *Am. J. Physiol.* **234,** H557-561.
Resnik, R., and Brink, G. W. (1980). *Am. J. Obstet. Gynecol.* **137,** 267-270.
Resnik, R., Killam, A. P., Barton, M. D., Battaglia, F. C. Makowski, E. L., and Meschia, G. (1976). *Am. J. Obstet. Gynecol.* **125,** 201-206.
Roberts, G. P., and Parker, J. M. (1974a). *J. Reprod. Fertil.* **40,** 291-303.
Roberts, G. P., and Parker, J. M. (1974b). *J. Reprod. Fertil.* **40,** 305-313.
Roberts, G. P., Parker, J. M., and Symonds, H. W. (1976). *J. Reprod. Fertil.* **48,** 133-141.
Robertson, H. A., Dwyer, R. J., and King, G. J. (1980). *J.Reprod. Fertil.* **58,** 115-120.
Roman-Ponce, H., Thatcher, W. W., Caton, D., Barron, D. H., and Wilcox, C. J. (1978). *J. Anim. Sci.* **46,** 175-180.
Sananes, N., Baulieu, E. -E., and Le Goascogne, C. (1976). *Mol. Cell. Endocrinol.* **6,** 153-157.
Sartor, P. (1977). *Acta Endocrinol. Copenhagen* **84,** 804-812.
Saunders, P. T. K., Ziecik, A. J., and Flint, A. P. F. (1980). *J. Endocrinol.* **85,** 25P.
Seamark, R. F., and Lutwak-Mann, C. (1972). *J. Reprod. Fertil.* **29,** 147-148.
Shelesnyak, M. C. (1957). *Recent Prog. Horm. Res.* **13,** 269-322.
Shemesh, M., Milaguir, F., Ayalon, N., and Hansel, W. (1979). *J. Reprod. Fertil.* **56,** 181-185.
Sherman, M. I., Atienza, S. B., Salomon, D. S., and Wudl, L. R. (1977). *In* "Development in Mammals" (M. H. Johnson, ed.), Vol. II, pp. 209-233. Elsevier, Amsterdam.

Short, R. V. (1969). *In* "Fetal Autonomy" (G. E. W. Wolstenholme and M. O'Connor, eds.), pp. 2–26. Churchill, London.
Singh, M. M., and Booth, W. D. (1978). *J. Reprod. Fertil.* **53**, 297–304.
Staples, L. D. (1980). *Biol. Reprod.* **22**, 675–685.
Staples, L. D., Lawson, R. A. S., and Findlay, J. K. (1978). *Biol. Reprod.* **19**, 1076–1082.
Stone, G. M., Wild, J., and Miller, B. G. (1979). *Biol. Reprod.* **21**, 273–280.
Study, R. E., and Greenguard, P. (1978). *J. Pharmacol. Exp. Ther.* **207**, 767–778.
Sundaram, K., Connell, K. G., and Passantino, T. (1975). *Nature (London)* **256**, 739–741.
Surani, M. A. H. (1977). *J. Reprod. Fertil.* **50**, 289–296.
Sylvan, P. E., Maclaughlin, D. T., Richardson, G. S., Scully, R. E., and Nikrui, N. (1981). *Biol Reprod.* **24**, 423–429.
Talley, T. J., Tobert, J. A., Armstrong, E. G., and Villee, C. A. (1977). *Endocrinology* **101**, 1538–1544.
Thatcher, W. W., Wilcox, C. J., Bazer, F. W., Collier, R. J., Eley, R. M., Stover, D. G., and Bartol, F. F. (1979). *Beltsville Symp. Agric. Res.* **3**, 259–275.
Thatcher, W. W., Lewis, G. S., Eley, R. M., Bazer, F. W., Fields, M. J., Williams, W. F., and Wilcox, C. J. (1980). *Proc. Int. Congr. Anim. Reprod. Artif. Insem., 9th, Madrid.* **1**, 9–22.
Tobert, J. A. (1976). *J. Reprod. Fertil.* **47**, 391–393.
Tseng, L., and Gurpide, E. (1974). *Endocrinology* **94**, 419–423.
Tzartos, S. J., and Surani, M. A. H. (1979). *J. Reprod. Fertil.* **56**, 579–586.
Wallace, G. I. (1981). *J. Reprod. Fertil. Suppl.* **29**, 173–181.
Ward, W. F., Frost, A. G., and Ward Orsini, M. (1978). *Biol. Reprod.* **18**, 598–601.
Wathes, D. C. (1980). *J. Reprod. Fertil.* **60**, 323–330.
Watson, J., and Patek, C. E. (1979). *J. Endocrinol.* **82**, 425–428.
Weitlauf, H. M. (1978). *J. Reprod. Fertil.* **52**, 321–325.
Weitlauf, H. M., and Kiessling, A. A. (1981). *J. Reprod. Fertil. Suppl.* **29**, 191–202.
Wide, L., and Hobson, B. (1978). *Upps. J. Med. Sci.* **83**, 1–6.
Wide, L., and Wide, M. (1979). *J. Reprod. Fertil.* **57**, 5–9.
Wiley, L. D. (1974). *Nature (London)* **252**, 715–716.
Wilmut, I., and Sales, D. I. (1981). *J. Reprod. Fertil.* **61**, 179–184.
Wimsatt, W. A. (1975). *Biol. Reprod.* **12**, 1–40.
Winkel, C. A., Gilmore, J., MacDonald, P. C., and Simpson, E. R. (1980). *Endocrinology* **107**, 1892–1898.
Wooding, F. B. P., and Wathes, D. C. (1980). *J. Reprod. Fertil.* **59**, 425–430.
Wooding, F. B. P., Chambers, S. G., Perry, J. S., George, M., and Heap, R. B. (1980). *Anat. Embryol.* **158**, 361–370.
Wu, J. T., and Chang, M. C. (1972). *Biol. Reprod.* **7**, 231–237.
Zavy, M. T., Mayer, R., Vernon, M. W., Bazer, F. W., and Sharp, D. C. (1979a). *J. Reprod. Fertil. Suppl.* **27**, 403–411.
Zavy, M. T., Bazer, F. W., Sharp, D. C., and Wilcox, C. J. (1979b). *Biol. Reprod.* **20**, 689–698.
Zavy, M T., Bazer, F. W., Thatcher, W. W., and Wilcox, C. J. (1980). *Prostaglandins* **20**, 837–851.
Zelinski, M. B., Hirota, N. A., Keenan, E. J., and Stormshak, F. (1980). *Biol. Reprod.* **23**, 743–751.

PROLACTIN AND PREGNANCY

Ulrich A. Knuth and Henry G. Friesen

DEPARTMENT OF PHYSIOLOGY
UNIVERSITY OF MANITOBA
WINNIPEG, MANITOBA, CANADA

I. Introduction 70
II. Effect of Prolactin on the Ovary 70
III. Prolactin in Normal Pregnancy 71
A. Maternal Prolactin Levels 71
B. Fetal Prolactin 74
C. Prolactin in Amniotic Fluid 76
D. Influence of Prolactin on the Immune System 78
E. Prolactin Heterogeneity 79
F. Factors Influencing Prolactin Secretion during Pregnancy 79
IV. Influence of Prolactin on Pregnancy-Specific Events 81
A. Role of Prolactin on Osmoregulation 81
B. Prolactin and Fetal Lung Maturation 83
V. Prolactin as a Marker in Pathological Pregnancy 84
A. Preeclampsia 84
B. Molar Pregnancies and Cholestasis of Pregnancy 84
VI. Lactation 85
A. Prolactin Levels and Profiles 85
B. Manipulation of Milk Production 86
C. Lactational Infertility as a Natural Contraceptive 88
VII. Prolactin-Secreting Tumors during Pregnancy 88
VIII. Summary and Future Research 90
References 91

Current Topics in
Experimental Endocrinology, Vol. 4

ISBN 0-12-153204-6

I. Introduction

The significance of hyperprolactinemia in the pathogenesis of secondary amenorrhea, anovulation, short luteal phase cycles, and infertility has been established in the past decade. In addition, the critical role of prolactin in the onset and maintenance of lactation has been elegantly demonstrated with the use of bromocriptine. It is now perhaps the treatment of choice as a lactation suppressant. Obstetricians are generally aware of these facts but have been less concerned with alteration in serum prolactin levels during pregnancy.

However, striking changes in prolactin (PRL) concentrations occur during the course of pregnancy and delivery with markedly different patterns of PRL in maternal and fetal circulation. The mechanisms by which these changes are brought about are still unclear and their physiological significance remains to be elucidated. It is unlikely that PRL concentrations in the amniotic fluid and decidual tissue (about 1000 times higher than normal serum values) have no purpose. Little is known about PRL effects on osmoregulation, lung maturation, and fetal membrane systems. In some areas relating to PRL in pregnancy contradictory information exists. Thus, the objective of this article is to provide a detailed analysis of the data available for PRL from conception to nursing, focusing especially on areas of controversy in order to encourage more well-designed clinical studies.

II. Effect of Prolactin on the Ovary

In rat and mouse PRL is the essential luteotropic factor required for the formation and function of the corpus luteum. In other species, including man, PRL participates with LH as part of the luteotropic complex. Although prolactin-deficient states have not been identified with ovarian dysfunction, it is clear that high serum PRL levels are associated with oligo/amenorrhea in females and are found in approximately 20% of all patients complaining of these symptoms (Franks *et al.*, 1975; Bohnet *et al.*, 1975). However, the gonadal effects of prolactin are complex and details of its precise effects remain sketchy and continue to be examined in a number of laboratories. Using human granulosa cells in culture McNatty *et al.* (1974) showed that prolactin concentrations of 25 to 100 ng/ml in the medium caused a significant decrease in progesterone production. A similar impairment of granulosa cell function was seen when prolactin was neutralized with excess antibodies present in the culture medium. Thus, both an excess and a deficiency of prolactin impaired progesterone synthesis by granulosa cells. A clinical counterpart of the *in vitro* experiments with high prolactin levels is found perhaps in patients with the so-called short luteal phase where serum prolactin levels are elevated (Seppala, 1978; del Pozo *et al.*, 1976) accompanied by low serum progesterone levels and immature endometrium. The clinical analogy to the absence of prolactin *in vitro* may be seen when prolactin oversuppression with bromocriptine leads to the formation of a nonfunctioning corpus luteum (Bohnet *et al.*, 1977). How prolactin can have both an obligatory permissive role on progesterone secretion and an inhibitory effect remains unexplained (McNeilly, 1980). In porcine granulosa cells in culture the action of prolactin is bipotential, depending critically on the degree of granulosa cell differentiation attained *in vivo*. Prolactin suppresses steroid production by cultured granulosa cells isolated from small (1–2 mm) immature follicles, but stimulates progesterone secretion by granulosa cells collected from large (6 mm) follicles. The response to prolactin is significantly altered by the concurrent presence of estradiol in the culture. Early (the first 48 hours) both estrogen and prolactin exert inhibitory effects, but from 48 hours onward estradiol stimulates steroidogenesis and more strikingly produces a switch in prolactin action from inhibitory to stimulatory. Thus estrogens may play an important part in regulating the divergent actions of prolactin in the ovary (Veldhuis and Hammond, 1980). Thus, although the species difference in this action has yet to be resolved, it seems that PRL may have an important regulatory role in granulosa cell development within the follicle (McNeilly, 1980). Although effects of prolactin on the gonad become obvious in the luteal phase of the cycle, the follicular phase is perhaps an even more critical period for the action of prolactin on the gonads. Direct evidence for this conclusion is provided by patients who are hyperprolactinemic in whom no effect is seen when serum prolactin levels are suppressed during the luteal phase only (Schulz *et al.*, 1976, 1978; Polatti *et al.*, 1978). In a complementary experiment Delvoye *et al.* (1974) showed that drug-induced hyperprolactinemia in the luteal phase had only slight effects on progesterone secretion from the granulosa cells whereas hyperprolactinemia induced during the follicular phase resulted in the formation of an inadequate corpus luteum.

III. Prolactin in Normal Pregnancy

A. Maternal Prolactin Levels

1. Serum Prolactin—Profiles until Term

Serum prolactin concentrations in normal pregnancy are in the same range as are found in the luteal phase until day 31 after the LH peak. At this time estradiol levels increase and within 1 to 3 days a marked increase of serum prolactin also occurs (Barberia *et al.,* 1975). PRL does not appear to be of major significance for implantation or maintenance of early pregnancy. This conclusion was based on observations in 30 women who had unprotected intercourse around ovulation and were subsequently treated with bromocriptine. Although PRL levels were lowered to 1.9 ng/ml, five women showed detectable hCG levels and three became pregnant (Ylikorkala *et al.,* 1979a). This rate of pregnancy is not different from that expected in women not receiving bromocriptine. From 10 weeks to term a 7- to 10-fold increase in circulating prolactin concentrations is observed (Tyson *et al.,* 1972a; L'Hermite and Robyn, 1972; Schenker *et al.,* 1975). In contrast to these earlier studies in which data from isolated random samples from individual patients were reported, Biswas and Rodeck (1976) analyzed 980 values from 839 patients with normal pregnancies between 8 and 40 weeks of gestation. Prolactin concentrations varied from 6 ng/ml during early pregnancy to 212 ng/ml at 34 weeks. Mean ± SD values at 8 weeks and between 34 and 40 weeks were 18.4 ± 6.5 ($n = 45$) and 117.4 ± 45.1 ($n = 164$) ng/ml, respectively. The highest mean values were found at 38 weeks (128.4 ± 41.5, $n = 34$), a sevenfold increase from the mean values at 8 weeks. A longitudinal study of four women from the fifth week of gestation until term with weekly blood sampling failed to show any decrease toward term; instead, prolactin concentrations increased progressively with advancing gestation until term (correlation coefficient of 0.956) (Rigg *et al.,* 1977) (Fig. 1).

The range of values for serum prolactin at various stages of pregnancy is very considerable. In individual patients serum prolactin under normal conditions also fluctuates somewhat. Prolactin, like a number of other pituitary hormones, is secreted in an episodic manner with nocturnal sleep induced values reaching a peak which may be 50 to 100% above the 24 hour mean (Sassin *et al.,* 1972, 1973; Parker *et al.,* 1973). The secretory pattern for a 24-hour period was studied by Boyar *et al.* (1975) in four patients during the twelfth, twentieth, and thirty-second week of gestation. Blood samples taken at 20-minute intervals displayed episodic prolactin secretion indistinguishable in character from normal subjects although at a higher set point.

2. PRL during Delivery

At term, serum prolactin concentrations undergo rapid changes during delivery, although the exact pattern is still not quite clear (Fig. 2). Rigg and Yen (1977) reported that serum prolactin levels began to decrease 5 hours before delivery reaching a nadir 2 hours prepartum. An abrupt increase then occurred with values exceeding those in early labor followed by a progressive fall during the next 5 hours and, finally, for the next 16-hour period, a

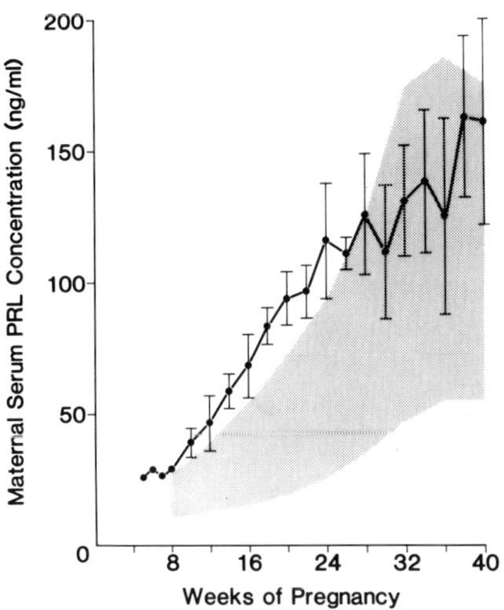

Fig. 1. Plasma prolactin levels in normal pregnancies. Shaded area shows range of 90th and 10th centiles based on 980 values from 839 patients (Biswas and Rodeck, 1976). Solid line represents mean ± SEM ($n = 4$) measured serially at weekly intervals as a function of duration of pregnancy (Rigg *et al.*, 1977). Redrawn with permission

plateau was established with only random fluctuations. Unfortunately, despite the detailed pattern noted with frequent blood sampling, only a very small number of patients were included in this study. In addition, no information was given about the degree of cervical dilatation and the time of spinal analgesia in some patients. In contrast to the findings of Rigg and Yen, Gregoriou *et al.* (1979) did not observe significant differences in prolactin levels, because of large individual variation when values were determined just before labor, during dilatation of the cervix at fixed intervals, 1–2, 5, and 10 cm, and at the time of delivery. None of the 15 patients received drugs or analgesia during labor. These results were confirmed by Jouppila *et al.* (1980) in eight patients receiving epidural anesthesia. However, the control group of patients who did not receive any analgesia had significantly lower prolactin concentrations when the cervix was dilated 6–8 cm. Objective evaluation is, however, difficult as the statistical analysis was not entirely appropriate, a criticism that also applies to the studies of de Gezelle *et al.*, (1977a,b) who reported that the lowest prolactin values occurred 60 minutes after delivery. No data seem to be available to explain the observed changes in PRL secretion during delivery. No correlations exist between PRL levels and prostaglandins, progesterone, or estradiol values (MacKenzie *et al.*, 1979; Laatikainen *et al.*, 1980). The administration of a β-sympathomimetic drug, Fenoterol, to inhibit labor did not cause a change in PRL levels

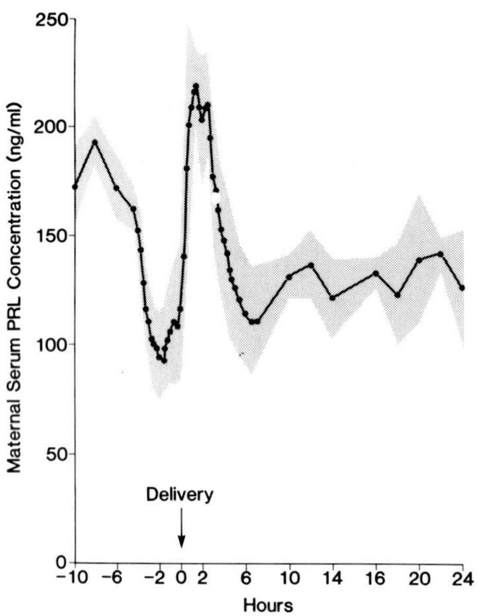

Fig. 2. Prolactin curve (mean ± SEM, $n = 4$) in the peripartum period centered around the time of delivery ($t = 0$). (Rigg and Yen, 1977). Redrawn with permission

(Bellmann *et al.*, 1979). Although induction of labor with oxytocin as well as administration of oxytocin during established labor leads to an increase in serum PRL, this mechanism does not seem to play a physiological role during spontaneous labor as there is little or no maternal release at the onset of contractions (Chard, 1975). Whether oxytocin of fetal origin or other fetoplacental factors are responsible for the paradoxical increase of maternal prolactin at the time of maximum stress during delivery remains unanswered. More well-designed and controlled studies will be necessary to establish more precisely the changes of PRL during the peripartum period, their extent and magnitude as well as the mechanisms which are operative.

B. Fetal Prolactin

1. Concentrations in Serum, Pituitary, and Umbilical Cord

In contrast to data available on maternal serum prolactin levels during pregnancy, information about fetal prolactin levels is perforce more limited. Fetal data are usually obtained on single specimens obtained following abortion or premature labor. Under these circumstances basal physiological conditions clearly do not prevail. Thus data obtained under these circumstances must be viewed and interpreted with considerable caution. Data obtained from nonhuman species may not necessarily be relevant because of different secretory patterns of many hormones during pregnancies among species. Even in rhesus monkeys marked differences in estrogen metabolism influence secretory patterns of prolactin to a great extent. In cord blood samples obtained from aborted fetuses after abdominal hysterectomy mean concentrations of serum prolactin were 53 ng–ml at 16 to 19 weeks, 233 ng/ml at 20 to 34 weeks, and 371 ng/ml at 35 to 42 weeks compared to 218 ng/ml in 1- to 8-day-old infants. In 314 fetal samples obtained during the thirty-fourth and forty-second week of pregnancy, prolactin levels seemed to be constant (Winters *et al.*, 1975).

In a detailed and comprehensive study Aubert *et al.* (1975) determined human prolactin content and concentration of 82 pituitary glands as well as serum levels in 47 fetuses of gestational age 68 days to term (Fig. 3). Siler-Khodr *et al.* (1974) reported detection of prolactin from pituitaries as early as 28–35 days (fifth week) when tissue samples were examined. Detectable prolactin concentrations were found in all but two pituitaries after 115 days of gestation with the earliest positive detection at 68 days. A marked increase in concentration as well as content of prolactin occurred between 100 to 160

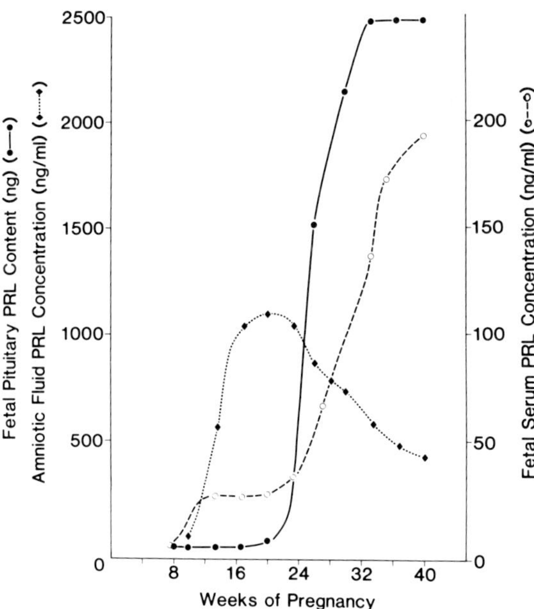

Fig. 3. Schematic summary of prolactin patterns throughout pregnancy in amniotic fluid (Clements *et al.*, 1977), fetal serum, and fetal pituitary (Aubert *et al.*, 1975). Redrawn with permission

days and all fetuses 88 to 165 days gestation had detectable serum prolactin. A progressive rise occurred after day 180 in serum prolactin concentrations (Fig. 3). There was no correlation between serum and pituitary prolactin levels. The mean concentration of prolactin in the umbilical vein was significantly higher than maternal values—results which were confirmed by Clements *et al.* (1977).

2. Mechanisms Regulating Fetal Prolactin

In an attempt to elucidate the mechanism regulating pituitary prolactin secretion during the first half of gestation, McNeilly *et al.* (1977) examined hypothalamic extracts for prolactin inhibitory factor activity. None was detected until the fifteenth week of pregnancy. On the contrary, prolactin-releasing activity equivalent to the effect of 10 ng TRH was found. After 15.5 weeks, fetal hypothalamic extracts primarily inhibited prolactin release.

C. Prolactin in Amniotic Fluid

1. Concentrations and Profiles

In 1972, Tyson *et al.* reported prolactin levels of 1.2 to 7 μg/ml in 28 samples obtained at amniocentesis during the first 20 weeks of gestation, while at term prolactin had decreased to 350 ng/ml. These initial results have been confirmed and extended by several other groups. Schenker *et al.*, (1975) and Clements *et al.* (1977) reported 2- to 10-fold greater amniotic fluid than maternal serum prolactin concentrations (Fig. 3). A sharp increase of prolactin levels was seen in fetuses of both sexes after 15 to 17 weeks reaching peak mean values of 1314 ng/ml with a gradual decline until term of 456 ng/ml. The ratio of amniotic fluid to fetal serum levels in paired specimens ($n = 9$) from 12 to 20 weeks gestation ranged from 9.1 to 35.2. At term, the mean ratio had decreased to 2.5:1. No significant correlation between prolactin levels in different compartments was found. On the other hand, Biswas (1976) after analyzing 319 amniotic fluid samples was not able to establish a typical pattern of change in prolactin during pregnancy. Values varied from 36 to 1800 ng/ml without any obvious rise or fall when pregnancy advanced. Only a poor correlation ($r = 0.1844$) among 203 pairs of maternal plasma and amniotic fluid prolactin values was shown. No significant correlation existed between plasma and amniotic fluid levels. In conclusion the 100- to 200-fold greater concentration of PRL in amniotic fluid compared to maternal or fetal levels and the lack of correlation in levels among the three compartments during pregnancy are striking (Soria *et al.*, 1977). Several suggestions for the source of amniotic fluid PRL were put forward but none seemed entirely satisfactory (Josimovich *et al.*, 1974; Schenker *et al.*, 1975;

Chochinov *et al.*, 1976; Fang and Kim, 1975) until it was recognized that the decidua secreted prolactin.

2. SOURCE OF AMNIOTIC PROLACTIN

With the unequivocal demonstration by Riddick and Kusmik (1977) that the decidua is a major source of PRL production a new and exciting field of PRL research emerged. In fact, Cassano *et al.* (1952) more than two decades earlier had reported lactogenic activity in extracts of sheep decidua when tested in the pigeon crop-sac assay. Friesen *et al.* (1972) also provided some suggestive evidence that the chorion synthesizes PRL. Subsequently to this first study Riddick *et al.* (1979) incubated amnion, chorion, and decidua from tissues obtained from term deliveries and reported that only decidua produced PRL with progressive increase in concentrations during the incubation period. Upon the addition of cycloheximide in concentrations sufficient to inhibit protein synthesis any further increase beyond the initial PRL content of the tissues was abolished. When [^{3}H]leucine was present in the incubation medium the specific synthesis of ^{3}H-labeled PRL could be demonstrated, which had the same elution volume on a Sephadex G-100 column as did iodinated pituitary PRL (Riddick *et al.*, 1978). Similar studies by Healy *et al.* (1979) and Frame *et al.* (1979a) also showed that the PRL synthesized by decidua in culture possessed immunological and chromatographic properties which were similar to human pituitary PRL.

Immunofluorescent localization studies have identified PRL in the cytoplasm of decidual tissue with less intensely fluorescent cells in the trophoblast (Frame *et al.*, 1979b). These results differ from the earlier report by Healy *et al.* (1977), who reported localization of PRL in the cytoplasm of amnion epithelial cells. The initial PRL content and *in vitro* production of PRL in samples of endometrial tissue obtained from women with ectopic pregnancies were similar to those of endometrial samples obtained from intrauterine pregnancies of similar gestational age. The synthesis of PRL was also demonstrable in endometrium taken at 26–27 days of the menstrual cycle from nonpregnant women (Maslar *et al.*, 1980).

The fact that the concentrations of PRL in decidual tissue follow a pattern similar to that of amniotic fluid PRL concentrations throughout gestation is compelling evidence to suggest that decidua is the source of amniotic fluid PRL. Both tissue content as well as the 24 hour PRL production *in vitro* is highly correlated with $r = 0.90$ and 0.96, respectively (Fig. 4) (Rosenberg *et al.*, 1980).

Although the origin of amniotic fluid PRL seems to be established the evidence of how PRL is transported from decidua to amniotic fluid is not available. The recent report by Riddick and Maslar (1981) has helped to

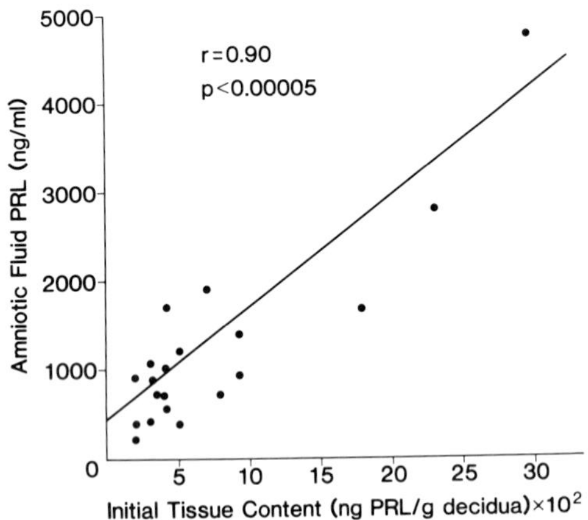

Fig. 4. Correlation of preincubation content of prolactin in decidual tissue and prolactin in amniotic fluid in the same patients (Rosenberg *et al.*, 1980). Redrawn with permission

clarify the situation. They noted that transport of radiolabeled PRL from the medium bathing the decidual surface of the membranes across the chorion to the amniotic side of the membrane in an *in vitro* system was less than 3%. In contrast to this low transport rate of labeled PRL 40% of the total radioimmunoassayable PRL originating from within the decidual tissue was released from the tissue and readily crossed the chorion to the medium bathing the amniotic surface.

The factors regulating PRL release from decidua remain unknown, but appear to differ from mechanisms controlling pituitary PRL secretion. Agents such as bromocriptine, dopamine, or TRH, which inhibit or stimulate PRL secretion by the pituitary, have no influence on PRL release by the decidua. Addition of fetal calf serum in a dose-related manner enhances the synthesis of PRL by explants of human decidua while addition of bovine serum albumin is without effect. Some PRL-stimulating activity was also present in human serum obtained from normoprolactinemic men or women. This activity could not be inhibited by heat treatment or dialysis (Luciano *et al.*, 1980).

D. *Influence of Prolactin on the Immune System*

The very high PRL concentrations at the line of demarcation between fetal and maternal tissues raises a question about a possible influence of PRL on inhibition of immunologic mechanisms. PRL decreases the reactivity of T lymphocytes *in vitro* (Contractor and Davies, 1973) and reduces the incorporation of radioactive thymidine into T cells after phytohemagglutinin (Karmali *et al.,* 1974). On the other hand PRL seems to stimulate the migration of immunocompetent cells (IgA producers) into the mammary gland (Weisz-Carrington *et al.,* 1978). In addition Berczi and Nagy (1981) have shown that PRL enhances antibody production and influences the development of delayed hypersensitivity, skin reactions, adjuvant arthritis, and graft rejection.

E. Prolactin Heterogeneity

In 1974 Suh and Frantz reported that after gel filtration of serum samples immunoreactive species of different molecular weight were recognized. The major species (75%) corresponded to monomeric or "little" PRL. Two other molecular species were recognized: "big" (a dimer of PRL) and a much larger form "big big" PRL. Fang and Kim (1975) subsequently found 16 to 31% big prolactin in sera of pregnant patients. When maternal, fetal, and amniotic PRL was separated by gel filtration notable differences in the proportion of big and little PRL were found. Size heterogeneity of PRL was also reported by Frame *et al.* (1979a) in incubation media from decidua or in milk samples obtained during lactation (Gala and van de Walle, 1977). The precise chemical nature of the different molecular weight species of prolactin has not been fully defined. Some have even argued that the different forms of PRL represent artifacts of the separation method. Ben-David *et al.* (1973) were not able to distinguish between amniotic fluid and serum PRL upon isoelectric focusing or acrylamide gel electrophoresis. On the other hand in some cases PRL of differing size might be generated by interchain disulfide linkages (Benveniste *et al.,* 1979), a situation which has also been reported for hPL (Schneider *et al.,* 1975).

F. Factor Influencing Prolactin Secretion during Pregnancy

The study of the mechanisms controlling PRL secretion during pregnancy in humans is restricted by a number of ethical considerations. The measurement of hormone concentrations serially in a well-designed longitudinal prospective study under control and experimental conditions is feasible in selected cases, when pregnancy is to be terminated for medical and/or social reasons; yet few studies of this kind have been done. Hertz *et al.* (1978) correlated serum concentrations of PRL, progesterone, estradiol, and estriol in 125 patients referred for legal abortion between the sixth and fourteenth week of pregnancy. A positive correlation between estrogens and prolactin was found, but ony during the twelfth week of gestation. This result is surprising in view of the general belief that the increase in PRL secretion is triggered by the rise in estradiol after week 12 (Barberia *et al.,* 1975). However, only single samples were evaluated in a cross-section of patients. Sadovsky *et al.* (1977) demonstrated a correlation between estradiol in 24-hour urine samples and serum PRL levels in 138 determinations ($r = 0.7$), a finding which was not confirmed by Ranta *et al.* (1980) although they reported a weak correlation between PRL and estriol serum levels ($r = 0.313$). No influence of estradiol on serum PRL was seen in patients with preeclampsia. Injection of dehydroepiandrosterone sulfate iv ($n = 10$) or into the amniotic sac ($n = 13$) in patients admitted for midtrimester abortions caused elevation of serum maternal PRL. No consistent change could be observed in amniotic fluid PRL levels, although the increase of amniotic fluid E_2 levels ranged between 10- and 22-fold (Ylikorkala *et al.,* 1979b). These data indicate the lack of responsiveness of the pituitary to additional stimulation by exogenous estrogens in midgestation. On the other hand the responsiveness of the pituitary to suppression by bromocriptine is demonstrated by a decrease of PRL levels from 21.5 ± 9.4 to 3.9 ± 1.8 ng/ml 6 hours after 5 mg was given orally. After 20 hours values rebounded to 107.9 ± 62.6 ng/ml with an accompanying decrease in FSH (correlation −0.893).

As in normal subjects release of PRL can be induced in pregnant women by TRH (Tyson *et al.,* 1972b) or drugs which interfere with dopamine metabolism. A fourfold increase in PRL concentrations was observed as early as the seventh week of gestation after 200 μg of TRH intravenously. A similar study by Hershman *et al.* (1973) in women between 8 and 22 weeks showed a mean maximum increase of 37.0 ± 7.4 ng/ml from baseline levels of 27.5 ± 4.5 ng/ml. These findings were extended in a longitudinal study between 9–15, 26–29, and 35–38 weeks in nine women (Ylikorkala *et al.,* 1979c). The mean maximal serum PRL concentrations at each of these periods were 163, 211, and 206 ng/ml with a relative peak increase of 45, 119, and 98%, respectively, demonstrating that there is no increased secretory reserve of the lactotrophs as pregnancy advances. Similar results were reported, when Sulpiride, a drug with strong dopamine antagonistic properties, was used (Guitelman *et al.,* 1978). In order to study the role of PRL in the regulation of 17β-estradiol, testosterone, and hPL, Sulpiride was administered orally at a dose of 50 mg three times daily for 2 weeks. Although PRL levels rose from 14.5 to 84 ng/ml after 1 week of therapy, no effect of increased PRL concentration was seen on the other hormones.

When chlorpromazine, a classical dopamine receptor inhibitor, is administered intramuscularly, an increase in maternal PRL levels of the same absolute magnitude as in nonpregnant women is seen, although the percentage increase is not as great (Freeman *et al.,* 1976). The effect of dopamine antagonistic drugs in elevating the already high PRL levels in pregnancy seems to prove that a dopaminergic inhibition is still operative, although some other factors might have changed the set point to a higher level. It is likely that this stimulating effect is brought about, at least to a certain extent, by estrogens (Ylikorkala *et al.*, 1979b; Seron-Ferre *et al.*, 1979; Friesen *et al.*, 1973). Although a 50% suppression of estradiol levels by administration of dexamethasone between 28 and 24 weeks for 2 to 3 days did not lead to any change in PRL levels (Kaupilla *et al.*, 1979). However, the period of suppression in this study might have been too short to cause significant effects; in addition dexamethasone itself may have had some effects. The possibility that the high PRL levels during pregnancy might be caused by an extrahypophyseal source was disproved by Riddick *et al.* (1979), who reported unchanged PRL levels during pregnancy in a patient who previously had undergone hypophysectomy for a chromophobe adenoma. Similary in a patient who had received radiation therapy for a presumed prolactin producing tumor no changes in serum prolactin were observed during pregnancy (Quigley *et al.*, 1976).

IV. Influence of Prolactin on Pregnancy-Specific Events

A. Role of Prolactin on Osmoregulation

As one of the oldest hormones phylogenetically PRL plays an important part in osmoregulation of submammalian vertebrates (for reference see Nicoll, 1974). When fish move from salt to fresh water it is necessary to regulate sodium and water movement across the gills. This change is modulated by PRL.

The closest humans come to living in salt water is *in utero* (Friesen *et al.*, 1972). Thus it was suggested that PRL might play a role in salt and water metabolism during fetal life. The demonstration of remarkably low PRL levels in amniotic fluid of some patients with hydramnios, seemed to support this theory. But the finding was not consistent as some patients showed normal PRL levels in spite of an increased volume of amniotic fluid.

In order to elucidate the action of PRL on amniotic fluid transfer different models were studied using guinea pig or human term amniotic membranes *in vitro*. Unfortunately the available results at times have been contradictory even in the same species.

Two different types of flow across the amniotic membrane have to be distinguished. The first, bulk flow, takes place as the organized movement of water and consists of the net flow through the amnion. The second component is diffusional flow which is the random movement of water usually measured as the rate of tritiated water passing the membrane in one direction.

The addition of purified PRL at 10 μg/ml to the fetal side of a guinea pig amnion preparation *in vitro* led to a fall in fetal–maternal diffusional water flow (average fall at 3 hours 9.7–17%) and reduced the net flow (bulk flow), measured gravimetrically, by 40% at 3 hours (Holt and Perks, 1975). Similar results were obtained using human membranes (Leontic and Tyson, 1977; Leontic *et al.*, 1979). PRL reduced the permeability in a dose-related fashion when added to the fetal side, an effect which was inhibited by neutralizing PRL with specific antibody. The maternal side was not responsive. No effect on bulk flow was seen. These observations favor an accumulation of amniotic fluid in the presence of high PRL values and are in contrast to the original clinical findings, in which low amniotic PRL was found in patients with hydramnios.

Using 50 to 10 times lower PRL concentrations Manku *et al.* (1975) reported just the opposite effect of PRL on bulk flow in guinea pig amnion with a dose-dependent increase of water movement to the maternal side.

The best model described so far to investigate the effects of PRL on fetal–maternal water exchange was presented by Josimovich *et al.* (1977) who used rhesus monkeys during the last third of gestation. Administration of 1 to 10 mg ovine PRL into the amniotic cavity consistently caused a decrease in amniotic fluid volume for 24 hours. When 60 to 87% of the normal amniotic fluid was replaced by PRL-free isotonic fluid in order to simulate the low intraamniotic PRL values, reported in patients with hydramnios, a rapid return to 65–72% of the original levels within 35–40 minutes occurred, thus making a meaningful study impossible.

In addition to these observations, which support a decrease of amniotic fluid volume with high PRL levels, evidence was presented that intraamniotic injection of PRL prevented or reversed a doubling of water and electrolyte content of the fetal extracellular fluid volume when an artificial hypertonic solution was substituted for the isotonic amniotic fluid. In the presence of hypotonic amniotic fluid efflux of water and electrolytes from the fetal extracellular fluid was similarly prevented by PRL in the artificial solution. Although this action of PRL may not be of physiological significance in humans it nevertheless provides evidence that PRL in amniotic fluid influences fetal handling of fluid and ions just as PRL influences the handling of salt when fish move from sea to fresh water or vice versa.

It is obvious that there is a need for further studies especially to resolve the opposite results obtained in the different models. With the decidua as the likely source of amniotic fluid PRL it might be interesting to see whether differences in decidual PRL production can be detected in patients with hydramnios. If a clear role were established for amniotic fluid PRL and definite changes were observed under pathological conditions attempts might be made to correct these by influencing decidual PRL production or by direct injection of PRL. Finally the placenta, fetal lung, and/or fetal gastrointestinal tract may be targets for PRL effects on water and electrolyte metabolism (Josimovich *et al.*, 1977).

B. Prolactin and Fetal Lung Maturation

There are several reports indicating PRL is involved in lung maturation and pulmonary surfactant production and, therefore by implication, in fetal respiratory distress syndrome (RDS). Hamosh and Hamosh (1977) reported that injection of fetal rabbits with 1 mg ovine PRL resulted in an increased concentration of lecithin within the fetal lungs 2 days later. Treatment of pregnant rabbits with bromocriptine for 2 days at 25 and 26 days of gestation (3 mg/kg im) decreased the phospholipid content by 31.02% (Mullon *et al.*, 1979). However, when the original experiment was repeated by Ballard *et al.* (1978) no effect of PRL on pulmonary surfactant was observed. No immediate explanation is available to clarify the discrepancies. The absence of effects of PRL on rabbit lung maturation was confirmed by van Petten and Bridges (1979) who found no change in pressure volume relationships after 2 days of PRL treatment. Infusion of PRL (1 mg/day iv) into fetal sheep continuously over five periods of 5–8 days did not affect the appearance of tracheal fluid surfactant even though supraphysiological concentrations of PRL were achieved with the infusion. It is, however, necessary to emphasize the great differences in the endocrinology of PRL secretion of rabbits, sheep, and man. In rabbits and sheep amniotic fluid PRL levels are low or absent and the increase in maternal serum PRL does not occur until the last days of pregnancy and even then the changes are modest. In contrast to these animal data, some clinical observations suggest that there might be a correlation between RDS and PRL levels in humans. Regression lines between gestational age and umbilical cord serum PRL levels differ significantly in control subjects and infants who develop RDS with lower PRL values in the later group (Gluckman *et al.*, 1978). Hauth *et al.* (1978) reported a lower incidence of RDS in newborns when PRL levels in cord serum were found above 200 ng/ml. It might, however, be argued that these correlations are incidental and do not indicate a cause and effect relationship. This possibility is even more likely as amniotic fluid PRL levels are relatively much higher than serum values and therefore amniotic PRL is likely to have a greater impact on development of PRL receptors in fetal lungs as well as on lung maturation than serum levels. However, no correlation between amniotic fluid PRL and lethicin/sphingomyelin ratio has been found (Bustos and Giussi, 1980).

V. Prolactin as a Marker in Pathological Pregnancy

A. Preeclampsia

As PRL causes sodium and water retention in some vertebrates and has some influence on vascular smooth muscle the hypothesis was advanced that PRL may be important in the pathogenesis of preeclampsia (Horrobin *et al.*, 1971; Horrobin, 1975).

Although Redman *et al.* (1975) described raised PRL levels in patients with preeclampsia no correlation was seen between blood pressure and PRL. A significant correlation was found between plasma urate levels and high PRL levels as is the case in nonpregnant patients with chronic renal failure (Frantz *et al.*, 1972). Other authors did not detect any correlation between PRL levels and hypertension in pregnancy (Dubowitz *et al.*, 1975; Ranta *et al.*, 1980). Findings by Jenkins and Perry (1978) claiming a significant correlation with the maximum increase in diastolic blood pressure were not confirmed by Yuen *et al.* (1978) who described lower than normal PRL levels in 78 women with preeclampsia and 30 women with essential hypertension. In studies using the rat mesenteric vascular bed the arterial vasoconstriction produced by norepinephrine and angiotensin was modulated by prolactin. Concentrations above 500 ng/ml inhibited the response while levels under 50 ng/ml potentiated the vasoconstriction of mesentric arterial vessels (Horrobin, 1974).

B. Molar Pregnancies and Cholestasis of Pregnancy

Mochizuki *et al.* (1976) reported higher levels of PRL in patients with molar pregnancies during week 13–19 of gestation. The increase in PRL levels after arginine infusion in these patients was significantly higher than in normal controls at the same stage of pregnancy even though estrogen levels were much lower in molar pregnancies. This rather unexpected finding was explained by a lack of feedback inhibition of hCS on pituitary lactotrophs as hCS levels were only 0.22 μg/ml in serum of normal pregnancies. In patients with cholestasis of pregnancy, high PRL levels (24 ± 38 vs 187 ± 23 ng/ml) as well as high concentrations of hPL were found (Ranta *et al.*, 1979). These findings suggest the liver may influence PRL secretion either by affecting metabolism of PRL or in some as yet undefined mechanism. In rats during pregnancy prolactin induces a major increase in the number of PRL receptors in the liver (Kelly *et al.*, 1974). PRL also causes an increase in ornithine decarboxylase (Richards, 1975) and somatomedin production (Francis and Hill, 1975) in liver tissue. An effect of PRL on bile acid metabolism during pregnancy also has been described by Moltz and Leidahl (1977).

VI. Lactation

A. Prolactin Levels and Profiles

PRL levels during the postpartum period and lactation were first reported by Tyson *et al.* (1972a). They reported a typical pattern of PRL release during the first postpartum week with an increase from 124 to 163 ng/ml after suckling. At subsequent periods the basal serum PRL levels were lower but with suckling increasing sixfold. The PRL response to suckling was much less marked beyond 80 days postpartum. TRH induced a considerable PRL surge even when administered after suckling (Tyson *et al.*, 1972b; Jeppson *et al.*, 1976).

Noel *et al.* (1974) studied the time course of PRL levels after initiation of suckling in patients between 8 and 41 days postpartum and 63 to 194 days as shown in Fig. 5. Comparison of responses to stimulation by suckling or breast pump in three women did not show any differences between the mean peak values. While the milk yield of three groups of lactating mothers did not depend on basal PRL levels (Aono *et al.*, 1977) the increase of PRL after suckling was correlated with milk production. As it was possible to stimulate

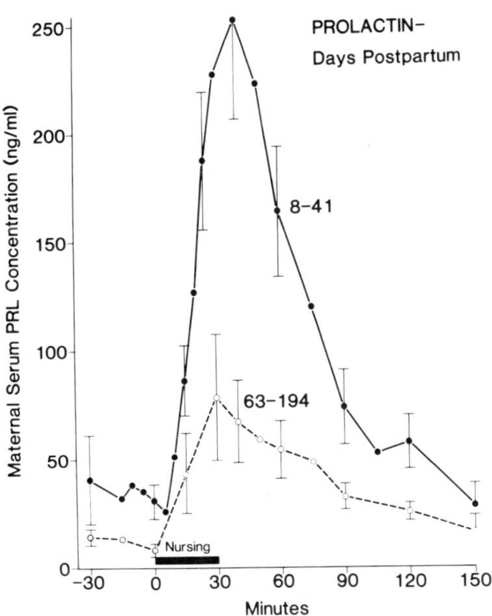

Fig. 5. Plasma prolactin concentrations (mean ± SEM) during nursing in postpartum women (Noel *et al.*, 1974). Redrawn with permission

PRL increase in all groups with a breast pump the authors stressed the importance of adequate nipple stimulation by the newborn to the process of lactation and PRL secretion. After 2 months postpartum only 9 out of 18 nursing episodes resulted in a rise of serum PRL levels and after 6 months only 5 of 27 exhibited an increase (Bunner *et al.*, 1978). Continued nursing even for more than a year is associated with elevated PRL levels above the nonpregnant range (Delvoye *et al.*, 1978; Thomson *et al.*, 1975). In lactating rats the vocalization of the pups which occurs at an ultrasonic frequency is a potent stimulus to PRL release (Terkel *et al.*, 1979), adding to the evidence that stimuli other than suckling, e.g., odor of the pups, can release PRL (Grosvenor, 1965; Mena and Grosvenor, 1971).

B. Manipulation of Milk Production

1. Increase in Volume

As suggested by Aono's data (1977, 1979), stimulation of PRL levels by TRH does not necessarily lead to higher milk production. Tyson *et al.* (1975) inferred from data obtained after 100 μ TRH iv that lactation and fat content increased, but no measurement of milk volume was performed and values are restricted to single examinations except for three cases. Hall and Kay (1977) followed a similar protocol and reported that TRH, while increasing PRL levels in five out of six women, actually decreased milk yields. A double blind study in which 16 patients received 20 mg of TRH orally three times daily 2 days after delivery for 4 weeks showed no effect of TRH on milk fat content and volume (Zarate *et al.*, 1976). A similar negative result was reported by Ylikorkala *et al.* (1980).

The failure to increase milk yield in some of these studies might result from inappropriate selection of patients, as no attention was paid to quality and adequacy of lactation before the onset of TRH administration. Another reason might be the mode of action of TRH, as PRL levels declined despite continued use of the drug suggesting that down-regulation of TRH receptors might have occurred. In another study in patients who had a history of insufficient lactation, metoclopramide was given twice daily at a dose of 10 mg. The milk yield was restored to a normal range over 4 weeks, and PRL levels remained four times higher than values from comparable controls. The diminution of milk production which occurred in the placebo-treated group with a similar history was corrected by metoclopramide (Guzman *et al.*, 1979). A similar augmentation of puerperal lactation was achieved by oral administration of sulpiride 50 mg twice daily to 66 mothers for 7 days starting immediately after delivery. The mean daily milk volume in the test group was 32.3% greater than in the controls (1211.7 versus 916.0 ml). Even more important only 21.1% of mothers produced insufficient amounts of milk after treatment with sulpiride compared to 46.9% in the control group. Follow-up after 1 month revealed that only 3.8% of 53 mothers were bottle feeding compared to 18.2% of 55 patients in the control group (Aono *et al.*, 1979). These results suggest that metoclopramide or sulpiride may be helpful therapy to patients with known lactational insufficiency and a strong desire to breastfeed. It should, however, be kept in mind that sulpiride was found in concentrations as high as 1.97 μg/ml in breast milk. No comparable data are available for metoclopramide.

2. Inhibition of Milk Secretion

The initiation of milk secretion during the postpartum period depends on a finely tuned integration of hormonal factors that include prolactin, GH, thyroxine, and insulin (for more extensive reviews of lactation the reader should consult Salazar and Tobon, 1974; Tulchinski, 1980; Spring-Mills *et al.*, 1980).

Since the initial studies of Varga *et al.* (1972) and Brun del Re *et al.* 1973), the effectiveness of bromocriptine in suppressing PRL and lactation has been repeatedly confirmed (for reference see de Gezelle *et al.*, 1979). Bromocriptine, 2.5 mg twice daily for 10 days, has become the method of choice to inhibit lactation. PRL levels fall immediately to normal levels after the first dose and onset of lactation is inhibited, thus showing the absolute necessity of PRL for lactation. The drug also suppresses lactation once it has been established even when PRL levels have already returned to normal levels.

A similar effect is achieved with lisuride, a semisynthetic ergot derivative (de Cecco *et al.*, 1979). In addition to its dopaminergic activity it also has antiserotoninergic activity. This property might help to block PRL release after suckling as there is some evidence that this response is mediated via serotoninergic mechanisms (Kordon *et al.*, 1974; Mena *et al.*, 1976). This hypothesis is supported by the effectiveness of metergoline, a serotoninergic antagonist, in inhibiting puerperal lactation in 69 women when given for 5 days at 8 mg/day (Delitala *et al.*, 1977). Some doubt about the mechanisms by which this agent acts has arisen because another serotoninergic antagonist cyproheptadine fails to lower plasma levels of PRL; moreover, methysergide, although highly effective in lowering PRL after suckling, was completely ineffective in inhibiting lactation (Crosignani *et al.*, 1979). This finding is surprising. Unfortunately, this observation is only briefly mentioned by the authors without presenting the original data. To our knowledge no detailed report has been published so far to allow a definite judgment to be made. If this preliminary report were confirmed it might suggest that different forms of PRL may be secreted. As pointed out by these authors other pharmacological effects in addition to the antiserotoninergic actions of this drug have to be considered as well.

In contrast to the central nervous system effects of the above mentioned substances, antiestrogens like tamoxifen and clomiphen do not interfere with PRL secretion (Zuckerman and Carmel, 1973; Masala *et al.,* 1977). Although effective in inhibiting lactation in 55 of 66 women after 10 mg four times daily, tamoxifen reduced PRL levels significantly only after 5 days. The release of PRL by the breast pump, however, was completely suppressed in all 15 postpartum women (Marsala *et al.,* 1978), so that one activity of these drugs might be to reduce the sensitivity of the breast to the suckling reflex (Robinson and Short, 1977).

C. Lactational Infertility as a Natural Contraceptive

In societies in which mothers breast feed for a prolonged time, lactation seems to be an effective natural contraceptive. Neuroendocrine changes during this period may be viewed as the control process regulating reproduction (Short, 1976). Women who breast feed have a much longer period of infertility after delivery than those who do not. With lactation proceeding for as long as 15 to 18 months mothers continue to be hyperprolactinemic. Serum hormone patterns in nursing amenorrheic mothers resemble those in infertile hyperprolactinemic patients with lowered estradiol and LH levels (Delvoye *et al.,* 1978). In addition to some action of elevated PRL levels on the ovary, already pointed out earlier, the suckling stimulus itself might be of importance, since the effectiveness of lactational contraception depends very much on the frequency of suckling, making demand feeding the most effective way to prevent new pregnancies. Although this approach to contraception does not seem to be acceptable generally in modern societies, in developing countries with other forms of contraception less readily available, spacing birth intervals by prolonged lactation seems to be an effective way of regulating population growth. Thus, besides its beneficial nutritional effect for the offspring, prolonged lactation should be encouraged as an effective means of regulating population growth in developing countries.

VII. Prolactin-Secreting Tumors during Pregnancy

Erdheim and Stumme (1909) first described the changes in the human adenohypophysis during pregnancy, documenting the increase in size and weight of the human pituitary. The increase in PRL cells in pregnancy has been well defined by Goluboff and Ezrin (1969). The increase in size of the pituitary during pregnancy carries with it a special risk for those patients harboring a pituitary adenoma. As major reports have been given on this topic, only a brief summary is presented here.

Microadenomas at random postmortem examination (Susman, 1933; Close, 1934) are found with a frequency of 20% in the age group of 20–30 years. A microadenoma by definition is less than 1 mm in diameter. In this group the incidence of pregnancy was lower than expected (Costello, 1936). In patients with established microadenomas only 2 of 91 pregnancies occurred spontaneously without treatment while in patients with macroadenomas 5 spontaneous pregnancies were noted in 56 patients (Gemzell and Wang, 1979). Therefore one should be especially aware of the possibility of pituitary adenomas in patients presenting with infertility or amenorrhea. The likelihood of a tumor increases if these symptoms are accompanied by galactorrhea, hyperprolactinemia, and a duration of symptoms longer than 2 years (Haesslein and Lamb, 1976; Jacobs *et al.,* 1976; Kleinberg *et al.,* 1977).

Although some controversy exists about diagnostic procedures necessary to establish the presence of a pituitary adenoma, opinion concerning appropriate treatment is also divided. As permanent blindness and fetal intracranial hemorrhage have been reported during pregnancies in patients harboring coexisting pituitary tumors it is critically important to observe these patients very carefully. Gemzell and Wang (1979) supplementing an earlier study by Magyar and Marshall (1978) described an uneventful pregnancy in 94.4% of 91 patients with previously untreated prolactin-producing microadenomas. In patients with an adenoma of more than 10 mm, 60% of 56 patients had to receive definite treatment either during or soon after pregnancy. Thus, the authors conclude that women with microadenomas could be treated with bromocriptine and in cases where pregnancy ensues should be monitored by monthly prolactin measurements and visual field testing. Should visual field defects appear, bromocriptine therapy must be reinstated or surgical intervention considered. Women with macroadenomas should be operated on before attempting pregnancy as the risk of some expansion of the large lesion is likely to have very serious consequences. Some studies indicate bromocriptine reduces mitotic activity and inhibits estrogen-induced proliferation of the pituitary (Lloyd *et al.,* 1975) and causes tumor regression in rats (MacLeod and Lehmeyer, 1973; Quadri *et al.,* 1972) and humans (Nillius *et al.,* 1978; Wass *et al.,* 1979). Therefore, this drug seems to offer an alternative to surgery.

In a prospective study eight of nine patients treated with 7.5 mg bromocriptine daily for 6 months showed lower PRL values, remodeling of the sella turcica, and/or reduction of tumor size. Symptoms rapidly returned after the drug was discontinued indicating that reduction in cell size is more probable than actual reduction of cell number (McGregor *et al.*, 1979; Thorner *et al.*, 1980; Sobrinho *et al.*, 1981). Administration of bromocriptine during early pregnancy seems to have produced few side effects and no teratological effects have been noted (Griffith *et al.*, 1978; del Pozo *et al.*, 1977). In a few patients bromocriptine has been given throughout pregnancy, again without adverse effects, although cord blood prolactin levels were low indicating the drug crossed the placenta into the fetal circulation. The influence of bromocriptine on the development of fetal neuroendocrine system has so far not been studied. However, the whole field of behavioral teratology is relatively new and subtle changes may go unnoticed for some time. This possibililty has to be kept in mind especially as some preliminary data indicate estrous irregularities in rats treated during fetal life with bromocriptine (Hoh and Havlicek, 1981.

VIII. Summary and Future Research

A considerable body of information has accumulated over the past decade on serum concentrations of prolactin during pregnancy. Ineresting differences in the pattern of levels in mother and fetus have emerged. Of particular interest are the very high concentrations of prolactin in amniotic fluid that occur early in pregnancy at a time when serum prolactin levels are still in the 10–20 ng/ml range. The source of amniotic fluid prolactin appears to be the decidua which is now recognized to be a special endocrine gland in its own right. The secretion of prolactin by the decidua appears to be under quite different regulatory mechanisms than secretion of prolactin by the pituitary, yet the structures of amniotic fluid and pituitary prolactin appear identical. In the peri- and postpartum period, rapid and major changes in prolactin secretion occur. In women who breast feed, prolactin levels remain elevated for a prolonged period while in those who bottle feed, prolactin concentrations return to nonpregnant levels within 2 weeks of delivery.

Thus far only a limited number of studies on prolactin have been conducted in pathological pregnancies. As yet they have not been especially rewarding, but given the limited number of studies performed this may not be entirely surprising. Of particular interest and practical importance is the management of patients with hyperprolactinemia who become pregnant often following treatment with bromocriptine. What is the optimal therapy for these patients and what particular risks may they encounter especially if they harbor prolactin-secreting microadenomas?

Although a mass of data on prolactin levels in various body fluids in mother and fetus have been generated, the physiological role of prolactin during pregnancy remains to be clarified. It is evident that hyperprolactinemia adversely affects ovarian function, and that in the postpartum period prolactin is essential for lactation but the precise mechanisms by which both of these actions are mediated remains to be elucidated. Suggestions have been made that the role of amniotic fluid is to influence salt and water transport across the amnion, but much more sophisticated physiological studies are necessary to establish this hypothesis. Prolactin in many species has important behavioral effects referred to as "mothering" or maternal instinct. Whether prolactin exerts similar effects in women has not been seriously examined, but it would be surprising if it did not have a similar significance. Finally, the interaction, if any, between placental lactogens and prolactin, two lactogenic hormones secreted in large amounts during pregnancy, is a likely fruitful area of research. Perhaps because lactation is of such biological importance a "fail safe" mechanism has evolved to ensure adequate mammary gland development during pregnancy.

Acknowledgments

This research was suppported by grants from MRC of Canada and USPHS HDO7843-09. UAK received a fellowship from MRC of Canada.

We thank Pam Meadows for typing the manuscript.

References

Aono, T., Shioji, T., Shoda, T., and Kurachi, K. (1977). *J. Clin. Endocrinol. Metab.* **44,** 1101–1106.

Aono, T., Shioji, T., Aki, T., Hirota, K., Nomura, A., and Kurachi, K. (1979). *J. Clin. Endocrinol. Metab.* **48,** 478–482.

Aubert, M., Grumbach, M. M., and Kaplan, S. L. (1975). *J. Clin. Invest.* **56,** 155–164.

Ballard, P. L., Gluckman, P. D., Brehier, A., Kitterman, J. A., Kaplan, S. L., Rudolph, A. M., and Grumbach, M. M. (1978). *J. Clin. Invest.* **62,** 879–883.

Barberia, J. M., Abu-Fadil, S., Kletzky, O. A., Nakamura, R. M., and Mishell, D. R. (1975). *Am. J. Obstet. Gynecol.* **121,** 1107–1110.

Bellman, O., Lang, N., and Schach, S. (1979). *Arch. Gynecol.* **228,** 155–158.

Ben-David, M., Rodbard, D., Bates, R. W., Bridson, W. E., and Chrambach, A. (1973). *J. Clin. Endocrinol. Metab.* **36,** 941–964.

Benveniste, R., Helman, J. D., Orth, D. N., McKenna, T. J., Nicholson, W. E., and Rabinowitz, D. (1979). *J. Clin. Endocrinol. Metab.* **48,** 883–886.

Berczi, I., and Nagy, E. (1981). *Fed. Proc. Fed. Am. Soc. Exp. Biol.* **40,** 1031.

Bigazzi, M., Pollicino, G., and Nardi, E. (1979a). *J. Clin. Endocrinol. Metab.* **49,** 847–850.

Bigazzi, M., Ronga, R., Lancranjan, I., Ferraro, S., Branconi, F., Buzzoni, P., Martorana, G., Scarselli, G. F., and Del Pozo, E. (1979b). *J. Clin. Endocrinol. Metab.* **48,** 9–12.

Biswas, S. (1976). *Clin. Chim. Acta* **73,** 363–367.

Biswas, S., and Rodeck, C. H. (1976). *Br. J. Obstet. Gynaecol.* **83,** 683–687.

Bohnet, H. G., Dahlen, H. G., Wuttke, W., and Schneider, H. P. G. (1975). *J. Clin. Endocrinol. Metab.* **42,** 132–143.

Bohnet, H. G., Mühlenstedt, D., Hanker, J. P. F., and Schneider, H. P. G. (1977). *Arch. Gynekol.* **223,** 173–178.

Boyar, R. M., Finkelstein, J. W., Kapen, S., and Hellman, L. (1975). *J. Clin. Endocrinol. Metab.* **40,** 1117–1120.

Brun del Re, R., Del Pozo, E., de Grandi, P., Friesen, H., Hinselmann, M., and Wyss, H. (1973). *Obstet. Gynecol.* **41,** 884–890.

Bunner, D. L, VanderLaan, E. F., and VanderLaan, W. P. (1978). *Am. J. Obstet. Gynecol.* **131,** 250–252.

Bustos, R., and Giussi, G. (1980). *Pediatr. Res.* **14,** 78.

Cassano, F., Chisci, R., and Tarantino, C. (1952). *Folia Endocrinol.* **5,** 69–74.

Chard, T. (1975). *Clin. Endocrinol.* **4,** 89–106.

Chochinov, R. H., Ketapanya, A., Mariz, I. K., Underwood, L. E., and Daughaday, W. H. (1976). *J. Clin. Endocrinol. Metab.* **42,** 983–986.

Clements, J. A., Reyes, F. I., Winter, J. S. D., and Faiman, C. (1977). *J. Clin. Endocrinol. Metab.* **44,** 408–413.

Close, H. G. (1934). *Lancet* **1,** 732–734.

Contractor, S. F., and Davies, H. (1973). *Nature (London) New Biol.* **243,** 284–286.

Costello, R. T. (1936). *Am. J. Pathol.* **12,** 205–215.

Crosignani, P. G., Lombroso, G. C., Mattei, A., Caccamo, A., and Trojsi, L. (1979). *J. Clin. Endocrinol. Metab.* **48,** 335–337.

De Cecco, L., Venturini, P. L., Ragni, N., Rossato, P., Maganza, C., Gaggero, G., and Horowski, R. (1979). *Br. J. Obstet. Gynaecol.* **86,** 905–908.

De Gezelle, H., Dhont, M., Parewyck, W., and Thiery, M. (1977a). *IRCS Med. Sci. Clin. Med.* **5,** 475.

De Gezelle, H., Dhont, M., Parewyck, W., and Thiery, M. (1977b). *Am. J. Obstet. Gynecol.* **130,** 736.

De Gezelle, H., Dhont, M., Thiery, M., and Parewyck, W. (1979). *Acta Obstet. Gynecol. Scand.* **58,** 469–472.

Delitala, G., Masala, A., Alagna, S., Devilla, L., Lodico, G., and Lotti, G. (1977). *Br. Med. J.* **1,** 744–746.

Del Pozo, E., Wyss, H. I., Lancranjan, I., Obolenski, W., and Varga, L. (1976). *In* "Ovulation in the Human" (P. G. Crosignani and D. R. Mishell, eds.), pp. 297–299. Academic Press, New York.

Del Pozo, E., Darragh, A., Lancranjan, I., Ebeling, D., Burmeister, P., Buhler, F., Marbach, P., and Braun, P. (1977). *Clin. Endocrinol.* **6,** (Suppl.), 47S–55S.

Delvoye, P., Taubert, H. D., Jurgensen, O., L'Hermite, M., Delogne, J., and Robyn, C. (1974). *C.R. Hebd. Seance. Acad. Sci. Ser. D* **279,** 1463–1466.

Delvoye, P., Demaegd, M., Nyampeta, U., and Robyn, C. (1978). *Am. J. Obstet. Gynecol.* **130,** 635–639.

Dubowitz, L., Strang, F., Hawkins, D. F., Blair, C. M., and Mashiter, K. (1975). *Br. Med. J.* **2,** 445.

Erdheim, J., and Stumme, E. (1909). *Beitr. Pathol. Anat.* **46,** 1–132.

Fang, V. S., and Kim, M. H. (1975). *J. Clin. Endocrinol. Metab.* **41,** 1030–1034.

Frame, L. T., Rogol, A. D., Riddick, D. H., and Baczynski, E. (1979a). *Fertil. Steril.* **31,** 647–640.

Frame, L. T., Wiley, L., and Rogol, A. D. (1979b). *J. Endocrinol. Metab.* **49,** 435–437.

Francis, M. J. O., and Hill, D. J. (1975). *Nature (London)* **255,** 167–168.

Franks, S., Murray, M. A. F., Jequier, A. M., Steele, S. J., Nabarro, J. D. N., and Jacobs, H. S. (1975). *Clin. Endocrinol.* **4,** 597–607.

Frantz, A. G., Kleinberg, D. L., and Noel, G. L. (1972). *Recent Prog. Horm. Res.* **28,** 527–590.

Freeman, R., Lev-Gur, M., Boyar, R. M., and Schylman, H. (1976). *Obstet. Gynecol.* **47,** 282–286.
Friesen, H., Hwang, P., Guyda, H., Tolis, G., Tyson, J., and Myers, R. (1972). *In* "Prolactin and Carcinogenesis" (A. R. Boyns and K. Griffiths, eds.), pp. 64–80. Alpha, Omega, Alpha, Cardiff.
Friesen, H., Fournier, P., and Desjardins, P. (1973). *Clin. Obstet. Gynecol.* **16,** 25–45.
Gala, R. R., and Van De Walle, C. (1977). *Life Sci.* **21,** 99–104.
Gemzelle, C., and Wang, C. F. (1979). *Fertil. Steril.* **31,** 363–372.
Gluckman, P. D., Ballard, P. L., Kaplan, S. L., Liggins, G. C., and Grumbach, M. M. (1978). *J. Pediatr.* **93,** 1011–1104.
Golander, A., Barrett, J., Hurley, T., Barry, S., and Handwerger, S. (1979). *J. Clin. Endocrinol.* **49,** 787–789.
Goluboff, L. G., and Ezrin, C. (1969). *J. Clin. Endocrinol.* **29,** 1533–1538.
Gregoriou, O., Pitoulis, S., Coutifaris, B., Varonos, D., and Batrinos, M. (1979). *Obstet. Gynecol.* **53,** 630–632.
Griffith, R. W., Turkalj. I., and Braun, P. (1978). *Br. J. Clin. Pharmacol.* **5,** 224–231.
Grosvenor, C. E. (1965). *Endocrinology* **76,** 340–342.
Guitelman, A., Aparicio, N. J., Mancini, A., and Debeljuk, L. (1978). *Fertil. Steril.* **30,** 42–44.
Guzman, V., Toscano, G., Canales, E. S., and Zarate, A. (1979). *Acta Obstet. Gynecol. Scand.* **58,** 53–55.
Haesslein, H. C., and Lamb, E. J. (1976). *Am. J. Obstet. Gynecol.* **125,** 759–767.
Hall, D. M. B., and Kay, G. (1977). *Br. Med. J.* **1,** 777.
Hamosh, M., and Hamosh, P. (1977). *J. Clin. Invest.* **59,** 1002–1005.
Haning, R. V., Jr., Barrett, D. A., Alberino, S. P., Lynskey, M. T., Donabedian, R., and Speroff, L. (1978). *Am. J. Obstet. Gynecol.* **130,** 204–210.
Hauth, J. C., Parker, C. R., Jr., MacDonald, P. C., Porter, J. C., and Johnston, J. M. (1978). *Obstet. Gynecol.* **51,** 81–88.
Healy, D. L., Muller, H. K., and Burger, H. G. (1977). *Nature (London)* **265,** 642–643.
Healy, D. L., Kimpton, W. G., Muller, H. K., and Burger, H. G. (1979). *Br. J. Obstet. Gynaecol.* **86,** 307–313.
Hershman, J. M., Kojima, A., and Friesen, H. G. (1973). *J. Clin. Endocrinol. Metab.* **36,** 497–501.
Hertz, J., Andersen, A. N., and Larsen, J. F. (1978). *Clin. Endocrinol.* **9,** 97–100.
Hoh, Y., and Havlicek, V. (1981). *Endocrinology* **108,** (Suppl.), 220.
Holt, W. F., and Perks, A. M. (1975). *Gen. Comp. Endocrinol.* **26,** 153–164.
Horrobin, D. F. (1974). "Prolactin." Medical and Technical Publ. Lancaster.
Horrobin, D. F. (1975). *Br. Med. J.* **1,** 629.
Horrobin, D. F., Lloyd, I. J., Lipton, A., Burstyn, P. G., Durkin, N., and Muiruri, K. L. (1971). *Lancet* **3,** 352–354.
Jacobs, H. S., Hull, M. G. R., Murray, M. A. F., and Franks, S. (1975). *Horm. Res.* **6,** 268–287.
Jenkins, D. M., and Perry, L. A. (1978). *Br. J. Obstet Gynaecol.* **85,** 754–757.
Jeppson, S., Nilsson, K. O., Rannevik, G., and Wide, L. (1976). *Acta Enodcrinol. (Copenhagen)* **82,** 246–253.
Josimovich, J. B., Weiss, G., and Hutchison, D. L. (1974). *Endocrinology* **94,** 1364–1371.
Josimovich, J. B., Merisko, K., and Boccella, L. (1977). *Endocrinology* **100,** 564–570.
Jouppila, R., Jouppila, P., Moilanen, K., and Pakarinen, A. (1980). *Br. J. Obstet. Gynaecol.* **87,** 234–238.
Karmali, R. A., Lauder, I., and Horrobin, D. F. (1974). *Lancet* **2,** 106–107.
Kauppila, A., Puukka, M., and Tuimala, R. (1979). *Am. J. Obstet. Gynecol.* **134,** 752–755.

Kelly, P. A., Posner, B. I., Tsushima, T., and Friesen, H. G. (1974). *Endocrinology* **95,** 532–539.

Khattab, T. Y., and Jequier, A. M. (1978). *J. Endocrinol.* **78,** 351–358.

Kleinberg, D L., Noel, G. L., and Frantz, A. G. (1977). *N. Engl. J. Med.* **296,** 589–600.

Kordon, C., Blake, C. A., Terkel, J., and Sawyer, C. H. (1973/74). *Neuroendocrinology* **13,** 213–223.

Laatikainen, T., Pelkonen, J., Apter, D., and Ranta, T. (1980). *J. Clin. Endocrinol.* **50,** 489–494.

Leontic, E. A., and Tyson, J. E. (1977). *Am. J. Physiol.* **232** R124–R127.

Leontic, E. A., Schruefer, J. J., Andreassen, B., Pinto, H., and Tyson, J. E. (1979). *Am. J. Obstet. Gynecol.* **133,** 435–438.

L'Hermite, M., and Robyn, C. (1972). *Ann. Endocrinol.* **33,** 357–360.

Lloyd, H. M., Meares, J. D., and Jacob, J. (1975). *Nature (London)* **255,** 497–498.

Lowe, K. C., Beck, N. F. G., McNaughton, D. C., Jansen, C. A. M., Thomas, A. L., Nathanielsz, P. W., Mallon, K., and Steven, D. H. (1979). *Q. J. Exp. Physiol.* **64,** 253–262.

Luciano, A. A., Maslar, I. A., Kusmik, W. F., and Riddick, D. H. (1980). *Am. J. Obstet. Gynecol.* **138,** 665–669.

McGregor, H. M., Scanlon, M. F., Hall, R., and Hall, K. (1979). *Br. Med. J.* **2,** 700–703.

MacKenzie, I. Z., Jenkin, G., and Bradley, S. (1979). *Br. J. Obstet. Gynaecol.* **86,** 171–174.

MacLeod, R. M., and Leymeyer, J. E. (1973). *Cancer Res.* **33,** 849–855.

McNatty, K. P., Sawers, R. S., and McNeilly, A. S. (1974). *Nature (London)* **250,** 653–655.

McNeilly, A. S. (1980). *Nature (London)* **284,** 212.

McNeilly, A. S., Gilmore, D., Dobbie, G., and Chart, T. (1977). *J. Endocrinol.* **73,** 533–534.

Magyar, D. M., and Marshall, J. R. (1978). *Am. J. Obstet. Gynecol.* **132,** 739–751.

Manku, M. S., Mtagji, J. P., and Horrobin, D. F. (1975). *Nature (London)* **258,** 78–80.

Masala, A., Delitala, G., LoDico, G., Slagna, S., and Devilla, L. (1977). *J. Endocrinol.* **74,** 501–502.

Masala, A., Delitala, G., LoDico, G., Stoppelli, I., Slagna, S., and Devilla, L. (1978). *Br. J. Obstet. Gynaecol.* **85,** 134–137.

Maslar, I. A., Kaplan, B. M., Luciano, A. A., and Riddick, D. H. (1980). *J. Clin. Endocrinol. Metab.* **51,** 78–83.

Mena, F., and Grosvenor, C. E. (1971). *Horm. Behav.* **2,** 107–116.

Mena, F., Enjalbert, A., Carbonell, L., Priam, M., and Kordon, C. (1976). *Endocrinology* **99,** 445–451.

Mochizuki, M., Morikawa, H., Kawaguchi, K., and Tojo, S. (1976). *J. Clin. Endocrinol. Metab.* **43,** 614–621.

Moltz, H., and Leidahl, L. C. (1977). *Science* **196,** 81–83.

Mullon, D. K., Smith, Y. F., Hamosh, M., and Hamosh, P. (1979). *Clin. Res.* **27,** A401.

Nicoll, C. S. (1974). *In* "Handbook of Physiology" (R. O. Greep and A B. Astwood eds.), Vol. IV, Part II, pp. 253–229. Williams & Dillon, Baltimore, Maryland.

Nillius, S. J., Berg, T., Lundberg, P. O., Stahle, J., and Wide, L. (1978). *Fertil. Steril.* **30,** 710–712.

Noel, G. L., Suh, H. K., and Frantz, A. G. (1974). *J. Clin. Endocrinol. Metab.* **39,** 413–423.

Parker, D. C., Rossman, L. G., and Vanderlaan, E. F. (1973). *J. Clin. Endocrinol. Metab.* **36,** 1119–1124.

Polatti, R., Bolis, P. F., Ravagni-Probizer, M. F., Baruffini, A., and Cavalleri, A. (1978). *Am. J. Obstet. Gynecol.* **131,** 792–796.

Quadri, S. K., Meites, J., and Lu, K. H. (1972). *Science* **176,** 417–418.

Quigley, M. M., Hammond, C. B., and Handwerger, S. (1976). *Fertil. Steril.* **27,** 1165–1170.

Ranta, T., Unnerus, H. A., Rossi, J., and Seppala, M. (1979). *Am. J. Obstet. Gynecol.* **134,** 1–3.

Ranta, T., Stenman, U. H., Unnerus, H. A., Rossi, J., and Seppala, M. (1980). *Obstet. Gynecol.* **55**, 428–430.

Redman, C. E. G., Bonnar, J., Beilin, L. J., and McNeily, A. S. (1975). *Br. Med. J.* **1**, 304–306.

Richards, J. F. (1975). *Biochem. Biophys. Res. Commun.* **63**, 292–299.

Riddick, D. H., and Kusmik, W. F. (1977). *Am. J. Obstet. Gynecol.* **127**, 187–190.

Riddick, D. H., and Maslar, I. A. (1981). *J. Clin. Endocrinol. Metab.* **52**, 220–224.

Riddick, D. H., Luciano, A. A., Kusmik, W. F., and Maslar, I. A. (1978). *Life Sci.* **23**, 1913–1922.

Riddick, D. H., Luciano, A. A., Kusmik, W. F., and Maslar, I. A. (1979). *Fertil. Steril.* **31**, 35–39.

Rigg, L. A., and Yen, S. S. C. (1977). *Am. J. Obstet. Gynecol.* **128**, 215–218.

Rigg, L. A., Lein, A., and Yen, S. S. C. (1977). *Am. J. Obstet. Gynecol.* **129**, 454–456.

Robinson, J. E., and Short, R. V. (1977). *Br. Med. J.* **1**, 118–119.

Rosenberg, S. M., Maslar, I. A., and Riddick, D. H. (1980). *Am. J. Obstet. Gynecol.* **138**, 681–685.

Sadovsky, E., Wienstein, D., Ben-David, M., and Polishuk, W. Z. (1977). *Obstet. Gynecol.* **50**, 559–561.

Salazar, H., and Tobon, H. (1974). *In* "Lactogenic Hormones, Fetal Nutrition, and Lactation" (J. B. Josimovich, M. Reynolds, and E. Cobo, eds.), pp. 221–227. Wiley, New York.

Sassin, J. F., Frantz, A. G., Weitzman, E. D., and Kapen, S. (1972). *Science* **177**, 1205–1207.

Sassin, J. F., Frantz, A. G., Kapen, S., and Weitzman, E. D. (1973). *J. Clin. Endocrinol. Metab.* **37**, 436–440.

Schenker, J. G., Ben-David, M., and Polishuk, W. Z. (1975). *Am. J. Obstet. Gynecol.* **123**, 834–838.

Schneider, A. B., Kowlaski, K., and Sherwood, L. M. (1975). *Endocrinology* **97**, 1364–1372.

Schultz, K. D., Geiger, W., Del Pozo, E., Lose, V. H., Kunzikg, H. F., and Lancranjan, I. (1976). *Arch. Gynecol.* **221**, 93–396.

Schultz, K. D., Geiger, W., Del Pozo, E., and Kunzig, H. J. (1978). *Am. J. Obstet. Gynecol.* **132**, 561–566.

Seppala, M. (1978). *Ann. Clin. Res.* **10**, 164–170.

Seron-Ferre, M., Munroe, S. E., Hess, D., Parer, J. T., and Jaffe, R. B. (1979). *Endocrinology* **194**, 1243–1246.

Short, R. V. (1976). *Proc. R. Soc. London Ser. B* **195**, 3–24.

Siler-Khodr, T. M., Morgenstern, L. L., and Greenwood, F. C. (1974). *J. Clin. Endocrinol. Metab.* **39**, 891–905.

Sobrinho, L. G., Nunes, M. C., Calhaz-Jorge, C., Mauricio, J. C., and Santos, M. A. (1981). *Acta Endocrinol.* **96**, 24–29.

Soria, J., Canales, E. X., Forsbach, G., Karchmer, S., Buzman, V., and Zarate, A. (1977). *Ann. Endocrinol.* **38**, 55–59.

Spring-Mills, E., Berg, N. B., and Hafez, E. S. (1980). *In* "Human Reproduction" (E. S. E. Hafez, ed.), 2nd Ed., pp. 355–370. Harper, New York.

Suh, H. K., and Frantz, A. G.(1974). *J. Clin. Endocrinol. Metab.* **39**, 928–935.

Susman, W. (1933). *Br. Med. J.* **2**, 1215.

Terkel, J., Damassa, D. A., and Sawyer, C. H. (1979). *Horm. Behav.* **12**, 95–102.

Thomson, A. M., Hytten, F. E., and Black, A. E. (1975). *Bull. WHO* **52**, 337–349.

Thorner, M. O., Martin, W. H., Rogol, A. D., Morris, J. L., Perryman, R. L., Conway, B. P. Howards, S. S.,Wolfman, M. G., and MacLeod, R. M. (1980). *J. Clin. Endocrinol. Metab.* **51**, 438–445.

Tulchinski, D. (1980). *In* "Maternal Fetal Endocrinology" (D. Tulchinski and V. J. Ryan, eds.), pp. 151–166. Saunders, Philadelphia, Pennsylvania.

Tyson, J. E., Hwang, P., Guyda, H., and Friesen, H. G. (1972a). *Am. J. Obstet. Gynecol.* **113** 14–20.
Tyson, J. E., Friesen, H. G., and Anderson, M. S. (1972b). *Science* **177,** 897–900.
Tyson, J. E., Khonjandi, M., Huth, J., and Andereasen, B. (1975). *J. Clin. Endocrinol. Metab.* **40,** 764–773.
Van Petten, G. R., and Bridges, R. (1979). *Am. J. Obstet. Gynecol.* **134,** 711–714.
Varga, L., Lutterbeck, P. M., Pryor, J. S., Wenner, R., and Erb, H. (1972). *Br. Med. J.* **2,** 743–744.
Veldhuis, J. D., and Hammond, J. M. (1980). *Nature (London)* **284,** 262–264.
Wass, J. A., Moult, P. J., Thorner, M. O., Dalie, J. E., Charlesworth, M., Jones, A. E., and Besser, G. M. (1979). *Lancet* **2,** 66–69.
Weisz-Carrington, P., Roux, M. E., McWilliams, M., Phillips-Quagliata, J. M., and Lamm, M. E. (1978). *Proc. Natl. Acad. Sci. U.S.A.* **75,** 2928–2932.
Winters, A. J., Colston, C., MacDonald, P. C., and Porter, J. C. (1975). *J. Clin. Endocrinol. Metab.* **41,** 626–629.
Ylikorkala, O., Huhtaniemi, I., Tuimala, R., and Seppala, M. (1979a). *Fertil. Steril.* **32,** 286–288.
Ylikorkala, O., Kaupilla, A., and Viinikka, L. (1979b). *J. Clin. Endocrinol. Metab.* **49,** 452–455.
Ylikorkala, O., Kivinen, S., and Reinila, M. (1979c). *J. Clin. Endocrinol. Metab.* **48,** 288–292.
Ylikorkala, O., Kivinen, S., and Kaupilla, A. (1980). *Acta Endocrinol.* **93,** 413–418.
Yuen, B. H., Cannon, W., Woolley, S., and Charles, E. (1978). *Br. J. Obstet. Gynaecol.* **85,** 293–298.
Yuen, B. H., Cannon, W., Lewis, J., Sy, L., and Woolley, S. (1980). *Am. J. Obstet. Gynecol.* **136,** 286–291.
Zarate, A., Villalobos, H., Canales, E. S., Soria, J., Arcovedo, F., and MacGregor, C. (1976). *J. Clin. Endocrinol. Metab.* **43,** 301–305.
Zuckerman, H., and Carmel, S. (1973). *Obst. Gynecol. Br. Commonw.* **80,** 822–823.

HUMAN CHORIONIC GONADOTROPIN IN EARLY PREGNANCY

*Brij B. Saxena** *and Premila Rathnam*†

DEPARTMENTS OF *MEDICINE AND †OBSTETRICS AND GYNECOLOGY
CORNELL UNIVERSITY MEDICAL COLLEGE
NEW YORK, NEW YORK

I. Introduction 98
II. Chemistry and Biosynthesis 98
A. Biological Properties 101
B. Immunological Properties 103
III. Measurement of hCG 105
A. Biological Pregnancy Tests 105
B. Hormonal Withdrawal Tests 105
C. Immunological Pregnancy Tests 107
D. Do-It-Yourself Pregnancy Tests 107
E. Radioimmunoassay 108
F. Radioreceptorassay 109
IV. Secretory Patterns of hCG during the Reproductive Cycle 110
A. The Preimplantation Phase 111
B. The Postimplantation Phase 113
V. Role of hCG in Early Pregnancy 118
VI. Role of hCG in Abnormal Conditions 118
A. Abnormal Pregnancies 119
B. hCG in Cancer 119
VII. Interaction of hCG with "Receptor" Site 121
A. Purification and Properties of the hCG–LH Receptor 121

Current Topics in Experimental Endocrinology, Vol. 4

ISBN 0-12-153204-6

B. Mechanism of Hormone–Receptor Interaction 121
References 122

I. Introduction

The development of sensitive and specific immuno-, receptor-, and microbiological assays has not only permitted early detection of human chorionic gonadotropin (hCG) in pregnancy, but also in a variety of tumors, normal tissue, placental extracts of the rat, mouse, hamster, and rabbit, and in bacteria (Saxena, 1981b; Saxena and Rathnam, 1981). Fifteen strains of bacteria isolated from the tissues of patients bearing malignant neoplasms exhibited the presence of a membrane-associated, immunoreactive protein similar to hCG (Acevedo *et al.*, 1977). The hCG-like antigen is, however, not present in every "cancer-associated bacteria." Many of these findings have still to be validated in terms of their physiological significance. The hCG in tissues other than those of placental and/or tumor origin is not glycosylated and is biologically inactive *in vivo*. It has been postulated that each cell may contain a gene for the synthesis of hCG, which is expressed by an appropriate stimulus. Recent studies on the presence of hCG-like material during the preimplantation phase (Saxena, 1979; Hertz, 1979) have suggested a role for this substance in the maintenance of corpus luteum function prior to implantation.The presence of hCG-like material in human spermatozoa and in the rabbit blastocyst has raised interesting biological speculations on the maintenance of corpus luteum of gestation prior to implantation and on the protection of the embryo from immunorejection by the mother. The quantitative determination of hCG has served as a marker for the early detection of pregnancy (Saxena *et al.*, 1974). The serial measurement of hCG permits early diagnosis and significantly improved management of abnormal pregnancy, gestational trophoblastic disease, and malignant ectopic tumors producing hCG (Saxena and Landesman, 1978).

II. Chemistry and Biosynthesis

Although chorionic gonadotropin has also been detected in nonhuman primates (Hobson and Wide, 1972), equidae (Allen, 1969), rodents (Haour *et al.*, 1976), sheep, and rabbits (Lacroix and Martal, 1979; Haour and Saxena, 1974b), etc., to date, only human chorionic gonadotropin has been extensively investigated chemically.

hCG has been isolated from first trimester pregnancy urine (Birken and Canfield, 1978; Bahl, 1972; Van Hell, 1974). It is a glycoprotein hormone containing approximately 30% carbohydrate; the molecular weight is 36,700 and the isoelectric point is 4.5 (Birken and Canfield, 1978). hCG consists of a hormone-nonspecific α subunit and a hormone-specific β subunit of molecular weights of 14,500 and 22,200, respectively. The subunits are of noncovalent (electrostatic and hydrophobic) linkage, and the primary amino acid sequences of the subunits have been elucidated (Figs. 1 and 2). The α subunit contains 92 amino acids, and the sequence is nearly identical to those of the α subunits of the other glycoprotein hormones, viz. hLH, hFSH, and hTSH. The complementary hCG-β subunit contains 145 amino acids, which is 80% similar to hLH-β subunit, except for the presence of a 30 amino acid peptide at the C-terminal of hCG-β. There are several regions of homology to the β subunits of hFSH and hTSH (Fig. 3). The amino acid sequences of the β subunits hFSH, hLH, hTSH, and hCG have been carefully compared by Stewart and Stewart (1977). The residues 1–15, 30–55, and 101 to the end of the hCG-β molecule represent hormone-specific variable regions, whereas residues 16–38 and 56–100 are constant or homologous. The variable regions may provide the conformation for the specific receptor recognition, whereas the constant may provide the areas of subunit–subunit interaction. Experimental studies have provided evidence that the α subunit may occupy an overlying position and allow the specific conformation of the β subunits (Ward, 1978; Saxena and Rathnam, 1978). The α subunit contains two and the β subunit contains five carbohydrate moieties attached to the protein chain. One carbohydrate moiety containing two branches is attached to asparagines in N-glycosidic linkage at residues 52 and 78 of the α subunit and to asparagine residues 13 and 30 of the β subunit of hCG. In contrast to all other oligosaccharide side chains, an additional four linear oligosaccharide carbohydrate moieties are attached via O-glycosidical linkages to serine residues 121, 127, 132, and 138 of the carboxyterminus of the hCG-β subunit. The monosaccharide sequences of the carbohydrate moieties are shown in Fig. 4 (Kessler *et al.,* 1979a,b).

Studies on the biosynthesis of hCG indicate that the α and β subunits are translated from separate messengers and that both are synthesized as percursors (Daniels-McQueen *et al.,* 1978). Due to the identity of the α subunits and the significant homology among the β subunits of the glycoprotein hormones hFSH, hLH, hTSH, and hCG, it is reasonable to assume that α and β subunits have separate genes which may lie in the same chromosome. The pre-hCGα NH_2-terminal signal peptide containing 24 amino acids has been sequenced (Birken *et al.,* 1978). The leader sequence is cleaved by a membrane-associated peptidase before alanine to release the α subunit from the precursor (Birken and Canfiled, 1980). The α subunit is synthesized in excess, whereas the β subunit is rate limiting in the production of the biologically active hormone and heralds cellular differentation and function.

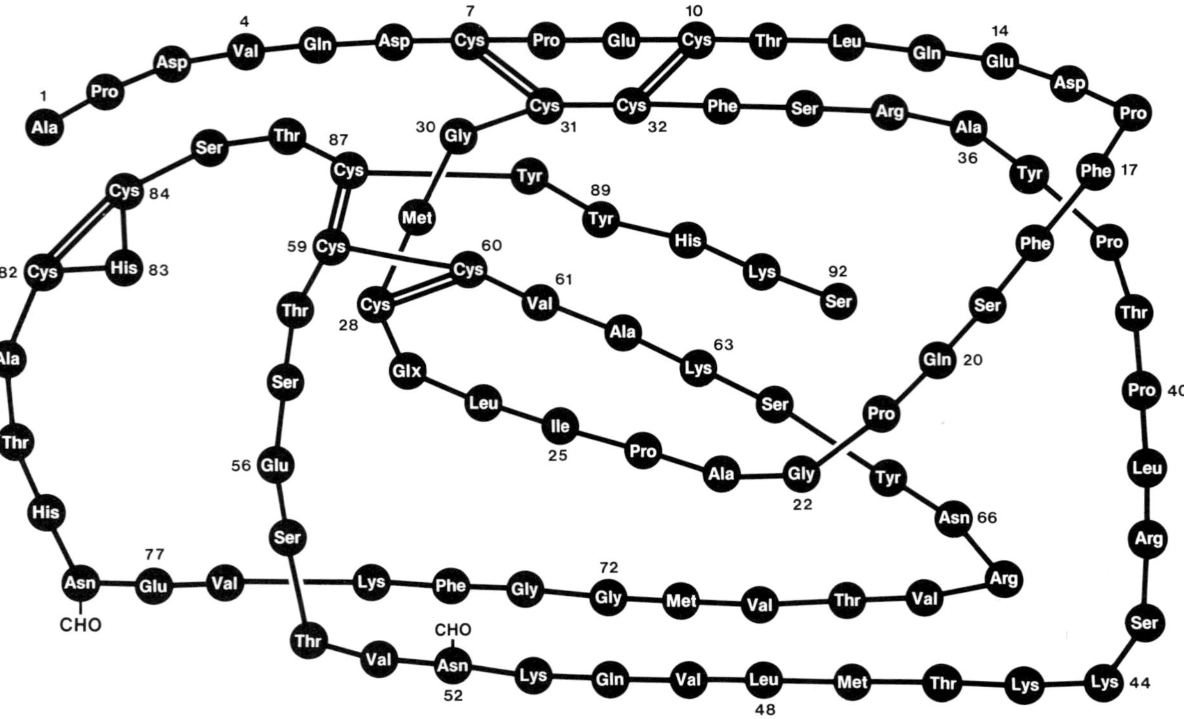

Fig. 1. Amino acid sequence of the hCG-α subunit, showing the disulfide bridges (as proposed by Mise and Bahl, 1980).

1 10 CHO
Ser - Lys - Glu - Pro - Leu - Arg - Pro - Arg - Cys - Arg - Pro - Ile - Asn - Ala - Thr - Leu -

20 CHO
Ala - Val - Glu - Lys - Glu - Gly - Cys - Pro - Val - Cys - Ile - Thr - Val - Asn - Thr - Thr -

40
Ile - Cys - Ala - Gly - Tyr - Cys - Pro - Thr - Met - Thr - Arg - Val - Leu - Gln - Gly - Val -

50 60
Leu - Pro - Ala - Leu - Pro - Gln - Val - Val - Cys - Asn - Tyr - Arg - Asp - Val - Arg - Phe -

70 80
Glu - Ser - Ile - Arg - Leu - Pro - Gly - Cys - Pro - Arg - Gly - Val - Asn - Pro - Val - Val -

90
Ser - Tyr - Ala - Val - Ala - Leu - Ser - Cys - Gln - Cys - Ala - Leu - Cys - Arg - Arg - Ser -

100 110
Thr - Thr - Asp - Cys - Gly - Gly - Pro - Lys - Asp - His - Pro - Leu - Thr - Cys - Asp - Asp -

120 CHO CHO
Pro - Arg - Phe - Gln - Asp - Ser - Ser - Ser - Ser - Lys - Ala - Pro - Pro - Pro - Ser - Leu -

130 CHO CHO 140
Pro - Ser - Pro - Ser - Arg - Leu - Pro - Gly - Pro - Ser - Asp - Thr - Pro - Ile - Leu - Pro -

Gln

Fig. 2. Amino acid sequence of the hCG-β subunit (Birkin and Canfield, 1978).

The hCG secretion during pregnancy is independent of any feedback controls; however, an autoregulation of hCG-mediated steriodogenesis has been postulated.

A. Biological Properties

Due to the structural similarites between hLH and hCG, the two hormones are similar in their primary biological and immunological activities. Since the 30 amino acid carboxy-terminal sequence is not present in the hLH-β subunit, it is reasonable to assume that this portion of the hCG molecule is not necessary for biologic activity. This is further suggested from the studies in which antibodies specific to the tail piece fail to neutralize the biological activity of hCG (Louvet *et al.,* 1974).

There is controversy concerning whether the secondary follicle stimulating hormone (FSH) and thyroid stimulating hormone (TSH) activities of the human chorionic gonadotropin (Siris *et al.,* 1977; Nisula *et al.,* 1974) are

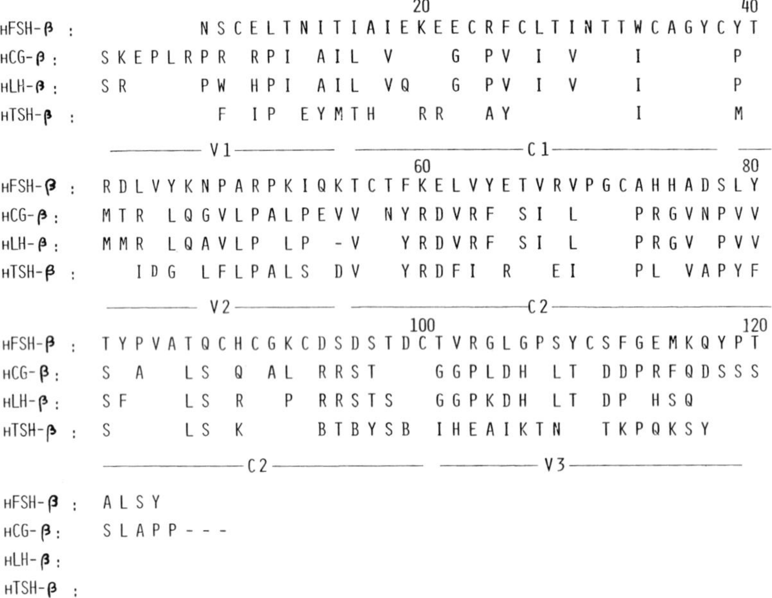

Fig. 3. Amino acid sequence of human glycoprotein hormone β subunits (Stewart and Stewart, 1977). S, Ser; K, Lys; E, Glu; P, Pro; L, Leu; R, Arg; C, Cys; I, Ileu; N, Asn; A, Ala; T, Thr; B, Asx; V, Val; G, Gly; Y, Tyr; M, Met; Q, Gln; D, Asp; F, Phe; H, His; W, Trp.

either of pituitary or placental origin. The evidence suggests that similar to luteinizing hormone activity, the FSH and TSH-like activities of hCG are due to a structural homology; hence, these activities are intrinsic to the hCG molecule. Observations of patients (Braunstein and Hershman, 1976) are consistent with the hypothesis that the hCG molecule is the thyrotropic factor which mediates the thyrotoxicosis with hyperthyroidism in late pregnancy and gestational trophoblastic disease. Recently an immunosuppressive activity of hCG which may inhibit the maternal processes of immunorejection of a fetus as a homograft, has also been implicated. hCG inhibits the response of lymphocytes to phytohemagglutinin in *in vitro* mixed lymphocyte cultures. However, the specificity of the inhibition of T lymphocyte activity of hCG is questionable since highly purified preparations were found to be without effect (Nisula *et al.*, 1974). Prolonged skin allograft survival and lower incidence of positive delayed hypersensitivity skin test (Finn *et al.*, 1972) during pregnancy have been attributed to hCG. However, immunosuppressive (Adcock *et al.*, 1973), porphyrin synthesis inhibitory (Rifkind *et al.*, 1976), and NAD-glycohydrolase activities (Moss *et al.*, 1978) are not copurified with hCG from crude commercial urinary hCG preparations.

N — Glycosidic Carbohydrate Units of hCG

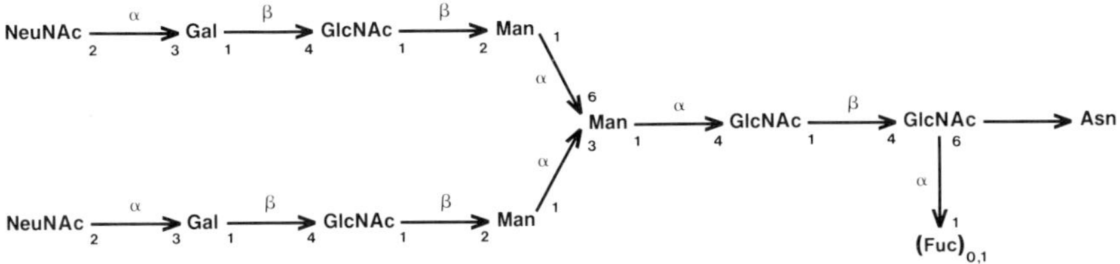

O — Glycosidically Linked Oligosaccharide Chains In β - Subunit of hCG

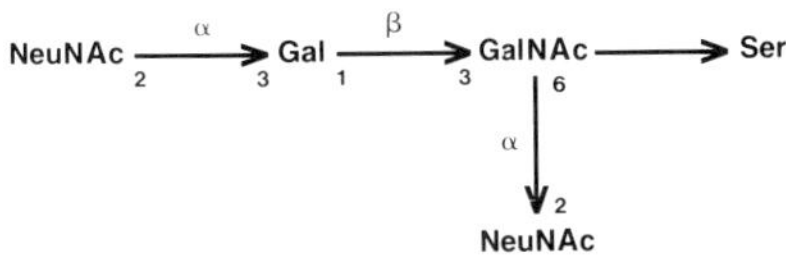

Fig. 4. The monosaccharide sequences of the carbohydrate moieties of hCG (Kessler *et al.*, 1979a,b).

B. Immunological Properties

hCG and both of its subunits are highly antigenic. The knowledge of the chemistry of hCG has opened new avenues of research in basic science and clinical application, for example, in the development of specific antisera for diagnostic and therapeutic use and in the effort to use hCG as an antifertility vaccine.

The identity of the α subunits among the glycoprotein hormones hFSH, hLH, hTSH, and hCG, the similarity of the β subunits of hLH and hCG, and the homology among the β subunits hFSH, hLH, hTSH, and hCG are of importance not only in the immunological measurement of hCG in the presence of hLH, hFSH, and hTSH, but also in the presence of biologically inactive but immunoreactive components circulating in the blood, such as the percursors and metabolites of hCG, which may bind to the heterogeneous population of antibodies in anti-hCG sera. The ubiquitous presence of immunoreactive hCG-like material, therefore, also needs stringent evaluation before a biologically valid basis for its existence is explained. The measurement of hCG by sensitive methods, at the limit of their sensitivity, is also likely to measure hCG components and metabolites even when present in small quantities, and thus amplify the nonspecificity in the measurement of biologically active intact hCG molecules. Swaminathan and Braunstein (1978) have determined that the major antigenic sites of hCG-β reside in the region of residues 21–23 with a disulfide bridge connecting cysteine-23 or cysteine-26 with a cysteine-72 or cysteine-110. Similarly, Birken and Canfield (1978) have shown that a thermolytic core portion of hCG-β, which contains the regions of peptide sequences identified by Swaminathan and Braunstein (1978), cross-reacts fully in the "conformation specific" Sb6–hCG antibody system. The main efforts toward the production of specific antisera have been possible by exploiting the structural differences between hCG and LH, although LH is immunologically identical to hCG. Antisera against purified hCG, for example, antisera H80 (Chen *et al.*, 1980), against hormone-specific hCG-β, for example, antisera Sb6 (Vaitukaitis *et al.*, 1972), against the unique chemically synthesized hCG-β COOH-terminal peptide, for example, antisera H93 (Chen *et al.*, 1980), and against the partially reduced and alkylated hCG-β (Pandian *et al.*, 1980) have been used to produce specific antisera. Such antisera are specific and yield hCG levels with a correlation coefficient close to the one with the radioreceptorassay. The immunization with hCG-β, therefore, generated antisera to conformational determinants, and, with the unique COOH-terminal peptide to sequential determinants, indicating two determinants, one specific to the intact biologically active molecule and the other limited to only the immunoreactive COOH-terminal amino acid sequence of hCG-β not present in hLH-β. Hence, the antisera are functionally more relevant to the first characteristic than to the second antigenic modality. The antisera raised to the reduced and alkylated hCG-β subunit did not cross-react with the native molecule, obviously due to the destruction of the conformational characteristics. However, these antisera cross-reacted with hCG precursors made by *in vitro* translation of mRNA in biosynthetic systems, indicating that native conformation of the hCG-β subunit is probably not achieved until the precursor piece is cleaved. H93 antiserum is produced against BSA conjugate of the carboxy-terminal tricosaglycopeptide (residues 123–145), isolated after digestion of an S-carboxymethylated, desialyated preparation of hCG-β, as well as against a chemically synthesized N^{α}-acetyl-tricontapeptide, analogous to residues 116–145, conjugated to bovine thyroglobulin. The H93 antiserum provides the highest immunological specificity; however, it has the following limitations: low titers, low K_d, low sensitivity, and interference from serum factors. Efforts have been made to extract the urine by the kaolin active procedure or the concanavalin A absorption method, to increase the sensitivity and specificity of the assay using the H93 antiserum.

Recently, the synthesis and secretion of hCG by a wide variety of neoplastic cells have been reported. These ectopic forms of hCG, unlike the placental hormones, may lack carbohydrate structures. Immunological recognition of these forms of hCG may require antisera which are sensitive to the presence or absence of terminal sialic acid residues of the carbohydrate moieties. Sialic acid containing β-COOH-terminal peptides perferred as immunogens to produce highly sensitive antisera that are also specific for hCG (Birken *et al.,* 1981).

III. Measurement of hCG

During the last century, four different techniques for the determination of hCG in blood and/or urine have been developed (Table I). These include (1) bioassays in intact laboratory animals and (2) immunological tube or slide methods with heme or latex agglutination inhibition, as well as the more recently developed competitive protein-binding method such as (3) radioimmunoassay (RIA) by the use of radioisotope-labeled hormones and specific antisera against hCG, and (4) radioreceptorassay (RRA) by the use of a radioisotope-labeled biologically active hormone and specific receptors as the binding proteins.

A. Biological Pregnancy Tests (Table I)

The bioassay of hCG as a pregnancy test was first described in 1927 by Aschheim and Zondek. The development of pregnancy tests in mice, rabbits, and rats, and their evaluation is described by Cabrera (1969), and by Hunt (1975). Urine or serum samples, when injected into the assay animals, resulting in ovarian hypertrophy, hyperemia (injected with blood), or hemorrhage, are used as a positive indication for the presence of hCG. The biological tests are accurate and qualitative, but are also time consuming, complicated, and expensive. They can detect 1 mIU of hCG/ml of urine and 0.4 IU hCG/ml blood (Delfs assay) and thus can detect pregnancy 14 days or earlier following a missed period. The bioassay may be used in the detection of a hydatidiform mole, chorioadenoma, and choriocarcinoma when levels of hCG are high, but fail to indicate ectopic pregnancies, threatened abortions, and other conditions associated with low production of hCG.

B. Hormonal Withdrawal Tests

This form of bioassay is based on the work of Zondek (1942) and uses the woman herself. The estrogen and progesterone are believed to simulate the normal hormonal increases that precede menstruation. Withdrawal of the hormones mimics the usual decrease in hormones typical of the normal menstrual cycle and results in menstrual bleeding in the nonpregnant woman. This diagnostic test takes at least 2 weeks for complete results and is occasionally used in women with amenorrhea with suspected pregnancy or positive hCG test without detectable clinical signs of pregnancy. The test in-

Table I

Techniques for the Determination of hCG in Blood and Urine

Type of test	Investigators	Endpoint	Time	Days of detection after ovulation	Specimen
Biologic	Aschheim and Zondek (1927)	Luteinization (mouse ovary)	5 days	25	Urine
	Friedman (1929)	Ovulation (rabbits)	48 hours	25	Urine
	Kupperman (1943)	Hyperemia (rat ovary)	2 hours	25	Urine
	Galli-Mainini (1947)	Ejection of sperm (frogs)	2 hours	25	Urine
Immunologic	Brody and Carlstrom (1960)	Latex particle slide test	2 minutes	25	Urine
	Wide and Gemzell (1960)	Hemagglutination inhibition	2 hours	25	Urine Serum
Radioimmunoassay	Wide (1969)	Competition with immunoreactive ^{125}I-labeled hCG for specific antibodies to hCG	24 hours	12	Serum
	Vaitukaitis (1972)	Competition with immunoreactive ^{125}I-labeled hCG for specific antibodies to the β unit of hCG	24 hours	8	Serum
Radioreceptorassay	Saxena (1974)	Competition with biologically active ^{125}I-labeled hCG for specific receptor sites	1 hour	8	Urine Serum

volves the administration of synthetic progestational and estrogenic compounds orally or by injection which is followed by observation for vaginal bleeding. In nonpregnant women, withdrawal bleeding occurs within 5 days. In pregnant women, the endometrium is already primed and maintained by elevated levels of both progesterone and estrogen produced endogenously by the corpus luteum and thus obviate bleeding despite withdrawal of steroids. The absence of bleeding within 10 days strongly suggests pregnancy. Recent findings implicate estrogen and progesterone as causes of adenocarcinoma of the endometrium, teratogenic effects, and multiple congenital malformation of the fetus. These anomalies are described by the acronym VACTEL (vertebral, anal, cardiac, tracheal, esophageal, and limb).

C. *Immunological Pregnancy Tests*

The second phase of the development of pregnancy tests in 1960 was possible due to further purification of hCG and the development of potent anti-hCG serum in rabbits, thus eliminating the need for maintaining an animal colony in each laboratory. The sensitivity of the agglutination inhibition tests did not improve over that of the bioassays, but the cost and time needed were considerably reduced. The biological and immunological tests provided a sensitivity of 500 to 1500 mIU/liter, which can detect pregnancy with 95% accuracy, 6 weeks after the last menstrual period (LMP). Long episodes of amenorrhea, delayed ovulation, and variability in urinary extraction of hCG may also complicate the detection of pregnancy by bioassays and by heme agglutination inhibition methods, and often result in false-negative results even 6 weeks after the LMP.

D. *Do-It-Yourself Pregnancy Tests*

Recent advances have made it possible for women to diagnose their pregnancy (or the lack of it) using a do-it-yourself test purchased at a pharmacy. Such tests are specially of interest to women with irregular periods, those whose periods have not returned after stopping oral contraceptives, those with infertility problems, those who do not wish to be pregnant, and adolescents who lose excessive weight and become amenorrheic. Obviously, a self-test detecting early pregnancy allows a woman simpler, quicker, and less traumatic means of termination such as menstrual extraction or mini-abortion if she decides not to remain pregnant. For women who desire pregnancy, a self-test can help protect the baby by prompting the mother to start proper prenatal care during the first month of pregnancy, when the risk of damage to the fetus is greatest. In spite of these advantages, the advisability, accuracy, and economy of self-tests for pregnancy have been debated; in many cases, the need to follow the result of a test with a visit to the physician has been deemed necessary.

Most of the do-it-yourself pregnancy tests are based on the modifications of the original heme agglutination inhibition principle, but claim different degrees of sensitivity and specificity. These can be used by women themselves, without the need for a doctor's prescription or access to a laboratory. These tests have some advantages, but need considerable care in performance and interpretation, and in dealing with the question of "what to do next?" If the laboratory tests, which use test tubes or slides, are performed about 2 weeks after a missed period, they can give, within a few hours, a highly accurate indication of the presence or absence of pregnancy. There are, of course, limitations to a woman doing her own pregnancy test. Pregnancy testing is a very emotional event, and there may be difficulty in following instructions and some impatience. One survey in Canada, where do-it-yourself pregnancy tests have been sold for years, shows that many women go back to the pharmacists to have the test repeated. Infrequently, a pregnancy test will give a positive result when in fact the woman is not pregnant. This could be due to contamination of urine, by, for example, detergent in the container, to blood or excessive protein in the urine, or more seriously, to the presence of a uterine growth, e.g., a hydatidiform mole or a chroiocarcinoma. Another cause for concern are women with ectopic pregnancies which occur in a fallopian tube instead of the uterus. If not removed surgically, ectopic pregnancies eventually rupture and could result in death. A self-test may give a negative result early in an ectopic pregnancy, giving the woman false assurance; or somewhat later, it could have a positive result, leading the woman to believe that she has a normal pregnancy or that she may need an abortion (which of course cannot remove an ectopic pregnancy). Any woman with a positive pregnancy test who has an intrauterine device (IUD) in place or who has had a sterilization operation should see a physician promptly to check for the possiblity of an ectopic pregnancy.

E. Radioimmunoassay

The standard hCG radioimmunoassay is nonspecific in that pituitary hormones, particularly LH, react with antiserum against hCG. The antisera raised against the β subunit of hCG or of chemically modified β subunit provide antigens with sites specific for each hormone and which produce hormone-specific antibodies. Such antibodies in the native state or after immunoaffinity purification can be used to measure hCG without cross-reaction with LH in the radioimmunoassay. These antisera are highly specific and provide a sensitivity as high as 6 mIU hCG/ml. Such radioimmunoassays are useful in the determination of lower levels of hCG and assist in the diagnosis of early pregnancy, ectopic pregnancy, management of all phases of trophoblastic disease including monitoring of therapy, and other ectopic (lung, pancreas, etc.) tumors which produce hCG in the form of prohormone, polymers, aggregates, and individual subunits in free states.

F. Radioreceptorassay

Circulating hCG is known to consist of several molecular species, some of which are low or negligible in *in vivo* biological activity (desialylated hCG, β subunit, α subunit, and hCG-like peptides), but still retain considerable immunological activity. For this reason, time consuming, expensive, and cumbersome bioassays are required if immunological tests are not compatible with the biological activity of the hCG. Radioreceptorassay provides a unique blending of the sensitivity of the radioimmunoassay and the specificity of the bioassay. This is a test that reliably detects pregnancy as early as 1 week after a normal contraception and is 98–100% accurate. In contrast to the antigen–antibody reaction which is immunological, the hormone–receptor interaction is biological; hence, the radioreceptorassay yields the estimates of the biological activity of the hormones. The radioreceptorassay is, therefore, a sensitive and specific test which detects hCG or luteinizing hormone (LH) due to the structural and biological similarity of the two hormones. However, two- to fivefold more LH than hCG would have to be present to match detection in the radioreceptorassay. The hCG-LH receptor does not detect follicle-stimulating hormone (FSH), prolactin (PRL), or human growth hormone (hGH). The quantitative receptorassay was first developed in our laboratory in 1974 (Saxena *et al.*, 1974). A sensitivity of 5 to 10 mIU hCG/ml allowed the diagnosis of pregnancy as early as 6 days after conception. The radioreceptorassay has also been useful in the diagnosis of ectopic pregnancy, spontaneous abortion, and in the follow-up of patients with trophoblastic disease and infertility problems (Saxena and Landesman, 1978). The radioreceptorassay is rapid enough for "stat" results in just 1 hour. Many medical and surgical procedures are contraindicated in pregnancy (extensive radiologic or diagnostic curettage). In trophoblastic disease, serial hCG assays are indicated for evaluation of therapeutic response. It should be emphasized that the radioreceptorassay has both the sensitivity of the radioimmunoassay and the specificity of the bioassay and, therefore, has greater sustained accuracy over the existing immunologic and biologic tests for pregnancy. A more accurate measurement of biologically active hCG and, hence, a significant contribution to improved patient care is offered by the radioreceptorassay.

The conventional pregnancy tests, immediately after the expected period, are so inaccurate that up to 30–50% of menstrual extractions are performed in women who are not pregnant. If a woman chooses to wait until conventional tests become reliable, i.e., 10–15 days after the missed period, more complicated procedures than the miniabortion are necessary which require hospitalization and increased costs. The early detection of pregnancy by the radioreceptorassay is beneficial in high risk pregnancy, in diabetes, or when a patient has been treated for infertility by ovulatory drugs and/or artificial insemination. The radioreceptorassay has been very useful in the differential diagnosis of ectopic pregnancy when only low levels of hCG are present in either the blood or urine. Radioreceptorassay can help diagnose 93–98% of ectopic pregnancies prior to rupture in all patients reporting to the physician soon after the first missed period or earlier. Other current uses of the radioreceptorassay are in the detection of multiple gestation, diagnosis and management of missed or threatened abortions, trophoblastic disease, and as a reliable screening test for all women of child-bearing age upon admission to the hospital. Such screening will protect the fetus from exposure to radiation and harmful drugs which may cause increased risk of congenital malformation, or surgical procedures which may be done in mothers who are either unaware of their pregnancy or fail to report it. The usefulness of pregnancy screening is obvious in adolescents prior to prescription of oral contraceptives, insertion of IUDs, administration of rubella vaccine, and use of drugs which may have deleterious side-effects in adolescent mothers.

IV. Secretory Patterns of hCG during the Reproductive Cycle

Maintenance of corpus luteum gestation is essential for the maintenance of pregnancy during periimplantation. The primary biological role of chorionic gonadotropin, thought to be secreted by the synctiotrophoblast at implantation (Wislocki and Streeter, 1938), is to extend the functional life span of the corpus luteum in the fertile menstrual cycle. There is increasing evidence to suggest the production of hCG by the blastocyst itself (Saxena, 1979). Since human trophoblast cells in tissue culture can produce ample amounts of hCG without involvement of any maternal factor, it would seem more likely that the 99 trophoblast cells present in the 107 cells of human blastocyst could already produce sufficient hCG to provide the necessary signal to the corpus luteum to persist (Hertz, 1979).

It seems clear that coincident with the initiation of implantation and detection of hCG in blood, the levels of progesterone are sustained at a time when the spontaneous demise of the corpus luteum has already begun. Evidence that progesterone is the essential hormone to secure implantation and avoid loss of the endometrium and the early conceptus is compelling (Goodman and Hodgen, 1979). Indeed, among women using a copper IUD, hCG-like activity has been detected transiently in the late luteal phase at a frequency indicative of normal conception rate (Landesman *et al.*, 1976). These observations, however, remain to be further confirmed. In the human, hCG rescues the corpus luteum from its declining phase and stimulates the luteinized cells to produce progestins that are necessary to support the endometrium (Goodman and Hodgen, 1979).

A. The Preimplantation Phase

1. Blastocyst

Indirect evidence for the presence of luteotrophic stimuli has existed and has been implicated in the rescue of the corpus luteum of pregnancy (Saxena, 1979). Recently, an hCG-like substance has been detected in the preimplanted blastocysts of mouse, rat, rabbit (Wiley, 1974; Chatterton and MacDonald, 1975; Varma *et al.*, 1979), and other species. The exact chemical nature, the time of appearance, and the role of the preimplanted gonadotropin, however, vary, and caution should be exercised in the interpretation of interspecies data. The absence of hCG-like material in unfertilized ova (Asch *et al.*, 1978) strongly suggests that the hCG-like substance is produced by the morulae themselves and is not a component of the uterine fluid that coats the early embryo. If an hCG-like substance is present in the blastocyst, its detection in blood suggests an active transport of material through the uterine wall before implantation and prior to the establishment of vascular connections. It is interesting that exogenous hCG introduced in the rabbit uteri and human reproductive tract appears in the peripheral circulation within 30 minutes (Saxen *et al.*, 1977). Recently hCG-like material was found in the serum and urine of 50–20% of the women using IUDs (Landesman *et al.*, 1976) suggesting the blastocyst as the source of the hormone. In a recent collaborative study (Beling *et al.*, 1976), however, a more specific radioimmunoassay of hCG and confirmatory bio- and radioreceptorassays detected transitory hCG-like activity in the urine of women with IUDs. The current disagreement about the presence of hCG in women with IUDs appears to be partly due to the use of nonspecific assays at the limit of their sensitivity.

2. Amniotic Fluid

The maximum levels of hCG are measurable in amniotic fluid prior to 12 weeks of gestation (Clements *et al.*, 1976). Recently, a determination of hCG was made following *in vitro* fertilization of human preovulatory oocytes from spontaneously ovulating women and did not detect hCG in the culture medium at any stage of embryo culture over the 3- to 4-day period (Shutt and Lopata, 1981). An hCG-like material has been detected in species including human (Asch *et al.*, 1979). The β subunit of chorionic gonadotropin was demonstrated by a fluorescent-labeled double-antibody technique in the spermatozoa of seven volunteers. The hCG-like substance is present in 5–7% of spermatozoa in all specimens analyzed. hCG-like material in the sperm (Acevedo *et al.*, 1977; Asch *et al.*, 1977) could provide the precursor for the production of a chorionic gonadotropin-like material by the conceptus prior to implantation. hCG has also been demonstrated in human testis and is present in carcinoma of the testes. The germ cells may be the source of hCG in the testis.

3. Regulation of Corpus Luteum Function and Luteoplacental Shift

On the basis of the current information, the regulation of the luteal function may be visualized in Diagram 1. Following the fertilization of the ovum, hCG acts as a stimulus to sustain the secretion of progesterone by the corpus luteum of gestation which is necessary for the growth and maintenance of the endometrium for implantation. In humans, the removal of the corpus luteum prior to 6 weeks resulted in abortion, suggesting a role of hCG in the maintenance of the progesterone secretion by the corpus luteum of pregnancy (Tulsky and Koft, 1957). Following 6 weeks of pregnancy, the placenta becomes the main site of progesterone production. Since, in contrast to the corpus luteum, the placenta contains little 17-hydroxlyase activity, the declining plasma levels of 17-hydroxy progesterone 4 weeks following ovulation reflects the transition of progesterone synthesis from the corpus luteum to the placenta. It has been proposed by Lauritzen and Lehman (1965) that hCG may control the synthesis of dehydroepiandrosterone (DHEA) as a precursor for the placental conversion to estrogen.

The issue of the time of the luteoplacental shift in women is of vital importance. However, prior to or coincident with the placental shift, a negative feedback mechanism between hCG production and progesterone synthesis has been observed to ensure the viability of the pregnancy; however, further study of the time of the luteoplacental shift in human pregnancy is necessary. With regard to application of "menstrual inducers" versus "abortifacients" for contraception, this time of luteoplacental shift is of paramount importance because in women, secretion of steroids by the corpus luteum declines rapidly about the fourth week after fertilization (Strott *et al.*, 1969), thus establishing the autonomy of the conceptus (Goodman and Hodgen, 1979). Further suppression of luteal progesterone during and after the luteoplacental shift may not lead to early abortion. The evaluation of antiluteal agents, for example, anti-hCG-sera, prostaglandins, and estrogens, should take into account the timing of the luteoplacental shift and the possible direct effects on the conceptus. In case of anti-hCG-sera, the pregnancy is intercepted only at high titers; hence, the mechanism of action of such antisera appears to be more like an abortifacient rather than a luteolytic contraceptive. If the hCG is produced as early as at the initiation of implantation or prior to implantation, low titers of antibodies should theoretically neutralize the luteotropic stimulus of hCG and cause inhibition of implantation and thus act as a menstrual inducer of contraception. However, this does not happen; and one possible explanation is the weak binding of the hormone to low titer and affinity antibody, which may protect the hormone from degradation and increase the metabolic half-life, thus making hCG available to high affinity receptors in the luteal cells for extended periods. This is a situation which may produce fertility rather than an antifertility effect. Further research should be directed to the above areas which will provide maximal value for the enhancement or suppression in humans.

B. The Postimplantation Phase

Normally, hCG is produced by the syncytiotrophoblast of the placenta and secreted in the blood of both mother and the fetus. Fetal serum contains maximum hCG levels from 60 to 5500 mIU/ml at 11–14 weeks and these are not influenced by the sex of the fetus (Clements *et al.,* 1976; Bruner, 1951). In fetuses of 12–29 weeks, the meconium contains the largest concentration of HCG (Clements *et al.,* 1976). However, immunoreactive α subunit is first identifiable in the fetal pituitary tissue during the eighth week of gestation (Dubois and Dubois, 1974) and is present throughout gestation (Kaplan *et al.,* 1976).

Pregnancy

The sensitivity and specificity of the radioimmuno- and radioreceptorassays have influenced our perception of secretory patterns of hCG during pregnancy. Generalizing, these observations suggest three patterns of hCG secretion. In humans, hCG is detectable in blood or urine virtually coincident with implantation, is maximum during the first trimester, and remains elevated continuously throughout gestation including a few weeks after delivery.

As shown in Fig. 5, during normal pregnancy, the primitive trophoblast produces hCG early. Serum concentrations of hCG rise to peak values by 8 to 12 weeks of gestation. Thereafter, there is a decrement in hCG levels to a plateau that is maintained throughout the remainder of the pregnancy (Ross, 1973). The blood and urine levels of hCG during a normal pregnancy are

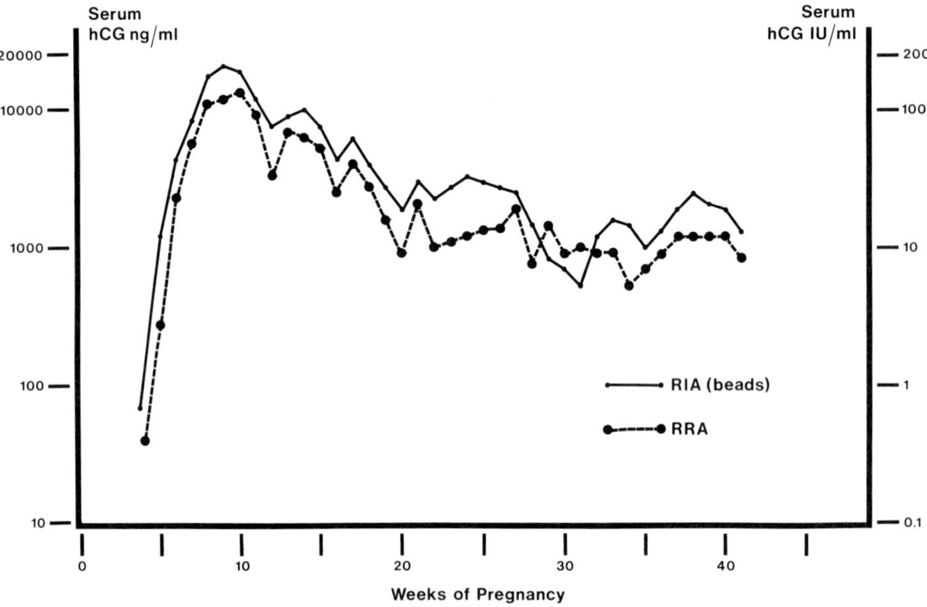

Fig. 5. hCG levels during normal pregnancy.

shown in Figs. 6 and 7 (Saxena and Rathnam, 1981; Post *et al.,* 1980). Plasma levels of hCG rise rapidly and double in concentration every 2 days. Between 40 and 90 days of pregnancy, the plasma hCG levels range from 160 to 200 IU hCG/ml. During the second trimester of the pregnancy, the hCG levels drop to approximately 10 IU/ml and remain constant until the occurrence of a slight rise during the third trimester. The peak immunologic activity of hCG usually plateaus at approximately 5 IU/ml, whereas its biological activity is two- to threefold higher. Normal placenta also produces free hCG-α. With the advancement of the pregnancy, the levels of hCG-α exceed that of hCG and after the eighth to tenth week of pregnancy, the hCG-α subunit is detected in the peripheral blood and urine, reaching blood levels of several hundred nanograms/milliliter in the thirty-sixth week of gestation and declines toward parturition. Large amounts of hCG and hCG-α and small amounts of hCG-β in serum indicate that circulating free hCG-α is not derived from spontaneous dissociation of hCG, but is directly secreted from the chorionic tissue (Vaitukaitis, 1978; Ashitaka *et al.,* 1974). The cytotrophoblast showed the presence of only hCG-α and not of hCg or hCG-β by immunofluorescence. In contrast, very low levels of hCG-β were found throughout the pregnancy (Fig. 8) (Ashitaka *et al.,* 1980). The trends of

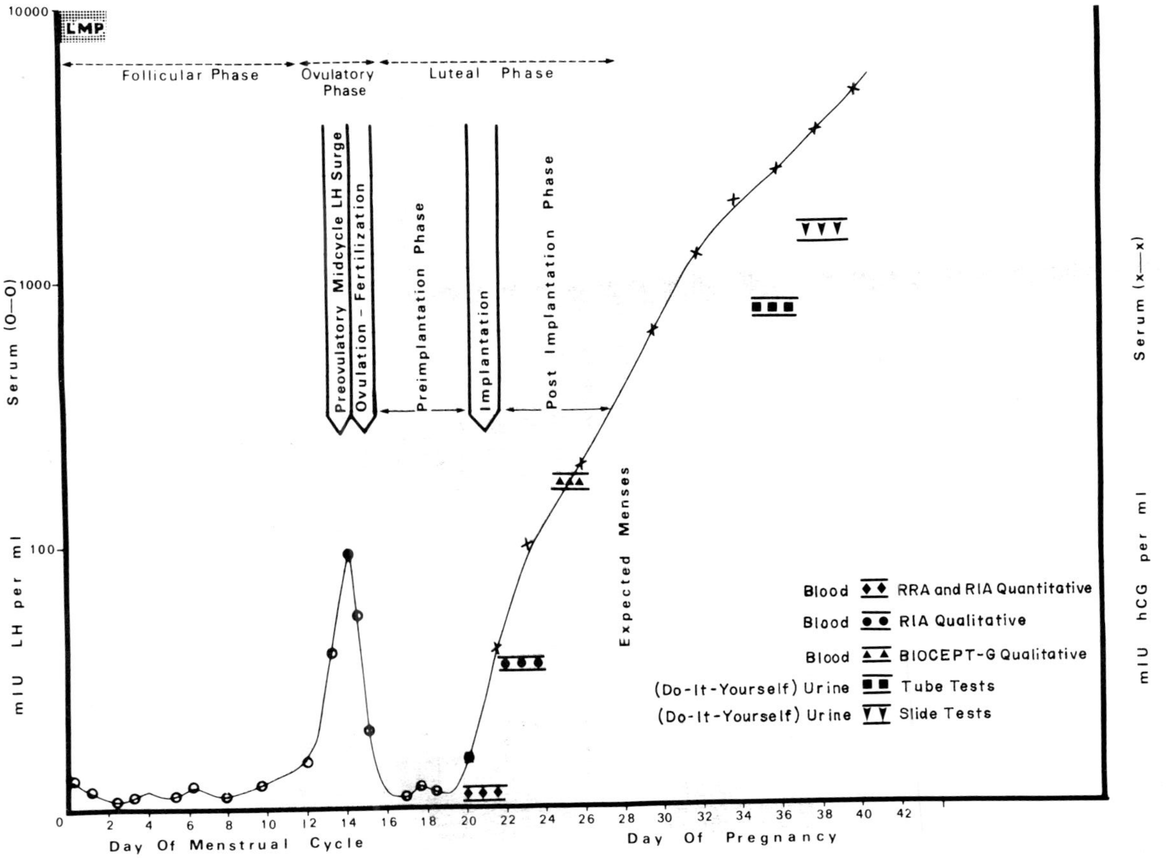

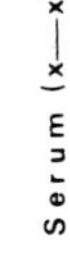

Fig. 6. Serum levels of hCG in early pregnancy, as measured by radioreceptorassay.

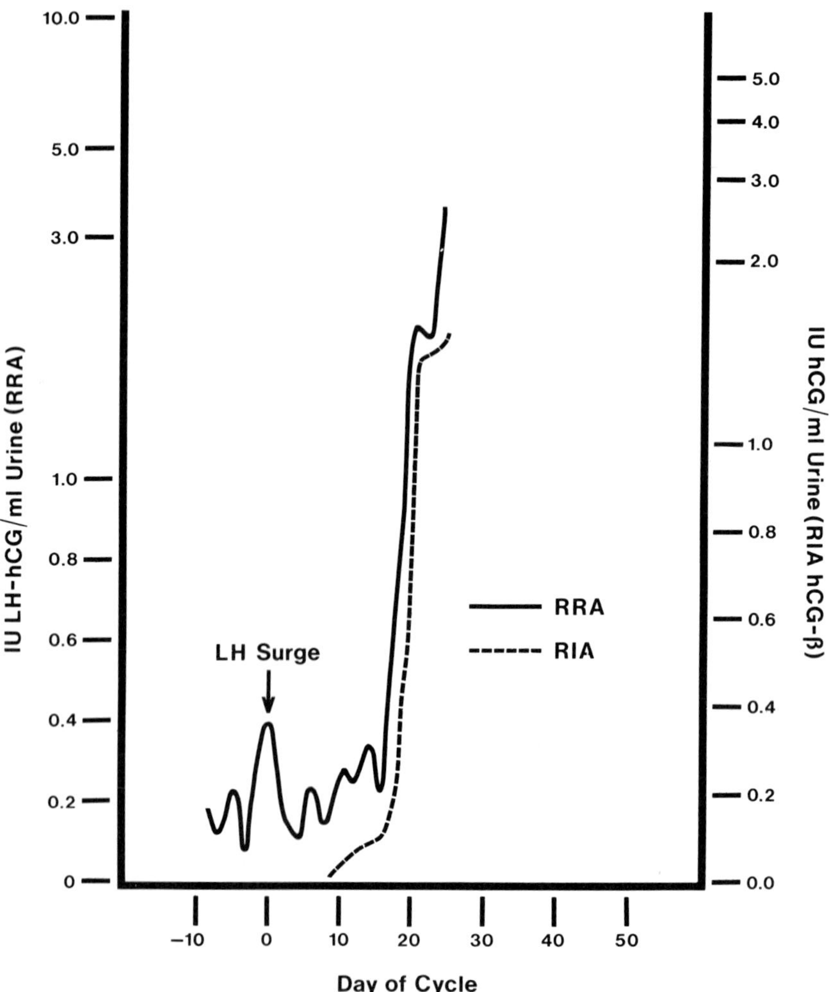

Fig. 7. Urine levels of hCG in early pregnancy (Post *et al.*, 1980).

hCG-β levels are similar to those of plasma hCG levels, although considerable within patient and patient-to-patient variation is found.

The levels of hCG-β at 4 to 16 weeks of gestation show an initial rise, a plateau at 7 to 9 weeks, and a further rise to a maximum at the eleventh week. The levels then dropped steadily to week 16 (Harrison *et al.*, 1980). The radioimmunoassays measure subunits of hCG as well as fragments of hCG which are not detected by bio- or receptorassay. This is reflected in the varying ratio of biological to immunological activities of hCG throughout gestation (Vaitukaitis, 1978) and by the levels of hCG-β during pregnancy.

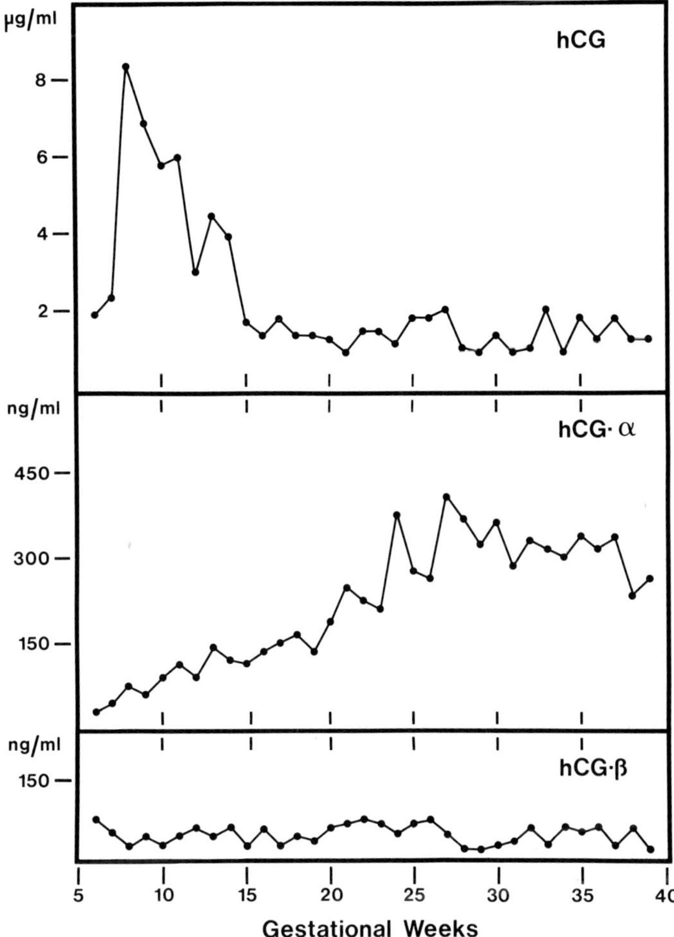

Fig. 8. Levels of hCG and its subunits during pregnancy (Ashitaka *et al.,* 1980).

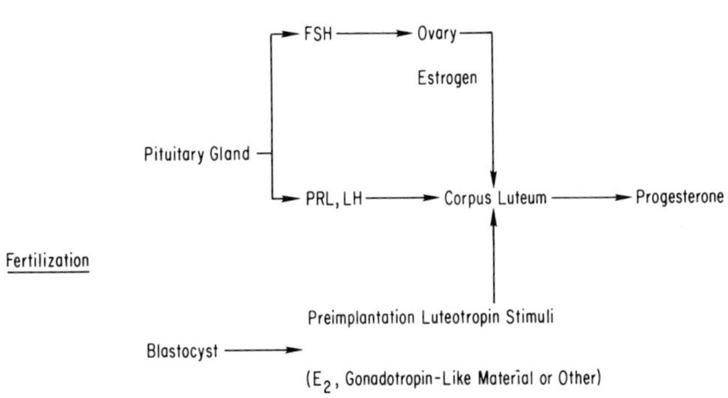

Diagram 1. Regulation of luteal function during preimplantation.

V. Role of hCG in Early Pregnancy

Hirono *et al.* (1972) showed that hCG has a direct effect on the median eminence in inhibiting the synthesis and release of FSH and LH, and thus hCG may play a role in the inhibition of ovulation during pregnancy. The evidence suggests that hCG may influence intrauterine immune privilege, fetal gonadal development, or placental metabolism. These additional effects of hCG remain tentative. The biological actions of chorionic gonadotropin upon the corpus luteum are imperative for early maternal recognition of pregnancy. The "rescue" of the corpus luteum (Neill *et al.*, 1969) is the subject of extensive study in relation to fertility regulation. hCG, similar to hLH, stimulates the interstitial cells of the preformed follicles converting them into a corpus luteum in the female and into the interstitial cells of the testes to secrete androgens in the male (Jutisz and Tetrin-Clary, 1974). hCG appears to be the primary stimulus to the fetal Leydig cell which results in testosterone synthesis and secretion with a maximum during 11 to 17 weeks and in the differentiation of the male genital tract (Clements *et al.*, 1976). The human fetal testis of 16 to 20 weeks can bind hCG and respond with maximal testosterone production to physiologic levels of hCG *in vitro* (Huhtaniemi *et al.*, 1977). hCG rescues the corpus luteum from its declining phase and stimulates the luteinized cells to produce progestins that are necessary to support the enodmetrium (Jutisz and Tetrin-Clary, 1974).

Braunstein *et al.*(1980) found a significant correlation between the concentrations of hCG, hPL, and PSBG during the first trimester of pregnancy indicating that the synthesis and secretion of these proteins are closely regulated and may be regulated by a common mechanism. The qualitative patterns of the concentrations of each of these proteins in serum during this period closely resemble the logarithmic increase of the estimated trophoblastic mass, suggesting that the secretary role of each of these processes is relatively constant per cell during early pregnancy. However, after the first trimester, the mechanisms which control the secretion of hCG by the syncytiotrophoblast are different from those which control the secretion of hPL and PSBG.

VI. Role of hCG in Abnormal Conditions

The quantitative determination of hCG has served as a marker for an early detection of pregnancy. The serial measurement of hCG permits an early diagnosis and significantly improved management of abnormal pregnancy is apparently not a metabolic waste since a decreased production of hCG results in a spontaneous abortion. Our studies, however, indicate that besides hCG, optimum concentrations of prolactin, estradiol, and progesterone are also vital to sustain a normal pregnancy (Jovanovic *et al.*, 1978). It has been shown that lower production of hCG can be compensated by enhanced corpus luteum and placental response.

A. *Abnormal Pregnancies*

Serum hCG levels that are twofold greater than those encountered in normal pregnancy at 4 to 8 weeks gestation indicate a twin pregnancy, which has been confirmed at 8 to 10 weeks by sonography (Jovanovic *et al.*, 1977; Harrison *et al.*, 1980). The hCG levels are lower in ectopic pregnancy and in spontaneous abortion (Saxena and Landesman, 1978).

Hydatidiform mole, a disorder of the human placenta, is characterized by hyperplasia of the trophoblast. Hydatidiform mole and choriocarcinoma can be distinguished from multiple pregnancy by sonography, and relevant symptoms. Most common symptoms of the molar pregnancy are uterine bleeding and enlarged uterus accompained with an excessive production of hCG by the syncytiotrophoblast (Choy *et al.*, 1979; Szulman and Surto, 1978). The levels of hCG-β are also considerably increased in hydatidiform mole and is proportionally greater than that of native hCG. At 10 to 18 weeks of gestation, the ratio of hCG-β to hCG is 3.68 in a patient with hydatidiform mole as compared to 1.79 in a normal patient; however, the increase in hCG-α is of lower magnitude (Franchimont *et al.*, 1978). In patients with choriocarcinoma, there is also an elevated production of hCG. These patients eventually develop widespread metastases and have increased production of hCG-α during periods when the concentration of hCG and hCG-β are low or undetectable (Rochman, 1978). Rutanen (1978) found free α subunits in three out of six patients with choriocarcinoma. These observations suggest that the monitoring of trophoblastic tumors can be considerably improved by assaying hCG as well as free α and β subunits.

B. *hCG in Cancer*

In general, excluding pregnancy, serum hCG levels over 1 ng/ml, serum hCG-β levels over 1.5 ng/ml, and serum hCG-α levels over 3.5 ng/ml are considered pathological (Franchimont *et al.*, 1978), in patients with adenocarcinoma of the ovary and in 51% of patients with testicular tumors (Rochman, 1978). In patients with nongonadal tumors, hCG is found in association with pancreatic carcinoma (33%), in gastric adenocarcinoma (22%), in hepatoblastoma (17%), in bowel tumors (13%), and in lung cancer (9%) (Hattori *et al.*, 1978; Javadpour, 1978b). The presence of hCG together with α-fetoprotein has been detected in testicular, ovarian, and extragonadal malignant germ cell tumors (Pederson, 1978).

1. Trophoblastic Tumors

There is evidence for the secretion of hCG and of either one or both subunits of hCG by a variety of ectopic tumors. Patients with gestational trophoblastic tumors have widely different ratios of hCG and its subunits in serum and tumor extracts (Vaitukaitis and Ebersole, 1976). In one study of trophoblastic disease, all hCG-positive serum samples also show α-subunit by RIA, without an exclusive α subunit elevation (Rutanen, 1978); but in another study, a tumor secreting exclusively hCG-α has also been reported (Birken and Canfield, 1978). No α or β subunits were detected in one study of patients responding to chemotherapy. The profile of hCG and its subunits found in patients who failed to respond to chemotherapy is indistinguishable from that found in patients with nongestational trophoblastic tumors as well as in patients with tumors ectopically secreting hCG and its subunits (Vaitukaitis, 1978).

2. Ectopic Endocrine Tumors

The hCG molecules are localized in the syncytiotrophoblastic component of the testicular choriocarcinoma and in the syncytiotrophoblastic giant cells which are occasionally found in association with embryonal carcinoma, teratoma, and seminoma (Javadpour, 1978a). In one study, 11 out of 130 patients with testicular seminoma show increased serum hCG levels (Javadpour *et al.*, 1978b), Schultz *et al.* (1978) have studied 67 patients with malignant germ cell neoplasia of the testis and found hCG elevation in 38% of 34 patients with nonseminoma. In 60 patients with seminoma, 4 had elevated serum hCG levels (Javadpour *et al.*, 1978a). After retroperitoneal lymph node dissection and chemotherapy, the hCG levels returned to normal.

3. Ectopic Nonendocrine Tumors

Gynecomastia has been associated with ectopic gonadotropin secretion in patients with carcinoma of the lung (Fusco and Rosen, 1966), adrenal gland (Rose *et al.*, 1968), and liver (Hung *et al.*, 1963). hCG, hCG-α, and hCG-β were detected in the blood, urine, and tissue from the malignant neoplasm of a patient with terminal bladder carcinoma and gynecomastia (Kawamura *et al.*, 1978). Tumors of the gastrointestinal tract have been among those associated with the highest circulating levels of ectopically secreted hCG. Vaitukaitis (1978) reported adenocarcinoma of the stomach in a postmenopausal woman producing quantities of hCG comparable to those observed in the first trimester of pregnancy. In studies of pineal tumors, the concentration of the subunits of hCG was increased, but was not sufficiently abnormal to provide a useful index of tumor activity (Barber *et al.,* 1978).

VII. Interaction of hCG with "Receptor" Site

The term target organ response has always implied the concept of the interaction of the hormone with the receptor site. Human chorionic gonadotropin (hCG) and luteinizing (hLH) hormone receptors are asymmetrical molecules of a hydrophobic nature which are located as partly exposed and mobile proteins in the basal region of the lipid bilayer of the intact cell membrane and plasma membranes of the endocrine responsive gonadal cells (Bretscher, 1975). The majority of hCG–LH receptors are present in the ovarian luteal and testicular Leydig cells (Catt *et al.,* 1976; Saxena, 1976). Human chorionic gonadotropin and hLH bind to the same receptor due to the similarity in their structure.

A. Purification and Properties of the hCG–LH Receptor

The LH–hCG receptor has been purified from rat testes (Catt and Dufau, 1978), rat ovaries (Ryan *et al.,* 1977), and bovine copora lutea (Dattatreyamurty *et al.,* 1981).

Characterization of gonadotropin receptor–hormonal receptor interactions has been performed in rats (Catt and Dufau, 1978; Means *et al.,* 1978), bovine corpora lutea (Haour and Saxena, 1974b; Dattatreyamurty *et al.,* 1981), porcine testes, and human ovaries (Wardlaw *et al.,* 1975; Rajaniemi *et al.,* 1981). The binding of the hormone to the receptor is of high specificity and affinity (K_a 10^9 to K_a 10^{10} moles/liter), saturable, reversible, and dependent upon time, temperature (rapid at 37°C and slower at 4°C), and ph (optimum at neutral pH) to reach equilibrium. There are two types of receptors, namely, high affinity, low capacity and low affinity, high capacity binding sites. There is a direct functional relationship between receptor occupancy and a characteristic biological response such as steroid secretion by gonadal cells. The hCG–LH receptors are macromolecules which consist of a major protein moiety and minor but essential lipid and carbohydrate components. The molecular weight of the hCG–LH receptor has been estimated to be 70,000 to 200,000 indicating a subunit nature and heterogeneity of the receptor.

B. Mechanism of Hormone–Receptor Interaction

The hCG–LH receptor consists of a regulatory subunit containing hormone binding sites and a catalytic subunit associated with adenylate cyclase activity which converts MgATP to cAMP. The two subunits are structurally independent (Dattatreyamurty *et al.,* 1981). Guanylyl nucleotide binding unit (G-protein), which activates the catalytic subunit, acts as an intermediate coupler for the two subunits and provides the functional entity of the receptor. The binding sites and adenylate cyclase interact only when hormone, the first messenger, binds to the receptor. Hence, the mere presence of hormone binding does not imply the presence of a functional receptor. The steroidogenic response to hCG–LH is mediated by the adenylate cyclase-stimulated cAMP, the second messenger. The cAMP binds to the regulatory subunit of the protein kinase and leads to the dissociation and activation of the catlytic subunit which then transfers a phosphate ion from ATP to yet unknown mitochondrial or nuclear proteins. The phosphorylated proteins function as metabolic regulators in the target cell to produce a specific steroid.

Recent studies (Wardlaw *et al.,* 1975; Rajaniemi *et al.,* 1981) in human ovarian homogenates during the menstrual cycle have shown that on days 5 and 6 of the cycle, the mean number of hCG binding sites is low, i.e., 0.32 ± 0.25 fmoles/mg protein. Following the postovulatory fall on days 14 to 16, the receptor concentration increases to a maximum of 4.23 ± 1 fmole/mg protein on day 17 and remains unchanged for the rest of the cycle. The affinity of the hormone–receptor binding does not change in granulosa cell and corpora lutea. In general, corpora lutea obtained during the follicular phase contain a significant number of receptor sites for hCG which tend to decrease with the approach of the ovulatory phase. Follicles during the luteal phase display low LH–hCG binding. The observation that the corpora lutea of the previous cycle display distinct binding may indicate that the disapperance of hCG–LH receptors is not the primary factor in luteolysis (Rajaniemi *et al.,* 1981). However, it is possible that the hormone binding subunit may be dissociated from the adenylate cyclase subunit, and the receptor is thus nonfunctional. This is consistent with the suggestion of Thomas *et al.* (1978) that luteolysis is related to the functional decoupling of the hormone binding and adenylate cyclase subunits of the functional receptor. The receptor concentration in corpora lutea is clearly lower during pregnancy than during the menstrual cycle and tends to increase toward the term.

References

Acevedo, H. F., Slifkin, M., Pouchet, G. R., and Rakhshan, M. (1977). *In* "The Testis in Normal and Infertile Men" (P. Troen and H. R. Nankin, eds.), pp. 185–192. Raven, New York.

Adcock, E. W., III, Teasdale, F., August, C. S., Cox, S., Meschia, G., Battaglia, F. C., and Naughton, M. A. (1973). *Science* **181,** 845.

Allen, W. R. (1969). *J. Endocrinol.* **43,** 593.

Asch, R. H., Fernandez, E. O., and Pauerstein, C. J. (1977). *Fertil. Steril.* **28,** 1258–1262.

Asch, R. H., Fernandez, E. O., Magnasco, L. A., and Pauerstein, C. J. (1978). *Fertil. Steril.* **29,** 444–446.

Asch, R. H., Fernandez, E. O., Siler-Khodr, T. M., and Pauerstein, C. J. (1979). *Am. J. Obstet. Gynecol.,* in press.

Aschheim, S., and Zondek, B. (1927). *Klin. Wochenschr.* **6,** 1322.

Ashitaka, Y., Nishimura, R., Ohashi, M., Futamuri, K., and Tojo, S. (1974). *Endocrinology (Jn.)* **21,** 429.

Ashitaka, Y., Nishimura, R., Takemore, M., and Tojo, S. (1980). *In* "Chorionic Gonadotropin" (S. Segal, ed.), pp. 147–175. Plenum, New York.

Bahl, O. P. (1972). *In* "Gonadotropins" (B. B. Saxena, C. G. Beling, and H. M. Gandy, eds.), p. 200. Wiley (Interscience), New York.

Barber, S. G., Smith, J. A., Cove, D. H., Smith, S. C. H., and London, D. R. (1978). *Lancet* **2,** 372–373.

Beling, C. G., Cederqvist, L. L., and Fuchs, F. (1976). *Am. J. Obstet. Gynecol.* **125,** 855–858.

Birken, S., and Canfield, R. E. (1978). *In* "Structure and Function of Gonadotropins" (K. W. McKerns, ed.), p. 47. Plenum, New York.

Birken, S., and Canfield, R. E. (1980). *In* "Chorionic Gonadotropin" (S. Segal, ed.), pp. 65–83. Plenum, New York.

Birken, S., Fetherstone, J., Desmond, J., Canfield, R. E., and Boime, I. (1978). *Biochem. Biophys. Res. Commun.* **85,** 1247.

Birken, S., Agosto, G., Canfield, R. E., Amr, S., and Nisula, B. (1981). *Annu. Endocrine Soc. Meet., 63rd, Cincinnati,* Abstr. No. 212.

Braunstein, G. D., and Hershman, J. M. (1976). *J. Clin. Endocrinol. Metab.* **42,** 1123.

Braunstein, G. D., Rasor, J. L., Engvall, E., and Wade, M. E. (1980). *Am. J. Obstet. Gynecol.* **138,** 1205.

Bretscher, M. S. (1975). *Nature (London)* **258,**43.

Bruner, J. A. (1951). *J. Clin. Endocrinol., Metab.* **11,** 360–374.

Cabrera, H. A. (1969). *Am. J. Obstet. Gynecol.* **103,** 32–38.

Catt, K. J., and Dufau, M. L. (1978). *In* "Receptor and Hormone Action" (L. Birnbaumer and B. W. O'Malley, eds.), Vol. 2, pp. 291–339. Academic Press, New York.

Catt, K. J., Detelslegers, J. M., and Dufau, M. L. (1976). *In* "Methods in Receptor Research" (M. Blecher, ed.), Part I, pp. 175–250. Dekker, New York.

Chatterton, R. T., and MacDonald, G. T. (1975). *Biol. Reprod.* **13,** 77.

Chen, H., Matsuura, S., and Ohashi, M. (1980). *In* "Chorionic Gonadotropin" (S. Segal, ed.), pp. 231–252. Plenum, New York.

Choy, Y. M., Lau, K. M., and Lee, C. Y. (1979). *J. Biol. Chem.* **254,** 1159–1163.

Clements, J. A., Reyes, F. I., Winter, J. S. D., and Faiman, C. (1976). *J. Clin. Endocrinol. Metab.* **42,** 9–19.

Daniels-McQueen, S., McWilliams, D., Birken, S., Canfield, R. E., Landefeld, T., and Boime, I. (1978). *J. Biol. Chem.* **253,** 7109.

Dattatreyamurty, B., Rathnam, P., and Saxena, B. B. (1981). *In* "Functional Correlates of Hormone Receptors in Reproduction" (V. Mahesh, T. J. Muldoon, B. B. Saxena, and W. A. Sadler, eds.). Elsevier, Amsterdam.

Dubois, P. M., and Dubois, M. P. (1974). *In* "Endocrinologe Sexuelle de la Période Périnatale," pp. 37–61. Editions Paris.

Finn, R. , St., Hill C. A., Govan, A. J., Ralfs, I. G., Gurney, F. J., and Denye, V. (1972). *Clin. Endocrinol.* **1,** 315.

Franchimont, P., Reuter, A., and Gaspard, U. (1978). *In* "Experimental Endocrinology" (L. Martini and V. H. T. James, eds.), Vol. 3, pp. 202–216. Academic Press, New York.

Fusco, F. D., and Rosen, S. W. (1966). *N. Engl. J. Med.* **275,** 507–515.

Goodman, A. L., and Hodgen, G. D. (1979). *J. Clin. Endocrinol. Metab.* **49**, 469.
Haour, F., and Saxena, B. B. (1974a). *J. Biol. Chem.* **249**, 2195.
Haour, F., and Saxena, B. B. (1974b). Science **185**, 444.
Haour, F.,Tell, G., and Sanchez, P. (1976). *C.R. Acad. Sci. Paris Ser. D* **282**, 1183.
Harrison, R. F., O'Moore, R. R., and McSweeney, J. (1980). *Br. J. Obstet. Gynecol.* **87**, 705–711.
Hattori, M., Fukase, M., Yoshimi, H., Matsukura, S., and Imura, H. (1978). *Cancer* **42**, 2328–2333.
Hertz, R. (1980). *In* "Chorionic Gonadotropins" (S. Segal, ed.), pp. 1–16. Plenum, New York.
Hirono, M., Igarashi, M., and Matsumoto, S. (1972). *Endocrinology* **90**, 1214–1219.
Hobson, B. M., and Wide, L. (1972). *J. Endocrinol.* **55**, 363.
Huhtaniemi, I. T., Korenbrot, C. C., and Jaffe, R. B. (1977). *J. Clin. Endocrinol. Metab.* **44**, 963–967.
Hung, W., Blizzard, R. M., Migeon, C. J., Camacho, A. M., and Nyhan, W. L. (1963). *J. Pediatr.* **63**, 895–903.
Hunt, W. R. (1975). *Popul. Rep. Ser. J.* pp. J109–J124.
Javadpour, N. (1978a). *Urol. Survey* **28**, 89–94.
Javadpour, N. (1978b). *Urology* **12**, 177–183.
Javadpour, N., McIntire, K. R., Waldman, T. A., and Bergman, S. M. (1978a). *J. Urol.* **120**, 687–690.
Javadpour, N., McIntire, K. R., and Waldman, T. A. (1978b). *Cancer* **42**, 2768–2772.
Jovanovic, L., Landesman, R., and Saxena, B. B. (1977). *Science* **198**, 738.
Jovanovic, L., Dawood, M. Y., Landesman, R., and Saxena, B. B. (1978). *Am. J. Obstet. Gynecol.* **130**, 274.
Jutisz, M., and Tetrin-Clary, C. (1974). *Curr. Top. Exp. Endocrinol.* **2**, 195–246.
Kaplan, S. L., Grumbach, M. M., and Aubert, M. L. (1976). *J. Clin. Endocrinol. Metab.* **42**, 1339–1343.
Kawamura, J., Machida, S., Yoshida, O., Oseko, F., Imura, H., and Hattori, M. (1978). *Cancer* **42**, 2773–2780.
Kessler, M. J., Mise, T., Ghai, R. D., and Bahl, O. P. (1979a). *J. Biol. Chem.* **254**, 7909.
Kessler, M. J., Reddy, M. S., Shah, R. H., and Bahl, O. P. (1979b). *J. Biol. Chem.* **254**, 7901.
Lacroix, M. C., and Martal, J. (1979). *C.R. Acad. Sci. Paris Ser. D* **288**, 771.
Landesman, R., Coutinho, E. M., and Saxena, B. B. (1976). *Fertil. Steril.* **27**, 1062.
Lauritzen, C., and Lehman, W. D. (1965). *Acta Endocrinol.* **100**, 112.
Louvet, J. P., Ross, G. T., Birken, S., and Canfield, R. E. (1974). *J. Clin. Endocrinol. Metab.* **39**, 1155.
Means, A. R., Dedman, J. R., Fakunding, J. L., and Tindal, D. J. (1978). *In* "Receptor and Hormone Action" (L. Birnbaumer and B. W. O'Malley, eds.), Vol. 3, pp. 363–392. Academic Press, New York.
Mise, T., and Bahl, O. P. (1980). *J. Biol. Chem.* **255**, 8516.
Moss, J., Ross, P. S., Agosto, G., Birken, S., Canfield, R. E., and Vaughan, M. (1978). *Endocrinology* **102**, 415.
Neill, J. D., Johansson, E. D. B., and Knobil, E. (1969). *Endocrinology* **84**, 45.
Nisula, B. C., Morgan, F. J., and Canfield, R. E. (1974). *Biochem. Biophys. Res. Commun.* **59**, 86.
Pandian, M. R., Mitra, R., and Bahl, O. P. (1980). *Endocrinology* **107**, 1564–1571.
Pederson, B. N. (1978). *Lancet* **2**, 8098–8042.
Post, K. G., Roy, A. K., Cederqvist, L. L., and Saxena, B. B. (1980). *J. Clin. Endocrinol. Metab.* **50**, 169–175.
Rajaniemi, H. J., Ronnberg, L., Kauppila, A., Ylostalo, P., Jalkanen, M., Saastamoinen, J., Selander, K., Pystynen, P., and Vihko, R. (1981). *J. Clin. Encodrinol. Metab.* **52**, 307.

Rifkind, A. B., Canfield, R. E., and Kappas, A. (1976). *Biochem. Biophys. Res. Commun.* **68,** 503.

Rochman, H. (1978). *Ann. Clin. Lab. Sci.* **8,** 167–175.

Rose, L. I., Williams, G. H., Jagger, P. I., and Lauler, D. P. (1968). *J. Clin. Endocrinol. Metab.* **28,** 903–908.

Ross, G. T. (1973). *In* "Methods in Investigative and Diagnostic Endocrinology" (S. A. Berson and R. S. Yalow, eds.), Part 2B, pp. 743–748. Amer. Elsevier, New York.

Rutanen, E. M. (1978). *Int. J. Cancer* **22,** 413.

Ryan, R. J., Birnbaumer, L., Lee, C. Y., and Hunzicker-Dunn, M. (1977). *Int. Rev. Physiol.* pp. 85–151.

Saito, T., and Saxena, B. B. (1976). *J. Clin. Endocrinol. Metab.* **43,** 1186–1189.

Saxena, B. B. (1976). *In* "Methods in Receptor Research" (M. Blecher, ed.), Part I, pp. 251–300. Decker, New York.

Saxena, B. B. (1979). *In* "Recent Advances in Reproduction and Regulation of Fertility" (G. P. Talwar, ed.), pp. 319–332. Elsevier, Amsterdam.

Saxena, B. B. (1981a). *In* "Endocrinology of Pregnancy" (F. Fuchs and A. Klopper, eds.). Harper, New York. In press.

Saxena, B. B. (1981b). *In* "Pediatric Clinics of North America" (L. C. Belfus, ed.), pp. 437–453. Saunders, Philadelphia, Pennsylvania.

Saxena, B. B., and Landesman, R (1978). *Am. J. Obstet. Gynecol.* **131,** 97.

Saxena, B. B., and Rathnam, P. (1978). *In* "Structure and Function of the Gonadotropins" (K. W. McKerns, ed.), pp. 183–212. Plenum, New York.

Saxena, B. B., and Rathnam, P. (1981). *In* "Hormones in Normal and Abnormal Human Tissues" (K. Fotherby and S. B. Pal, eds.), Vol. 1, pp. 167–206. De Gruyter, Berlin.

Saxena, B. B., Hasan, S. H., Haour, F., and Schmidt-Gollwitzer, M. (1974). *Science* **184,** 793.

Saxena, B B., Kaali, S., and Landesman, R. (1977). *Eur. J. Obstet. Gynecol.* **7,** 1–4.

Schultz, H., Sell, A., Norgaard-Pederson, B., and Arends, J. (1978). *Cancer* **42,** 2182–2186.

Shutt, D. A., and Lopata, A. (1981). *Fertil. Steril.* **35,** 413.

Siris, E. S., Nisula, B. C., Catt, K. J., Horner, K., Birken, S., Canfield, R. E., and Ross, G. T. (1977). *Endocrinology* **102,** 1356.

Stewart, M., and Stewart, F. (1977). *J. Mol. Biol.* **116,** 175.

Strott, C. A., Yoshimi, T., and Ross, C. T. (1969). *J. Clin. Endocrinol. Metab.* **29,** 1157.

Swaminathan, N., and Braunstein, G. D. (1978). *Biochemistry* **17,** 5832.

Szulman, A. E., and Surto, U. (1978). *Am. J. Obstet. Gynecol.* **131,** 665–671.

Thomas, J. P., Dorflinger, L. J., and Berham, H. R. (1978). *Proc. Natl. Acad. Sci. U.S.A.* **75,** 1344.

Tulsky, A. S., and Koff, A. K. (1957). *Fertil. Steril.* **8,** 118.

Vaitukaitis, J. L., (1978). *In* "Structure and Function of the Gonadotropins" (K. W. McKerns, ed.), pp. 339–360. Plenum, New York.

Vaitukaitis, J. L., and Ebersole, E. R. (1976). *J. Clin. Endocrinol. Metab.* **42,** 1048–1055.

Vatiukaitis, J. L., Braunstein, G. D., and Ross, G. T. (1972). *Am. J. Obstet. Gynecol.* **113,** 751.

Van Hell, H. (1974). *In* "Gonadotropins and Gonadal Function" (N. R. Moudgal, ed.), pp. 66–78. Academic Press, New York.

Varma, S. K., Dawood, M. Y., Haour, F., Channing, C. P., and Saxena, B. B. (1979). *Fertil. Steril.* **31,** 68.

Ward, D. N. (1978). *In* "Structure and Function of the Gonadotropins" (K. W. McKerns, ed.), pp. 31–46. Plenum, New York.

Wardlaw, S., Laursen, N. H., and Saxena, B. B. (1975). *Acta Endocrinol.* **79,** 568.

Wiley, L. D. (1974). *Nature (London)* **252,** 715.

Wislocki, G. B., and Streeter, G. L. (1938). *Carnegie Contrib. Embryol.* **27,** 1–66.

Zondek, B. (1942). *J. Am. Med. Assoc.* **118,** 705–708.

SPECIFIC PREGNANCY PROTEINS

Arnold Klopper

DEPARTMENT OF OBSTETRICS AND GYNAECOLOGY
UNIVERSITY OF ABERDEEN
ABERDEEN, SCOTLAND

I. Introduction 128
II. Schwangerschaftsprotein 1 (SP_1) 129
A. Historical Note 129
B. The Chemistry of SP_1 130
C. SP_1 in Other Anin.als 133
D. The Origin of SP_1 133
E. The Measurement of SP_1 134
F. The Metabolism of SP_1 136
G. SP_1 in Normal Pregnancy 137
H. Pathological Pregnancy 141
I. The Function of SP_1 146
III. Pregnancy-Associated Plasma Protein A (PAPP-A) 147
A. Historical Note 147
B. The Chemistry of PAPP-A 148
C. The Assay of PAPP-A 149
D. The Origin of PAPP-A 150
E. The Metabolism of PAPP-A 151
F. PAPP-A in Normal Pregnancy 151
G. PAPP-A in Pathological Pregnancy 153
H. The Function of PAPP-A 154
IV. Pregnancy-Associated Plasma Protein B (PAPP-B) 155
A. Historical Note 155
B. Chemistry of PAPP-B 155
C. The Physiology of PAPP-B 156

Current Topics in Experimental Endocrinology, Vol. 4

ISBN 0-12-153204-6

D. Future Studies on PAPP-B 156
V. Placental Protein 5 (PP5) 156
A. Historical Note 156
B. Chemistry of PP5 157
C. Origin of PP5 157
D. PP5 in Normal Pregnancy 157
E. PP5 in Abnormal Pregnancy 158
F. The Function of PP5 158
VI. Other Pregnancy-Associated Proteins 159
VII. Envoy 160
References 160

I. Introduction

A woman with a hydatidiform mole is pregnant but carries no fetus. A placenta, or at least trophoblastic tissue, is more essential to the definition of pregnancy than a fetus. By the same reasoning specific pregnancy proteins are proteins produced only by the placenta. For our purposes this is still too embracing a definition, although it conveniently excludes nonplacental proteins such as sex hormone binding globulin or pregnancy-associated globulin, both of which increase greatly during pregnancy but are not of placental origin. By the same token pregnancy-associated proteins such as ∝-fetoprotein are also excluded. The exclusively placental protein is itself no more than a convenient fiction. Probably all cells carry the code for the full range of proteins which the organism is capable of synthesizing. In the case of the specific pregnancy proteins it is repressed in all but the placenta and certain primitive tissues such as fibroblasts and some tumors. In the final analysis the definition of a pregnancy protein is quantitative, not absolute. But the difference in the amount of specific pregnancy protein produced by the placenta and the traces produced by nontrophoblastic tumors or fibroblast cultures is so great that there is no difficulty in operating the distinction in practice.

I propose to operate two further exclusions for reasons of convenience rather than logic. This survey will be confined to proteins secreted by the trophoblast into the maternal circulation in increasing amounts as pregnancy advances. This excludes interesting newly isolated proteins such as the proteins of the syncytial microvilli which sit at the interface between mother and conceptus, the structural proteins of the placenta and functional proteins such as ferritin receptors engaged in transplacental transport. Lastly, established placental hormones such as hCG and hPL are also excluded. This leaves a number of proteins such as Schwangerschafts protein 1 (SP_1), pregnancy-associated plasma proteins A and B (PAPP-A and PAPP-B), and placental protein 5 (PP5), all of which are presumed to be synthesized in the trophoblast and released into the maternal blood stream. Even so the list is open ended—new ones are being added month by month. For our purposes the list will be restricted to those placental proteins about which a sufficient body of clinical data has accumulated to be worthy of comment.

II. Schwangerschaftsprotein 1 (SP_1)

When Bohn (1971) isolated this protein, he called it Schwangerschaftsprotein 1 (SP_1). It has also variously been called pregnancy-specific β_1-globulin (Tatarinov *et al.*, 1976a), pregnancy-associated plasma protein C (Lin *et al.*, 1974a), and pregnancy-specific β_1-glycoprotein (Towler *et al.*, 1976a). For a while the last designation, contracted to PSβ_1G, held sway as it seemed a more specific chemical description. Then other pregnancy-specific β-glycoproteins were recognized and the name PSβ_1G had to be abandoned. At a meeting in 1979, it was agreed by investigators working on this protein to revert to Bohn's term SP_1 until a functional description could be derived (Halbert, 1979).

A. Historical Note

During the 1960s a number of new proteins with β_1 electrophoretic mobility were recognized in the sera of pregnant women. Possibly the protein now called SP_1 was among them, but it was not sufficiently characterized, chemically or immunologically, for it to be identified with the protein known today. The credit for the first description of SP_1 goes by a narrow margin to two Russian investigators, Tatarinov and Masyukevich, who in 1970 demonstrated a new β_1 from the sera of pregnant women. They were followed in short order by Hans Bohn who independently isolated from human placentas a β_1-glycoprotein in 1971. Bohn characterized his protein so clearly that subsequent investigators had little difficulty in recognizing it when it appeared in placental extracts or in the purification of pregnancy plasma. A somewhat different approach did in fact lead to another independent recognition of SP_1. This was the technique used by Gall and Halbert (1972) who injected whole pregnancy serum into rabbits. By doing so they of course raised a spectrum of antibodies to the proteins in the serum of a pregnant woman. By absorbing out such an antiserum with serum from a nonpregnant individual, they were able to remove all the antibodies to normal serum proteins, leaving behind only antibodies to the proteins peculiar to pregnancy. In this fashion they raised antibodies to SP_1 and used the antiserum to identify SP_1 during various steps in their procedure for the purification of pregnancy plasma. They were thus able to isolate a protein which they called pregnancy-associated plasma protein C (PAPP-C) which was later, by immunological techniques, shown to be the same as the SP_1 isolated by Bohn a year earlier.

In late pregnancy the blood of a pregnant woman contains a high concentration of SP_1. There is so much that it can be measured by simple techniques such as immunodiffusion. Not surprisingly, therefore, a spate of studies on the changes of SP_1 in pathological pregnancies followed its isolation. Soon, however, investigators began to be uneasy about what they were measuring. The immunoprecipitation patterns were pleomorphic and some workers began to talk of "variants" of SP_1 (Horne *et al.,* 1979a). The breakthrough came when Teisner *et al.* (1978) demonstrated that the serum of pregnant women carried not one, but two different molecular species each having SP_1 determinants. It transpired that the smaller of these two molecules was the protein originally isolated by Bohn, and shown to have β_1 electrophoretic mobility. The second, much larger molecule, had an α_2 electrophoretic mobility. The two have therefore become known as $SP_1\beta$ and $SP_1\alpha$. Both molecules occur in all pregnancy sera (Ahmed and Klopper, 1981a) but have different affinities for the antisera. Measurements of SP_1 by any technique are not simply the sum of $SP_1\alpha + SP_1\beta$. The $SP_1\beta$ component is present in higher concentration but its apparent value is much affected by the proportion of $SP_1\alpha$. Doubts as to the validity of previous clinical studies done by such nonspecific methods are now being entertained. It is not difficult to design specific methods of measurement and it might be wise to withhold judgment on the clinical usefulness of SP_1 measurements until these methods have been used.

B. The Chemistry of SP_1

The immunological techniques of the early 1970s picked out a number of plasma proteins with strong pregnancy associations, notably hPL, hCG, pregnancy-associated globulin, sex hormone binding globulin, and SP_1. The pioneer groups of Bohn and Halbert both wrote of four such proteins in the serum of pregnant women, albeit not the same four in each case (Bohn, 1971; Gall and Halbert, 1972). The one protein common to both groups was SP_1. By 1972, Bohn had already begun the large scale extraction and workup of human placentas at the Behring factory in Marburg, which was to lead to the identification of a long series of new placental proteins over the next decade (Bohn, 1972a,b).

The findings in his laboratory on the chemical characteristics of SP_1 were reviewed by Bohn in 1978. They are summarised in Table I and contrasted with the immunologically similar metabolite found in human urine and the related protein in the blood of pregnant monkeys.

Table I
Chemical Characteristics of SP_1

Characteristic	Human SP_1 placenta and blood	Rhesus SP_1 placenta	Human SP_1 urine
Sedimentation coefficient	4.5 S	3.8 S	2.9 S
Molecular weight	90,000	80,000	65,000
Subunits	—	—	—
Extinction coefficient			
1%	12.1	9.6	10.2
E_1 cm 278 nm			
Isoelectric point	4.1	3.8	3.8
Electrophoretic mobility	β_1	β_1–α_2	β_1

The protein is apparently composed of a single peptide chain as reduction with mercaptoethanol did not reduce the molecular size. The amino acid composition is not exceptional; aspartic acid, serine, and leucine being the most abundant residues. The N-terminal amino acid is histidine. The analysis done by Lin *et al.* (1974a) did not differ greatly. Both groups comment on the heterogeneity of the protein. Lin *et al.* found two isoelectric points, the major component having a p*I* of 3.8 and the lesser a p*I* of 6.0.

A noteworthy feature of SP_1 is its high carbohydrate content. Bohn found the carbohydrate to compose 29.3% of the weight, with hexoses, hexosamines, fucose, and neuraminic acid all represented. Treatment of SP_1 with neuraminidase greatly changes the electrophoretic mobility of the protein; it becomes much slower running. The sedimentation coefficient also changes from 4.5 S to 5.6 S. The antigenic properties are, however, not changed by neuraminidase. The sera of other pregnant animals such as dogs or rats do not react with antisera to human SP_1 although it is likely that such animals produce a related placental protein of their own (Lin *et al.*, 1974b). On the other hand certain primates, notably cyanomologus monkeys and baboons, do produce a cross-reacting protein (Stevens *et al.*, 1976).

In the late 1970s various investigators, including Bohn himself, began to voice doubts about the chemistry of SP_1 (Towler *et al.*, 1978; Bohn and Sedlacek, 1975). Teisner *et al.* (1978) found two shapes of rocket on Laurell-type immunoelectrophoresis and showed that, on crossed immunoelectrophoresis, two antigen populations could be detected. There is a general consensus about $SP_1\beta$, the protein of 90,000 MW characterized by Bohn. On immunoelectrophoresis it has an immunoprecipitation pattern with a rounded peak. The second protein precipitates much less readily with SP_1 antisera and has a sharply pointed peak on immunoelectrophoresis, the immunoprecipitation line becoming visible only if polyethylene glycol has been added to the agarose of the immunoelectrophoresis plate. The two types of immunoprecipitation patterns are shown in Fig. 1.

Although it is generally agreed that the second SP_1 determinant has an α_2 electrophoretic mobility (Westergaard *et al.*, 1979a), investigators differ about its molecular weight, how it is formed, and indeed whether it is a single molecular species. The Odense group originally estimated the molecular weight of this second protein, $SP_1\alpha$, as 200,000 (Teisner *et al.*, 1978). Later they identified two proteins other than $SP_1\beta$, one having a molecular weight around 200,000 and the other more than 400,000 (Westergaard *et al.*, 1979b; Hindersson *et al.*, 1981). Ahmed and Klopper (1981b) also identified a protein with SP_1 determinants having a molecular weight of 430,000 and α_2 electrophoretic mobility but failed to find the 200,000 MW molecular species. While the existence of this intermediate molecular species is open to doubt, the 430,000 MW molecule is generally accepted and is the entity designated as $SP_1\alpha$. A surprising recent development has been the claim by Griffiths and Godard (1981) that the native serum SP_1 is a molecule of 280,000 MW composed of two dissimilar subunits of equal molecular size which are bonded together by covalent bonds. Chromatography on hydroxylapatite resulted in the formation of two dissociation and/or degradation products, one of 69,000 and the other of 23,000 MW and both having γ electrophoretic

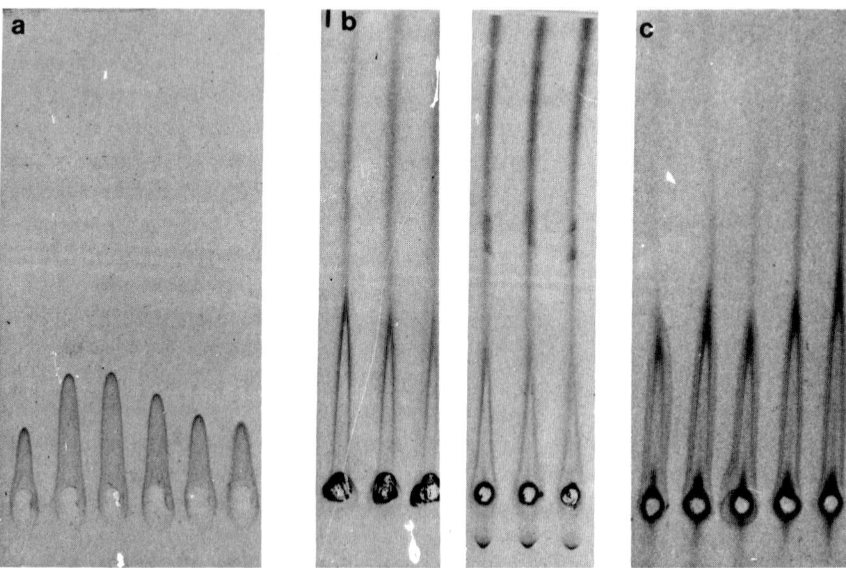

Fig. 1. Precipitation patterns of SP_1 immunoelectrophoresis. (a) Pure $SP_1\beta$; (b) pure $SP_1\alpha$; (c) a mixture of $SP_1\beta$ and $SP_1\alpha$. (Reproduced with permission from Ahmed and Klopper, 1980.)

mobility. These findings are very difficult to reconcile with the previous data on SP_1 and will have to be confirmed.

C. SP_1 in Other Animals

It is clearly important to establish whether other animals produce a protein equivalent to SP_1. It could be a chance phenomenon, peculiar to the human and not a manifestation of pregnancy common to all mammals. An animal model would be of great value to investigations concerning the physiology of the protein. Not surprisingly the search turned first to those familiar laboratory mammals, rats and mice. Lin *et al.* (1974b) found four pregnancy-associated antigens in the blood of these rodents but were unable to identify them with particular human pregnancy proteins as they did not cross-react with antisera to SP_1 or other human placental proteins. For the most part attention has been directed at the primates, but interest in mice has recently revived (Hau *et al.,* 1980) and the Odense workers may have found the murine equivalent of SP_1 (Hau *et al.,* 1982).

The search for SP_1 equivalents in primates has been energetically pursued (Bohn and Sedlacek, 1975; Stevens *et al.,* 1976). Proteins which resemble SP_1 and show partial cross-reaction with antisera to it were found in rhesus and cyanomolgus monkeys, various macaque species,and in squirrel monkeys. Baboon SP_1 was studied in more detail by Stevens *et al.* (1976). Among the higher primates, chimpanzees and orangutans produce an SP_1 which seems to be the same as that of humans (Lin and Halbert, 1978).

Much of the interest in primate SP_1 springs from the use of these animals as models to study the effects of immunizing the females against SP_1. When rabbit antisera to human SP_1 are injected into pregnant cyanomolgus monkeys, abortions are caused (Bohn and Weinmann, 1974), and when non-pregnant monkeys are actively immunized by injection of human SP_1, their fertility is much reduced (Bohn and Weinmann, 1976).

D. The Origin of SP_1

There is plenty of evidence that SP_1 occurs in the syncytiotrophoblast. Bohn (1971) originally isolated the protein from placental extracts and by 1973 Bohn and Ronneberger had shown that it could be detected in the cytoplasm of the syncytiotrophoblast. One of the earliest localizations of SP_1 came from the Moscow group. Tatarinov *et al.* (1976a) demonstrated it in the syncytiotrophoblast and in the cytotrophoblast of early and mature placentas and in chorioepithelioma, by direct immunofluorescence. Using the same technique Sedlacek *et al.* (1976) found SP_1 not only in human but also in monkey placentas. The matter was clinched by the study of Lin and

Halbert (1976) who found an even layer of SP_1 in the cytoplasm of the villous trophoblast by immunofluorescence.

Localization is not proof of synthesis. This nettle was grasped by Horne *et al.* (1976a). They used a superior technique—the immunoperoxidase bridge method—which enabled them to do ultrastructural studies. By this means they found SP_1 in the cisternae of the rough endoplasmic reticulum within the syncytiotrophoblast, suggesting strongly that the protein was indeed synthesized in the trophoblast. They went on to supply more definitive evidence of synthesis by showing that placental explants incorporated radioactive amino acids into SP_1.

For the moment the matter rests there; but doubts have already begun to creep in. The model of the trophoblast synthesizing SP_1 and secreting it actively into the intervillous maternal blood does not fit all the facts. Klopper *et al.* (1979) showed that the concentration of SP_1 did not show the gradient from retroplacental blood to uterine vein and thence to peripheral vein which might be expected if the protein was flowing from the placenta to the maternal peripheral circulation. They suggested that, although SP_1 might be produced in the trophoblast, it made its way into the maternal circulation mainly by the dissolution of embolic or migrating trophoblast. The hypothesis of trophoblastic synthesis and secretion also takes no account of the suggestion of Bohn (1979a) and of Ahmed and Klopper (1980) that $SP_1\alpha$ consists of placental $SP_1\beta$ combined with a normal nonpregnancy serum protein. An alternative scenario which deserves consideration is that $SP_1\beta$ is a resident protein of the syncytiotrophoblast which binds a maternal serum protein to form $SP_1\alpha$ and that the latter is released into the maternal circulation by the dissolution of embolic trophoblast, forming an equilibrium mixture, 80% $SP_1\beta$ and 20% the original $SP_1\alpha$. Certainly SP_1 can be found in tissues other than the trophoblast. It has been isolated from maternal decidua and also appears to be synthesized in the amnion (Koh and Cauchi, 1981).

E. The Measurement of SP_1

1. Methods of Assay

SP_1 is present in relatively high concentration in late pregnancy blood and it is not difficult to measure it by insensitive but simple and well-established methods such as radial immunodiffusion (Mancini *et al.*, 1965). Commercial kits for these measurements were soon developed and the early clinical studies were all done by this method. It is, however, slow (3 days for the assay) and insensitive: measurements are not possible earlier than 20 weeks gestation and unreliable before 30 weeks. An improvement, both in speed and in sensitivity, resulted from the use of Laurell-type "rocket" immunoelectrophoresis (Bruce and Klopper, 1978). This method has proved its value in late pregnancy clinical studies but the attractions of greater sensitivity and adaptability to large-scale turnover led to the publication of a number of radioimmunoassay methods, differing from one another only in matters of detail (Grudzinskas *et al.,* 1977; Sørenson *et al.,* 1977; Towler *et al.,* 1977a). There are disadvantages in radioimmunoassay, notably the use of isotopes and the difficulty of obtaining pure radioactive tracers. This led on one hand to the development of an immunofluorometric assay (Sykes and Chard, 1980) and on the other to an enzyme immunoassay (Grenner, 1978). The former has not met with a great deal of success but enzyme immunoassay methods bid fair to bridge the sensitivity gap between immunoelectrophoresis and radioimmunoassay without involving the use of radioactive materials. Laser nephelometry, although insensitive, has the attraction of being readily adaptable to automation, and a method using this approach has been put forward (Wood *et al.,* 1978). At present not all the problems connected with nephelometric methods for SP_1 have been solved, but this is a technique which is gaining ground elsewhere in clinical chemistry and more may be heard of it in the context of SP_1 measurements.

2. The Influence of Methodology upon the Results

The development of several methods for the assay of SP_1 led to a comparison of the results by different techniques. It was soon found that in some sera radioimmunoassay methods gave much lower values than did immunoelectrophoresis (Schultz-Larsen *et al.,* 1979a). Nor was it only a question of the difference between radioimmunoassay and immunoelectrophoresis. One publication reached the alarming conclusion that there was no correlation of the results between radial immunodiffusion, immunoelectrophoresis, and nephelometry (Schultz-Larsen *et al.,* 1979b). It gradually became clear that the essential difference lay between immunoprecipitation methods, such as immunoelectrophoresis on the one hand, and competitive protein binding methods, such as radioimmunoassay on the other hand. The reason for this became clear when it was found that there was not one, but at least two antigens reacting with SP_1 antisera. It is likely that the affinity of $SP_1\beta$ for the antibody is more than that of $SP_1\alpha$ (Teisner *et al.,* 1979a). This led the Odense group to conclude that, when measuring mixtures of $SP_1\beta$ and $SP_1\alpha$ as in pregnancy serum, the antiserum would react exclusively with $SP_1\beta$ in radioimmunoassay methods (Teisner *et al.,* 1979b). This can hardly be true for all mixtures of $SP_1\beta$ and $SP_1\alpha$. Displacement of tracer will depend not only on the avidity of the antiserum for the antigen but also on the relative populations of $SP_1\beta$ and $SP_1\alpha$ molecules competing for the binding sites. Whatever the reason for the discrepancy, it is clear that radioimmunoassay, immunoelectrophoresis, and laser nephelometry give different results (Anthony *et al.,* 1980a).

One way out of the impasse is to say, as Teisner *et al.* (1979b) have done, that radioimmunoassay measures only $SP_1\beta$ and immunoelectrophoresis measures $SP_1\beta + SP_1\alpha$, i.e., total SP_1. This is less than satisfactory because it assumes that $SP_1\alpha$ has no effect on the measurement of $SP_1\beta$ by radioimmunoassay and that $SP_1\beta$ and $SP_1\alpha$ react equally and are additive on immunoelectrophoresis.

On account of these methodological difficulties Ahmed and Klopper (1980) have suggested that many of the recorded measurements of SP_1 may be seriously in error and that it would be well to build a fresh body of data based on the separate measurement of each component. There are two ways to achieve specific measurements of $SP_1\alpha$ and $SP_1\beta$. One is to adsorb out the present generation of antiserum which reacts with both $SP_1\alpha$ and $SP_1\beta$ with one of these two proteins until only antibodies to the other is left. Hindersson *et al.* (1979) claimed to have done this, adsorbing the mixed antiserum with $SP_1\alpha$ until only $SP_1\beta$ antibodies were left. Ahmed and Klopper (1982) failed to achieve this and chose instead the alternative method of separating the variants biochemically and then measuring the separated proteins with an antiserum which did not distinguish between them.

F. The Metabolism of SP_1

1. The Placental Content of SP_1

Both $SP_1\beta$ and $SP_1\alpha$ are present in placental tissue and can be extracted from it (Ahmed *et al.*, 1981). Although $SP_1\beta$ is readily extracted by physiological saline, $SP_1\alpha$ is much more difficult to solubilize. As Bohn's first isolations were made from saline extracts of placentas it is not surpising that he found only $SP_1\beta$. In view of its larger size and tight binding in the placenta, Ahmed *et al.* (1981) surmised that $SP_1\alpha$ was a placental precursor molecule which gave rise to a secretory product—$SP_1\beta$. The subsequent discovery that $SP_1\alpha$ was a combination of $SP_1\beta$ with a widely distributed serum and tissue protein (Bohn, 1979a; Ahmed and Klopper, 1980) makes this hypothesis unlikely. Lee *et al.* (1979) have studied the placental concentration of a number of trophoblastic proteins and compared this with their blood concentration in early and late pregnancy. Curious differences in pattern emerged. Proteins not specific to pregnancy such as ferritin showed no real change as gestation advanced and the maternal serum:placental tissue ratio stayed unchanged. It is well known that serum levels of hCG are high in early pregnancy and fall later, and the placental tissue levels follow the same pattern. As might be expected hPL and SP_1 showed the opposite pattern with placental concentration increasing in late pregnancy. As the extractions were done with phosphate-buffered saline their findings apply only to $SP_1\beta$, not $SP_1\alpha$. Surprisingly PP5 did not show the same late pregnancy increase in placental concentration as did hPL and SP_1. Lee *et al.* (1979) point out that this differential pattern of serum and placental concentration change is evidence that the mechanism of secretion of trophoblast-specific proteins varies from one protein to the other.

There is very little SP_1 in the liquor amnii or the cord blood and all investigators are agreed that it passes almost entirely from the placenta into the maternal circulation (Grudzinskas *et al.,* 1978). The manner in which it does so is open to some argument. If it were simply a matter of direct secretion from the trophoblast into the retroplacental blood, there would be a higher concentration of SP_1 in the retroplacental blood than in the peripheral circulation. Smith *et al.* (1979a) found, however, that the retroplacental concentration of SP_1 was less than in the uterine vein or peripheral veins, not more. Other placental products such as hPL and estriol, measured in the same patients at the same time, showed the expected gradient from retroplacental blood to uterine vein blood. This curious finding was confirmed by Grudzinskas *et al.* (1979a) who used hPL and PP5 as controls. Although both groups had taken care to avoid the contamination of the retroplacental blood with liquor, Grudzinskas *et al.* (1979a) suggested that this was the reason for this otherwise irreconcilable finding.

Once present in maternal blood SP_1 is slowly removed, at least in part by excretion as a urinary metabolite (Bohn and Kraus, 1977). Lin *et al.* (1976a) on the basis of rather haphazard sampling in five women after delivery said that SP_1 became undetectable 2–3 weeks after delivery. Klopper *et al.* (1978) who studied 10 women found a half-life for SP_1 of 21.53 hours when hPL in the same patients had a half-life of 13.33 minutes. The logarithmic plots of the decline in plasma concentration of SP_1 after delivery of the placenta suggested that the protein was distributed through only two compartments in the mother. Menabawey *et al.* (1979) using a design similar to that of Klopper *et al.* (1978) found that the half-life of SP_1 ranged from 17 to 45 hours. It must be emphasized that all these investigators simply studied the decline in SP_1 after delivery of the placenta. If any of the protein is produced or stored in the maternal organism these half-lives may be greatly overestimated.

G. *SP_1 in Normal Pregnancy*

1. Early Pregnancy

The immunodiffusion methods first used are inadequate for the measurement of SP_1 in pregnancy before about 10 weeks gestation. Immunoelectrophoresis is somewhat more sensitive, but it was not until radioimmunoassay techniques were evolved that it became possible to explore the sequence of events just after conception. Grudzinskas *et al.* (1977) were the first group to develop such a method and they use it to good effect in early pregnancy.

They could not detect the protein in the blood of males or nonpregnant women but were able to pick it up as early as 7 days after ovulation, i.e., 2 or 3 days after implantation. With more experience of early pregnancy levels it became clear that SP_1 could be securely measured 18–23 days after the LH surge (Grudzinskas *et al.*, 1979b). At this time the concentration is at the detection limit of the method, (0.02 mg/liter). Thereafter it rises exponentially, the concentration doubling every 2–3 days. Such a rise suggests that one is measuring cell multiplication. At 40 days after ovulation the slope decreases but, unlike hCG, SP_1 continues to rise in later pregnancy.

Grudzinskas *et al.* (1977) working with a sensitivity limit of 20 μg/liter did not find SP_1 in nonpregnancy blood, but Searle *et al.* (1978) and Wurz (1979) found SP_1 in the 3–20 μg/liter range in some nonpregnant subjects. This aspect has not been pursued very far but it is generally accepted that traces of SP_1 can be produced by tissues other than the placenta—most likely fibroblasts. The protein is therefore pregnancy associated, not pregnancy specific. As radioimmunoassay measures mainly $SP_1\beta$, it must be assumed that these early pregnancy findings apply to this protein, although it is likely that it is accompanied by $SP_1\alpha$, undetectable at these low levels.

Early pregnancy studies were carried a stage further by Anthony *et al.* (1980b). They designed a radioimmunoassay with a working range of 3–400 μg/liter. An undefined proportion of nonpregnant subjects gave positive readings up to 6 μg/liter. They were unable to determine whether these represented true SP_1 or methodological noise and accepted 6 μg/liter as the cut-off point for the diagnosis of pregnancy. They studied women being treated in an infertility clinic with a variety of agents for the induction of ovulation, taking blood on day 21 and again between days 22 and 40 of their menstrual cycle. They recorded 16 instances in which the SP_1 concentration exceeded 6 μg/liter 21–40 days from the last menstrual period. In 11 of these, pregnancy was confirmed. They surmised that in the remaining 5, fertilization had occurred but implantation had not succeeded or a very early abortion had occurred. It is evident from other studies on induced ovulation (Seppälä *et al.*, 1979; Grudzinskas *et al.*, 1979b) that SP_1 concentration starts to rise soon after implantation and by the time of the first missed period is above 20 μg/liter. Whether values between 6 and 20 μg/liter can be taken as indicative of fertilization is doubtful. It is probable that some nonpregnant subjects produce detectable amounts of SP_1; it is certain that there is some blank reading in all methods.

2. Late Pregnancy

All the pioneers who independently isolated SP_1 endeavored to measure the concentration of the protein in late pregnancy blood. Their methods were crude and they did not have pure standards. Bohn (1972a), using radial immunodiffusion, suggested that the concentration rose with advancing gestation to reach values of 5–20 mg/liter in the last trimester.

The first definitive study of SP_1 levels in late pregnancy was published by Tatra *et al.* in 1974. They found that the levels rose from a mean of 33.5 mg/liter at 20 weeks to 150.3 mg/liter at 40 weeks. The concentration rose steadily up to 37 weeks after which it flattened out. Other surveys of normal pregnancy followed thick and fast as methods were refined. They confirmed the general pattern, i.e., a steep rise to 37 weeks and then a plateau with a tendency to fall after 40 weeks. The mean values at 37 weeks found by various investigators are listed in Table II. They vary from 95 to 250 mg/liter, a disappointingly large range for mean values. There does not appear to be any consistent difference related to the assay technique. If the extreme values below 95 and above 200 mg/liter are ignored most of the other findings cluster closely about a mean peak value of 150 mg/liter.

Many of the authors listed in Table II give enough detail for the spread of values from one normal subject to another at the same stage of gestation to be calculated. The coefficients of variation cluster closely about 30%. The methodological variation of simple techniques such as radial immunodiffusion or immunoelectrophoresis is only 2–3%. The rest represents real variability from one person to another. Nor can the large spread be accounted for in terms of rapid fluctuations from time to time in the same subject. Masson *et al.* (1977) found the mean day to day variability of SP_1 to be 4.8%, perhaps a third of that a placental steroid like estriol. Such a large normal range does not augur well for the use of SP_1 assays as a parameter of placental function. There is bound to be considerable overlap between the lower normals and the higher pathological pregnancies.

Table II

Concentration of SP_1 in Late Pregnancy (± 37 Weeks)

Reference	Mean SP_1 (mg/liter)	Method of assay
Tatra *et al.* (1974)	139	RID
Towler *et al.* (1976a)	199	DRID
Gordon *et al.* (1977a)	250	RIA
Klopper *et al.* (1977)	159	IEA
Sørensen (1978)	199	IEA
Chapman and Jones (1978)	225	DRID
Higuchi *et al.* (1978)	141	RID
Karg *et al.* (1978)	189	IEA
Pluta *et al.* (1979)	168	RIA
Heikenheimo *et al.* (1978)	95	RIA
Wurz *et al.*	140	RIA

SP_1 is a placental product and the shape of its mean concentration curve during pregnancy closely resembles that of placental weight. It might be thought that a major factor in determining the difference in SP_1 concentration between one woman and another lies in placental weight. Some investigators have sought, and found, a correlation between SP_1 concentration and placental weight (Tatra, 1979). As fetal and placental weights are related it is to be expected that SP_1 concentration would also be related to the weight of the newborn. This aspect was explored in the study of Schultz-Larsen (1978) who found the correlation coefficient between SP_1 concentration and placental weight to be 0.39. There was also a positive correlation with fetal weight, albeit a weaker one (0.28). A search for other factors in mother and baby which might be related to SP_1 concentration proved unavailing except for the curious finding that SP_1 was negatively related to the age of the mother. There might, in this odd finding, be a clue to the factors which determine SP_1 production and it should be further explored.

By and large the levels of SP_1 in normal pregnancy fit well with the model proposed by Gordon and Chard (1979), in particular their hypothesis that its production is solely related to trophoblast mass and placental blood flow.

3. Relation of SP_1 to Other Placental Proteins

As hCG and SP_1 are both produced by the trophoblast very early in pregnancy, it is of interest to determine whether their secretion is regulated by the same factors. This is very unlikely as their mean curves during gestation have greatly different patterns. Also *in vitro* their secretion by tumors was discordant and followed different time courses (Rosen *et al.*, 1980). Generally, but not invariably, β-hCG can be detected a day or two before SP_1 in very early pregnancy but this difference is as likely to be a reflection of the greater sensitivity and reliability of hCG assay, as it is an indication that hCG is produced before SP_1. The detection of hCG has long been established worldwide as a pregnancy test. It is not likely to be replaced by SP_1, although SP_1 is more readily detected during the luteal phase of the cycle in women wearing an intrauterine contraceptive device and may be a better test for occult pregnancy (Seppälä *et al.*, 1978). Of course SP_1 assay is also useful for the detection of implantation in women being treated with hCG (Seppälä *et al.*, 1979).

The curves for hPL and SP_1 run parallel until 37 weeks and it is likely that the same processes govern the production of both proteins. Indeed a good many investigators have found that SP_1 and hPL are correlated (Gordon *et al.*, 1977a: Sørensen, 1978). It is not so certain that they run together in the last few weeks of pregnancy. Towler *et al.* (1976b) found that hPL fell after 37 weeks while SP_1 continued to rise, and both Towler *et al.* (1976a) and Klopper *et al.* (1977) found that they were not correlated in late pregnancy.

H. Pathological Pregnancy

1. Abnormalities of Early Pregnancy

As SP_1 appears in the circulation of pregnant women almost as early as hCG, investigators have looked to see whether SP_1 assays would give information any different from that by hCG assay, particularly in ectopic pregnancy and abortion. Initial studies indicated that there was very little to choose between the two proteins in the diagnosis of ectopic pregnancies (Seppälä *et al.*, 1980). All the patients who were found to have ectopic pregnancy also had pregnancy levels of both SP_1 and hCG. In these days of laparoscopic examination it is not difficult to make a positive diagnosis of ectopic pregnancy. The difficulty arises with overlapping conditions such as incomplete or threatened abortion, occult pregnancy, or corpus luteum cyst. For these SP_1 assay, like hCG, is useful but not definitive. Not surprisingly, the enthusiasts for SP_1 assay have found it more useful than hCG in the difficult cases with corpus luteum cysts.

In studies on abortion the pace was set by Schultz-Larsen and Hertz (1978). They addressed themselves to the question of the predictive value of SP_1 assays when patients are admitted to hospital with threatened abortion. They found that a low SP_1 value occurred in 89% of patients who eventually aborted, much the same predictive value as other authors noted for hPL, hCG, estradiol, and progesterone measurements. When one considers that patients present at all stages of the abortion process, and that very different causes may be operative, this is a remarkable finding for any diagnostic process across the field of medicine. When it comes to predicting which pregnancies would continue SP_1 assays were even more successful—94% of such patients had values within the normal range. This figure could be even further improved by serial assays which gave the correct result in 100% of cases. Time is of the essence in the prediction of threatened abortion, and serial assays which take several days to produce a clear answer have little practical value. It appears from the work of Schultz-Larsen and Hertz (1978) that SP_1 assays are rather better at predicting a successful outcome of pregnancy than are other parameters. If so, they may be particularly valuable in preventing the disaster of evacuating a normal pregnancy.

The results of Schultz-Larsen and Hertz (1978) for the predictive value of SP_1 in patients who were going to abort were confirmed by Jandial *et al.* (1978), but their study was based on a group of patients who, on examination, were thought to have an inevitable incomplete or missed abortion. A substantial proportion of such patients can be securely diagnosed on clinical grounds. Jandial *et al.* (1978) were less successful than Schultz-Larsen and Hertz (1978) in predicting which pregnancies would continue. They claimed a correct prediction in 75% of cases and thought that serial SP_1 assays would be advisable before 10 weeks, but concluded that single SP_1 assays were more reliable than single hPL assays.

Investigators may invest a great deal of their time and resources in developing and applying a particular technique. Without conscious intent to deceive they may design and interpret experiments in a manner which puts their assay in the best light. This applies to assay as much as anything else. It is not possible to set and operate clinical criteria rigidly from place to place or even from time to time in the same place. SP_1 assays make a better showing the more clinically obvious cases are included, either by way of those well advanced in the abortion process, or those where the disturbance of pregnancy is so slight that the likelihood of a successful outcome is high. In studies of placental function the criteria evolved by Gordon *et al.* (1978) are a useful tool. They should properly be applied to the screening of an unselected population but were used to good effect by Jouppila *et al.* (1980) in a group of 145 patients who presented with bleeding in the first trimester of pregnancy. Once again SP_1 assays proved to be most useful in identifying those pregnancies which would continue to term. In 107 samples from 84 pregnancies which continued, only two were below the 10th centile. Over the group as a whole, the sensitivity was 65%, the predictive value 96%, and the specificity 98%. Three separate groups of workers have therefore viewed SP_1 assays in threatened abortion with approval.

In view of the fact that SP_1 was first detected by workers in a cancer institute in Moscow, it is not surprising that SP_1 production by trophoblastic tumors was one of the first clinical applications of SP_1 assay to be explored. Indeed this line of investigation followed from the publication of Tatarinov *et al.* (1976b) which demonstrated the presence of SP_1 in trophoblastic tumors and showed that a large proportion of patients with such tumors had SP_1 in their circulation. The introduction of radioimmunoassays for SP_1 made it possible to examine the use of SP_1 measurements, both for the diagnosis of trophoblastic tumors and for the monitoring of their treatment. Seppälä *et al.* (1978) found SP_1 in the serum of all the patients they examined (eight subjects with choriocarcinoma), and that the concentration decreased *pari passu* with chemotherapy. The matter was set on a quantitative footing by the work of Searle *et al.* (1978) who took a cutoff point of 2 μg/liter. At this level all patients with trophoblastic tumors were positive, but so were a number of normal subjects (12 out of 94). In view of this it may be wiser to use the cutoff point of 12 μg/liter later advocated by Tatarinov (1979).

The demonstration that SP_1 assays had a useful function in the diagnosis and treatment of trophoblastic tumors led to comparison of SP_1 with other tumor markers. It fairly soon became obvious that SP_1 assays were superior to hPL and alkaline phosphatase measurements, which have indeed been largely discarded. A report by Lee *et al.* (1981a) suggests that there may be a place for PP5 estimations in that measurements of this protein, like those of SP_1, may discriminate between benign and malignant gestational trophoblastic tumors. The critical comparison, however, is with hCG assays. Searle *et al.* (1978) at first concluded that SP_1 and hCG were synchronized in their behavior but that SP_1 assays might have a particularly useful place in monitoring patients where fluctuating barely detectable β-hCG levels suggest residual disease. They eventually came down fairly firmly in favor of hCG (Searle *et al.*, 1978) and presently the concensus of opinion is that SP_1 assays are a useful backup to β-hCG measurements, which remain the first line in the control of treatment.

The studies of SP_1 in trophoblastic tumors also raised the question of whether SP_1 measurements could be useful in other, nontrophoblastic malignancies. It was first posed by the publication of Horne *et al.* (1976b) who found SP_1 by an enzyme-bridge immunoperoxidase technique in 76% of the tumors from women with carcinoma of the breast, and suggested that women without this protein in the tumor tissue had a better prognosis. The work of Tatarinov (1979) indicates that some patients with lung or testicular tumors will have SP_1 levels somewhat higher than the occasional positive normal subjects, and overlapping the lower end of the trophoblastic tumor range. Later work by Horne *et al.* (1979b) puts the SP_1 levels in nontrophoblastic tumors somewhat nearer the normal nonpregnant range than this and it is clear that SP_1 estimations are of little use either in the diagnosis or in the treatment of malignant nontrophoblastic tumors. There is, however, no doubt that certain nontrophoblastic tumors have the capacity to produce SP_1 as it has been identified in the culture medium from an ovarian cystadenocarcinoma (Azer *et al.*, 1980).

In view of the fact that SP_1 appears in the circulation so soon after pregnancy, the assays have been undertaken in cases of suspected ectopic pregnancy (Seppälä *et al.*, 1980; Tatra *et al.*, 1981a). The introduction of enzyme immunoassay techniques has enlarged the number of centers doing SP_1 assays in early pregnancy and some investigators have found SP_1 assays to be preferable to hCG estimation in the diagnosis of ectopic pregnancy (Tatra *et al.*, 1981b). With the widespread use of laparoscopy it is unlikely, however, that either assay will be of more than occasional interest.

2. Abnormalities of Late Pregnancy

A simple technique such as radial immunoassay can be set up anywhere in the world, and provided one can wait several days for the result, the assays are adequate for late pregnancy studies. Not surprisingly there have been a great many published studies on the changes in SP_1 concentration in various diseases of pregnancy. There are notable shortcomings in many of these studies. The first has been inadequate categorization. Generalizations embracing very diverse pathological entities are unlikely to be sensible and even more restricted categories, such as placental insufficiency and fetal distress, are still heterogeneous and embrace different diseases likely to have very different effects on SP_1 production. Often too, investigators have failed to define what constitutes clinical usefulness. In clinical practice SP_1 assays could be used in one of three ways. First, as a control measure, that is, determining SP_1 concentration day by day and observing the trend of change. It is assumed that a falling level indicates deteriorating placental function. There are only occasional, poorly documented, observations on serial SP_1 assays used in this sense. In view of its long half-life it is unlikely to show rapidly or clearly such changes and this type of application for SP_1 assays will not be examined. Second, the assay might be used in a diagnostic sense. Preeclampsia, fetal death, and other obstetric pathologies are better diagnosed by other means, but given an established disease, single SP_1 assays might be used to indicate fetal state, e.g., the degree of growth retardation or the likelihood of fetal distress in labor. But in view of their simplicity and relative cheapness these assays bear the promise of another useful clinical application, that is as a screening process applied to an unselected obstetric population. It is this aspect of the use of SP_1 assays which is most worthy of examination. Unfortunately very few studies on a whole population have been done and for the most part we shall have to look at the outcome of pregnancy in groups loaded with known or suspected pathology.

a. Retarded Fetal Growth. One of the earliest published papers on the clinical aspects of SP_1 assay purported to show a relationship between SP_1 concentration and fetal weight (Tatra *et al.*, 1975). Many subsequent studies were devoted to examining how accurately SP_1 could predict fetal growth retardation, generally defined as a baby with a birthweight less than the 10th centile of birthweight for its stage of gestation. Towler *et al.* (1977a) found that 60% of patients giving birth to a growth-retarded baby had an SP_1 level below 2 standard deviations from the mean for the stage of gestation, but this finding has little bearing on the prognostic value of SP_1 assay for retarded fetal growth. The data of Gordon *et al.* (1977b) apply not to a single screening assay, but to at least one low value in a series of an unspecified number of assays. On this basis they concluded that SP_1 values were low in over 70% of women carrying a growth-retarded fetus. Gordon *et al.* (1978) later published most pertinent criteria for evaluating parameters of placental function and it is a pity these were not applied to their data. The figure of 60% or more of patients giving birth to growth-retarded babies having a low SP_1 value occurs again in the study of Chapman and Jones (1978). It is not possible to deduce any figure from the study of Pluta *et al.* (1979) although the generalization is made that serial studies on severe growth retardation showed SP_1 values below the 10th centile throughout. A similar conclusion is drawn in the study of Viala *et al.* (1980). Although Wurz *et al.* (1981) concluded that there was a "marked tendency" toward reduced SP_1 values with retarded fetal growth only 45% of patients with fetal growth retardation had values lower than the 10th centile and Hughes *et al.* (1980a) failed to find a significant reduction in the mean SP_1 value of women with a growth-retarded baby as compared to the mean value in normal pregnancy. It might be concluded that, although there is some tendency for SP_1 to be low in women carrying a growth-retarded baby, there is as yet no definitive study showing how reliable SP_1 assays applied as a screen to a whole obstetric population would be as a means of categorizing patients at risk of producing a growth-retarded baby.

b. Preeclamptic Toxemia. Almost all the studies of SP_1 in preeclamptic toxemia have been directed to the question of whether the concentration is normal or reduced in the established disease, and there are few data on whether SP_1 assays give any indication of fetal prognosis in preeclampsia. Some of the more thoughtful analyses have also attempted to correlate the SP_1 value with the severity of the disease and whether or not there was a coexistent fetal growth retardation. Towler *et al.* (1977b) found that SP_1 concentration "tended to fall in the lower part of the normal range" with severe preeclampsia only if there was concomitant fetal growth retardation, while Gordon *et al.* (1977a) found little difference. Siekmann and Heilmann (1979) also found SP_1 values reduced "in the majority" of cases when preeclampsia was coexistent with fetal growth retardation, while Wurz *et al.* (1981) found "predominantly" low values in preeclampsia with growth retardation. It is questionable whether preeclampsia by itself has any effect on SP_1 concentration. Although Tatra *et al.* (1979) found significantly increased urinary values in severe toxemia and Weber *et al.* (1980) found an "extreme decrease" in plasma, most other authors have concluded that there is no real change (Chapman and Jones, 1978; Pluta *et al.*, 1979). It would appear therefore that, although SP_1 assays may be of some small help in deciding whether a patient with preeclamptic toxemia has a growth-retarded baby, they have otherwise no clinical use in this disease.

c. Other Abnormalities of Late Pregnancy. SP_1 assays have been rather haphazardly recorded in a variety of other pathologies of pregnancy. They fall within the normal range in diabetic pregnancy (Tatra *et al.*, 1974; Grudzinskas *et al.*, 1979c; Siekmann and Heilmann, 1979) while they are raised in cholestasis of pregnancy (Heikenheimo *et al.*, 1978) and in twin pregnancy (Pluta *et al.*, 1979).

Many authors have compared the value of SP_1 assays with other parameters of placental function in a variety of pathologies of pregnancy. In the case of a steroid like estriol or of other placental proteins such as PAPP-A and hCG, such comparisons have little meaning as the factors operating on their synthesis are quite different, and the effect of different diseases on their concentration is liable to be different. In the case of hPL, the comparison is more real. It might be expected that, in terms of the hypothesis advanced by Gordon and Chard (1979), there is nothing to choose between hPL and SP_1, but surprisingly Gordon *et al.* (1977a) found SP_1 assays to be marginally better; so did Chapman and Jones (1978), Viala *et al.* (1980), and Weber *et al.* (1980). Pluta *et al.* (1979) found hPL and SP_1 assays equally useful and all authors are agreed that a combination of both assays is superior to either alone.

I. The Function of SP_1

We have got nearly as far as direct measurements of SP_1 will take us. Simply measuring blindly on the assumption that SP_1 is a placental product, at best provides a cracked mirror held up to the placenta, and an even poorer reflection of the fetus. The way forward is to relate SP_1 concentration to its function. That assumes two wholly unproven propositions. The first is that SP_1 concentration in peripheral blood bears some relation to its function. If, as seems probable, this function is exerted in the placenta, this is unlikely. The second is that it has any function at all. There is very little to set against Gordon and Chard's (1979) disconcerting hypothesis that none of the placental proteins has a function. To which must be added the evidence that SP_1, like hPL, may not be essential in pregnancy (Grudzinskas *et al.*, 1979c).

There have been only three suggestions regarding the function of SP_1: one is discredited, the other unlikely, and the third a mere speculation. It has been proposed that SP_1 might be a carrier protein for steroid hormones such as estradiol-17β but *in vitro* tests show much less affinity than the accepted carrier protein, SHBG (Bohn and Kranz, 1973). The suggestion that SP_1 might be concerned in carbohydrate metabolism has been investigated by measuring SP_1 following administration of either insulin or glucose to pregnant women (Tatra *et al.*, 1976). The results were not convincing and have never been followed up. One thought crops up again and again in discussions on the possible function of SP_1 (Stimson, 1980). This is that SP_1 may have an immunosuppressive function—be part of the mechanism which prevents the rejection of the trophoblast. Although Stimson's experiment did not show any immunosuppressive effect of SP_1, an earlier one by Cerni *et al.* (1977) did indicate that SP_1 could inhibit mitogen-induced lymphocyte transformation. The possible immunosuppressive role of SP_1 remains to be explored by more discriminating experiments.

III. Pregnancy-Associated Plasma Protein A (PAPP-A)

A. Historical Note

We owe our awareness of the existence of this protein, and others, to the researches of S. P. Halbert at the University of Miami in the early 1970s. Halbert developed hyperimmune rabbit antisera by injecting the animals with pooled late pregnancy human serum. These antisera were then adsorbed out with nonpregnant human sera, leaving only antibodies to proteins peculiar to pregnant women. By this technique Gall and Halbert (1972) found four antigens in the sera of pregnant women which could not be detected in the blood of men or nonpregnant women. Two years later the Miami team had purified three of these antigens (Lin *et al.,* 1974c). The fourth one was to prove much more difficult to purify and to this date has only been roughly characterized and no pure specimen exists. They named their proteins pregnancy-associated plasma proteins (PAPPs) as they had been isolated from the blood of pregnant women. Two of the PAPPs turned out to be proteins which had already been isolated and named: PAPP-C was SP_1 and PAPP-D was hPL, but the remaining two, PAPP-A and PAPP-B, were immunochemically different from other known pregnancy-associated proteins (Lin and Halbert, 1975). This is still true to the present day and we are stuck with the ponderous full designation or mysterious initials until they can be assigned proper names indicating their function.

In the middle 1970s all the work on PAPP-A came from the Miami team. They showed that it was present in the placenta (Lin *et al.,* 1976c) and devised means to measure it in blood during pregnancy (Lin *et al.,* 1974d). They found that the concentration increased steeply as gestation advanced (Lin *et al.,* 1976b), and produced evidence that assays of the protein were a useful parameter of placental function (Lin *et al.,* 1977). Early in the development of their work, the Miami team realized that it would be very useful to have an animal model which could be used to study the function of PAPP-A. They examined the sera of pregnant mice and rats and were able to detect four pregnancy-associated antigens analogous to the ones they had found in the human (Lin *et al.,* 1974b), although there was no immunological cross-reaction with antisera to the human antigens. Lin and Halbert (1978) extended their search for pregnancy-associated proteins to the primates. In the chimpanzee and the orangutan they found an antigen immunologically identical to human PAPP-A and in other old world monkeys an antigen which gave a partial cross-reaction with PAPP-A. There was no such antigen in the blood of pregnant new world monkeys such as the squirrel monkey. Lin and Halbert have not pursued their search for an animal model but recent work (Hau *et al.,* 1980) has shown that mice produce a species specific equivalent of SP_1 and there is reason to hope that an animal model for PAPP-A may yet be found.

Halbert was generous with gifts of PAPP-A antisera and with his help groups working on PAPP-A came into being in Aberdeen, Odense, Sydney, and Geneva. International meetings on placental proteins which featured work on PAPP-A were held in Aberdeen in 1978 and 1981, in Siena in 1979, and in Sydney in 1981. They have fired interest in many quarters and the 1980s are likely to see an explosion of publications on this protein.

B. The Chemistry of PAPP-A

Using their antiserum to locate the PAPP-A in various fractions Halbert and Lin (1979) put pregnancy serum through a variety of standard purification procedures. They used ammonium sulfate precipitation, ion exchange chromatography, molecular size filtration, and hydroxylapatite chromatography and were able to produce material which gave a single band on SDS–polyacrylamide electrophoresis. To this Paul Bischof (1980) added chromatography on concanavalin A and affinity chromatography. Affinity chromatography was also used to great effect by Sutcliffe *et al.* (1979), who introduced the idea of negative affinity chromatography, i.e., putting pregnancy serum through an affinity column with immobilized nonpregnant antiserum which would not adsorb the PAPP-A but would remove a great many other proteins. The most favorable conditions for positive affinity chromatography were worked out by Sutcliffe *et al.* (1979) and subsequent workers came to rely on this step more and more in the purification of PAPP-A (Folkersen *et al.,* 1979). Recently a further useful step has been added to purification techniques for PAPP-A. This arises from the fact that PAPP-A complexes with heparin and will be adsorbed by a column of heparin immobilized on Sepharose (Sinosich *et al.,* 1981).

Lin *et al.* (1974a) published a set of findings on the biochemical characteristics of PAPP-A which were a template for all subsequent investigations. They noted that the electrophoretic mobility was that of an α_2-globulin and by gel filtration studies suggested a molecular weight of 750,000, a finding supported also by ultracentrifugation in a sucrose density gradient. The isoelectric point was at a pH of 4.4. Exposure of PAPP-A to neuraminidase decreased the anodic mobility of the protein, and they proposed that it was a glycoprotein with some content of sialic acid (Lin and Halbert, 1975). The p*I* of PAPP-A was confirmed by Sutcliffe *et al.* (1980a) who found the total carbohydrate content to be 19.2%. Major studies on the biochemical characterization of PAPP-A were published by Bischof (1979) and by Sutcliffe *et al.* (1980a). These confirmed and extended the findings recorded by Lin *et al.* (1974a), e.g., by determining the amino acid composition. Two important aspects of the biochemistry of PAPP-A brought out by these studies were its close similarity to α_2-macroglobulin, and its structure. It was found that PAPP-A was a dimer of around 800,000 MW, with each monomer of 400,000 MW composed of sulfhydryl-linked chains of 200,000 MW.

C. *The Assay of PAPP-A*

The measurement of PAPP-A in the studies of the Miami school were done by crossed immunoelectrophoresis (Lin *et al.*, 1974a). This was too clumsy for large-scale routine measurements and was replaced by a Laurell rocket immunoelectrophoresis technique designed by Bischof *et al.* (1979). This method has a very good precision (4.4%), is specific, and simple to operate. Provided a good supply of antiserum is available the assays can be done in the most modestly equipped laboratories. It is, however, not sensitive enough to measure plasma PAPP-A in pregnancies earlier than 20 weeks. For this reason attempts to develop a radioimmunoassay for PAPP-A were set in train in other centers. The first to be published was by Bischof *et al.* (1981). This proved to be sufficiently sensitive for measurements in very early pregnancy, but somewhat surprisingly showed measurable amounts of PAPP-A in the blood of nonpregnant subjects. This is a controversial finding which may cast some doubt on the method. It would be advisable to wait and see when other radioimmunoassay methods devised elsewhere are available whether they produce similar results.

The standards constitute a problem in the assay of PAPP-A. The Miami group used pooled late pregnancy serum to which they assigned an arbitrary value in units per milliliter. Bischof found that a pool of late pregnancy plasma contained 120 μ/ml of PAPP-A as measured against his pure preparation. An international reference pregnancy serum pool has been prepared under WHO auspices and is available from Dr. P. Sizaret, International Agency for Research on Cancer, 150 Cours Albert Thomas, Lyon, France. Pure PAPP-A is very difficult to prepare, and the concentration in pregnancy pools is probably very similar if sufficient subjects contribute to the pool. At present it is advisable to use a pregnancy serum pool, standardized against the international reference pool.

Until recently it was assumed that PAPP-A readings would be the same in serum or plasma, and that the anticoagulant would have no effect on the PAPP-A value of plasma. This is not the case, at least as far as measurements by immunoelectrophoresis are concerned (Klopper and Toop, unpublished observations). Serum gives readings, on average, 8% less than heparinized plasma from the same patient. This could be accounted for by the fact that PAPP-A complexes with heparin (Sinosich *et al.*, 1981), but it is more difficult to account for the finding than anticoagulation with EDTA results in a reading 12% higher than heparin plasma, while oxalate or citrate result in PAPP-A readings significantly lower than serum. In order to make PAPP-A measurements in different centers strictly comparable, they should be done by the same method on the same type of serum or plasma. It should not be necessary to standardize methods provided they are all read against the WHO standard, but we are in a dilemma about anticoagulants: heparinized plasma is used in Aberdeen, EDTA in Geneva, and serum in Sydney. As the international reference preparation is serum it would be reasonable to adopt this for future studies.

D. The Origin of PAPP-A

Lin and Halbert (1976) studied the localization of PAPP-A by immunofluorescence and found that it was confined to the trophoblast. This technique is liable to nonspecific effects, and they might be faulted for having used an undiluted antiserum, but such criticisms cannot be leveled against the work of Wahlström *et al.* (1981) who used an immunoperoxidase method. They showed that PAPP-A occurred as a thin intracytoplasmic rim on the apical border of the syncytiotrophoblast and presumed that this reflected an intensive secretion of PAPP-A into the maternal intervillous blood. But localization is not necessarily synthesis. Doubts were expressed by Klopper *et al.* (1979) who did not find the regular falling gradient of concentration from retroplacental blood to uterine vein, to peripheral vein, which might be expected if the protein were being secreted by the trophoblast. They thought it possible that, if PAPP-A were being produced in the trophoblast, it was not being secreted into the intervillous blood but was making its way into the maternal circulation by dissolution of trophoblastic emboli. This explanation was espoused by Smith *et al.* (1980) to account for their finding that PAPP-A showed a higher increase when labor was induced. The area of doubt was further expanded by Bischof *et al.* (1981) who found PAPP-A in nonpregnancy blood. They have now produced the heretic suggestion that PAPP-A is not a fetal product at all, but is produced in the mother, probably by the endometrium, and is simply taken up and bound in the trophoblast (Bischof *et al.*, 1982). This bold suggestion puts quite a different complexion on studies of PAPP-A. The established belief that it is a placental product is by no means destroyed. It should be possible to prove, or disprove, Bischof's hypothesis with the means at our command. To do so is clearly the essential next step in the investigation of the physiology of this protein.

E. The Metabolism of PAPP-A

Whatever its origin, PAPP-A does not penetrate into the fetus beyond the trophoblast basement membrane to any extent. There are only traces in the liquor amnii or the fetal circulation, although it can be found in the chorion and the amnion (Klopper and Thomson, unpublished observations). In the maternal circulation it probably passes from the intravascular compartment to the interstitial fluid as it can be found in the peritoneal fluid of pregnant women (Smith *et al.*, 1979a).

In the maternal circulation PAPP-A levels are remarkably stable. Smith *et al.* (1979b) found the coefficient of variation from day-to-day to be only 7.3%. This does not necessarily mean that the input is equally steady. PAPP-A has a remarkably long half-life for a placental protein, the average being 51 hours (Smith *et al.*, 1979b). This figure is founded on a study of the decline in plasma PAPP-A concentration after delivery and therefore assumes that the placenta is the only source of PAPP-A. If any secretion can occur from the decidua the estimated half-life may be a great deal too long.

F. PAPP-A in Normal Pregnancy

As radioimmunoassay is a recent introduction to the PAPP-A field there are few data on PAPP-A in early pregnancy except for an unsupported statement that it can be identified in the circulation of pregnant women 28 days after conception (Sinosich *et al.*, 1981). The early studies of Lin *et al.* (1974a) laid down the shape of the mean pregnancy curve and it has not been seriously modified since. The concentration mounts slowly until about 30 weeks after which it rises more steeply right up to term. The continued steep rise in the last few weeks of pregnancy is an unusual feature. The placental weight curve and other placental parameters, such as SP_1, flatten off in the last few weeks of pregnancy. Subsequent studies have confirmed that PAPP-A continues to rise, not only right up to term but even into labor (Smith *et al.*, 1979b), an odd finding for which there has as yet been no adequate explanation.

Although there is agreement about the shape of the mean curve during pregnancy, when one sets out to compare actual values in late pregnancy, discrepancies appear which are difficult to explain. Of course in the early stages there was no common unit and in recent years the values have been derived by a variety of assay techniques—immunoelectrophoresis (Bischof *et al.*, 1979), radioimmunoassay (Bischof *et al.*, 1981), and radiorocket line immunoelectrophoresis (Folkersen *et al.*, 1981). All the investigators are using pooled late pregnancy serum and the PAPP-A concentration should not differ much. By definition, taking each pool as having a PAPP-A concentration of 100 units/ml, the normal term values did not differ much. Table III shows the values recorded by various authors.

The Aberdeen group whose results are recorded in Table III used the same standard in these studies. It follows that in a number of investigations their term value clusters around 138 units. Their standard was later found to contain 1.5063 μg of Bischof's PAPP-A preparation per unit which would give a figure of 207 μg/ml. Bischof himself later recorded a figure of 389 μg/ml (Bischof *et al.*, 1981). This is 10 times greater than the figure of 38 μg/ml which can be calculated from the data of Folkersen *et al.* (1981). It is true that PAPP-A concentration varies greatly from one subject to another. Investigators have generally recorded standard deviations over half the mean value. It is to be expected that average figures would differ, but not as widely as between the Geneva and Odense groups. Both cannot be right. It is essential that there should be a basis for comparison between the groups. With an international standard now available it is urgent that comparative studies on the same material should be done in order to determine whether there is a real methodological difference.

The reason for the large normal range has always been a point of interest. Why should one normal women have two or three times the concentration of PAPP-A of another normal women at the same stage of gestation? Is there any difference between the women that can account for this? Investigators have matched various characteristics of pregnancy against the PAPP-A concentration to see if this gave any clue to the factors determining PAPP-A concentration. Lin *et al.* (1976b) did PAPP-A assays on 187 normal women within a week before delivery. They found a positive correlation with placental weight ($r = 0.23$) and fetal birthweight ($r = 0.145$). They also found that PAPP-A levels were related to hPL concentration ($r = 0.23$) and to SP_1 ($r = 0.18$). PAPP-A was higher in primigravidae than in multipara and there was a marginally significant negative correlation with parity.

Table III
Mean PAPP-A at Term[a]

Reference	PAPP-A (units/ml)
Lin *et al.* (1977)	136
Klopper *et al.* (1979)	150
Smith *et al.* (1979b)	137
Hughes *et al.* (1980b)	97
Bischof *et al.* (1980)	168

[a] Measured in units per milliliter taking a late pregnancy plasma pool as having a concentration of 100 units/ml.

Bischof *et al.* (1980) measured PAPP-A in 176 normal women at 34 weeks and again in early labor. Their material is therefore not strictly comparable with that of Lin *et al.* (1976b) but even allowing for this there were surprising differences in their conclusions. They found no correlation with placental weight or birthweight. They agreed with Lin *et al.* (1976b) that PAPP-A was higher in primigravidae and declined with parity. They also found a decline in PAPP-A with increasing age which they ascribe to the effect of parity. Heavier women tended to have lower PAPP-A, perhaps a dilution effect. The mother's weight gain in pregnancy was not related to her PAPP-A concentration nor did the sex of the fetus have any effect. There was a tendency for patients with low PAPP-A values in labor to have low Apgar scores. Some of the differences between Lin *et al.* (1976b) and Bischof *et al.* (1980) are important and should be resolved as the findings may bear on the physiological role of the protein. If PAPP-A concentration is an expression of placental mass and, less directly, of fetal growth, it may have no specific function as suggested by the hypothesis of Gordon and Chard (1979). If it is not related to placental mass it may be an essential feature of pregnancy, and its correlations with other obstetric parameters may give a clue to its function. Bischof *et al.* (1980) surmised that the reason for the undoubted relationship with parity was immunological. If so, the function of PAPP-A is to be sought somewhere in the region of the immunological privilege of the fetal allograft.

G. PAPP-A in Pathological Pregnancy

For methodological reasons all the studies of PAPP-A in complications of pregnancy have been done on late pregnancy. There is thus no information concerning PAPP-A levels in abortion, ectopic pregnancy, or hydatidiform mole. The late pregnancy studies have been few and haphazard but have yielded some very interesting results which may cast some light on the function of the protein. Lin *et al.* (1977) assayed PAPP-A in patients with twin pregnancies, with diabetes and with preeclamptic toxemia. In twin pregnancy, the PAPP-A concentration was more than double the corresponding normal value, a finding which speaks in favor of the placental origin of the protein. Diabetic pregnancy showed no notable change but preeclamptic toxemia was surprisingly accompanied by a significant rise in PAPP-A. If the change in preeclampsia were the consequence of placental damage, one would expect PAPP-A to fall, not rise. An increase in PAPP-A associated with preeclampsia has been noted by the Odense group (Westergaard *et al.*, 1980) and extensively documented by the Aberdeen group (Hughes *et al.*, 1980a,b; Klopper and Hughes, 1980; Klopper, 1980, 1981b; Toop and Klopper, 1981). The Aberdeen group have examined PAPP-A levels in relation to the severity and duration of preeclampsia and whether or not it was accompanied by fetal growth retardation. They could not demonstrate any difference in PAPP-A concentration with regard to the presence or absence of fetal growth retardation in preeclampsia, but did find that the rise of PAPP-A tended to be higher in severe preeclampsia with albuminuria. Of interest was the finding that PAPP-A rises tended to be most marked when the preeclampsia occurred relatively early in pregnancy. This led them to examine patients before overt symptoms of preeclampsia developed and it was found that the rise in PAPP-A often preceded the onset of preeclampsia (Toop and Klopper, 1981). This raises the possibility of using PAPP-A measurements to isolate a group of patients at risk of subsequently developing preeclampsia. Preliminary analysis of the results of such a screen trial shows promise (Toop and Klopper, 1982).

The role of PAPP-A in pathological pregnancy will not be understood until more is known of the function of the protein. It is already clear that it is quite a different kettle of fish from traditional parameters of placental function such as hPL or SP_1. PAPP-A is not affected by fetal growth retardation, and in toxemia, it changes early in the genesis of the disease, and in the wrong direction. There is some indication of rises in PAPP-A preceding abruptio placentae and premature labor (Hughes *et al.*, 1980a). This may be related to the same process as is involved in preeclampsia and indicates that PAPP-A (and probably PP5) are to be regarded in quite a different light from other placental proteins such as hPL and SP_1.

H. The Function of PAPP-A

There are few hard facts but much speculation on the function of PAPP-A (Bischof *et al.*, 1982; Klopper, 1982). Much of the evidence indeed is negative or controversial. Although there is no doubt that PAPP-A increases right up to term and even more in early labor, Smith *et al.* (1981), in a careful study of spontaneous and induced labor, came to the conclusion that there was no reason to suppose that changes of PAPP-A were involved in the onset of labor. Bischof (1979) adduced evidence that PAPP-A was an inhibitor of plasmin and deduced that it might be concerned with the restraint of fibrinolysis *in vivo*. This would fit with its resemblance to α_2-macroglobulin and its surprising change in preeclampsia, a condition associated with disseminated intravascular coagulation. Unfortunately Klopper (1982) was unable to confirm Bischof's finding and the antifibrinolytic role of PAPP-A must be held in abeyance until more evidence is available. The resemblance to α_2-macroglobulin may be misleading as Sutcliffe *et al.* (1980b) found marked differences between the two proteins on peptide mapping.

Although some aspects of its role in the immunology of pregnancy are in dispute, it is in the area of immunosuppression that the best evidence for the role of PAPP-A can be found. Bischof *et al.* (1982) adduced evidence of a suppressive effect of PAPP-A on the response of lymphocytes to stimulation with phytohemagglutinin, but McIntyre *et al.* (1981) concluded that PAPP-A did not have a suppressive effect on cellular immune responses. There is, however, no disagreement about its activity as a complement inhibitor (Bischof, 1981; Klopper, 1982). If, therefore, it plays a part in allowing the survival of the trophoblast as an allograft this function is likely to be bound up with its ability to inhibit complement fixation.

IV. Pregnancy-Associated Plasma Protein B (PAPP-B)

A. Historical Note

PAPP-B was one of the antigens detected by the Miami group in their early investigations into the antigenic constituents of pregnancy plasma which could not be found in nonpregnancy serum (Gall and Halbert, 1972). At first their efforts were directed at making sure that PAPP-B was not one of the known pregnancy-associated proteins such as hPL or α_2PAG. PAPP-B proved to be more difficult to detect than the other pregnancy-associated proteins and their early publications merely noted the presence of PAPP-B in late pregnancy plasma but not in nonpregnant blood (Lin *et al.,* 1974d). They succeeded in purifying enough PAPP-B to give some chemical characterization (Lin *et al.,* 1974a) but to the present time the methods for measuring PAPP-B are in an early stage of development and are too insensitive to give more than a rough indication of the changes in late pregnancy. The Miami group are the only investigators who have looked at PAPP-B. They ceased work on placental proteins in 1979 and no publications have appeared since their review in that year (Halbert and Lin, 1979).

B. Chemistry of PAPP-B

Most of what is known about the chemistry of PAPP-B is contained in two publications (Lin *et al.,* 1974a, 1978b). PAPP-B is a protein with β_1-globulin electrophoretic mobility. It is a glycoprotein which contains sialic acid. It has an estimated molecular weight of 1,000,000 and an isoelectric point of 4.6–5.0. Halbert and Lin (1979) have detailed various ways in which it can be separated from other serum proteins. It proved too difficult to estimate quantitatively in pregnancy serum, perhaps because the concentration is a good deal less than that of SP_1 or PAPP-A. Lin *et al.* (1978b) have briefly described a rocket immunoelectrophoresis technique which is adequate for late pregnancy studies. As with SP_1 and PAPP-A, other mammals produce an equivalent of PAPP-B and the protein has been detected in the circulation of pregnant chimpanzees and orangutans (Lin and Halbert, 1978).

C. The Physiology of PAPP-B

As far as present insensitive methods allow, PAPP-B is not present in non-pregnant serum. It can be extracted from the placenta (Lin *et al.,* 1976c) and disappears from the circulation soon after delivery of the placenta (Lin *et al.,* 1976a). It is therefore surmised that it is a protein synthesized in the placenta and released into the maternal circulation. Its physiology resembles that of hPL or SP_1 more that that of PAPP-A. Like hPL it has a short half-life and the plasma concentration comes to a plateau in late pregnancy. Its concentration correlates with placental and neonatal weight (Lin *et al.,* 1978b). The concentration is greatly increased in twin pregnancy, but is lowered in diabetic pregnancy and preeclamptic toxemia.

D. Future Studies on PAPP-B

It will be obvious that very little is known about PAPP-B. We are fairly sure of its existence as a separate entity and know something of its chemical characteristics. It is probably a pregnancy-associated placental protein. We know almost nothing of the clinical applications of its measurement or of its function. It presents a challenge to the reproductive physiologist and a rare opportunity for fruitful research. Were it not for the severe financial restraints presently put upon original research, this article would have had much more to say about PAPP-B.

V. Placental Protein 5 (PP5)

A. Historical Note

Since the early 1970s Hans Bohn's laboratory in Marburg has been engaged in working up placentas on a large scale. The placental extracts are fractionated by a variety of physicochemical techniques; each crude fraction is numbered and when a protein is isolated it is numbered accordingly. Many of these proteins proved to be ones which had been previously described and others turned out to be proteins which were present in other maternal or fetal tissues. Some were structural proteins of the placenta which were not secreted, but PP5 was one of a small number of proteins which like hPL, hCG, and SP_1 was released into the maternal circulation. Although Bohn isolated it in 1972 (Bohn, 1972a) and demonstrated that a closely related protein existed in the placentas of apes (Bohn and Sedlacek, 1975) it was not until 1977 that it was fully characterized (Bohn and Winckler, 1977) following a preliminary report in 1976 (Bohn and Weinmann, 1976). Bohn presented samples of his protein and antisera to Professor T. Chard who set up a radioimmunoassay (Obiekwe *et al.*, 1979a). It is from his laboratory at St. Bartholomew's Hospital in London that a series of publications have flowed which has focused attention on the physiological role of this interesting protein.

B. Chemistry of PP5

It is a β_1-glycoprotein with a molecular weight of 36,000 and an isoelectric point of 4.6. The sedimentation coefficient is 2.8 S. It has 19.8% carbohydrate and according to the amino acid analysis published by Bohn and Winckler (1977) aspartic acid, glutamic acid, leucine, and alanine are the chief constituents. Although these workers were able to measure the placental content of PP5 by immunoelectrophoresis, the serum concentration is too low for such measurements and pregnancy studies could not be done until Obiekwe *et al.* (1979a) set up a radioimmunoassay. With similar help from Bohn, a second, solid phase, radioimmunoassay was developed by Nisbet *et al.* (1981).

C. Origin of PP5

Bohn and Winckler (1977) found an average of 12 mg of PP5 per placenta, much more than could be accounted for in terms of the blood content of the placenta. In the earlier studies using immunofluorescence, PP5 was localized mainly in the stromal cells of the placenta. More recently immunoperoxidase methods have shown PP5 in both the syncytiotrophoblast and in the villous stroma (Sedlacek *et al.*, 1976; Seppälä *et al.*, 1979). No PP5 could be detected in the blood of nonpregnant subjects (Grudzinskas *et al.*, 1979a).

D. PP5 in Normal Pregnancy

PP5 concentration has been determined in the blood of pregnant women from 8 weeks gestation to term (Grudzinskas *et al.*, 1979a; Obiekwe *et al.*, 1979a, 1980b; Nisbet *et al.*, 1981). As values are different in serum and heparinized plasma, investigators have standardized on serum measurements. The levels rise from less than 10 μg/liter in early pregnancy to peak at a mean level of 32 μg/liter at 36 weeks, by no means as steep a rise as other placental parameters. Like hPL and SP_1 the levels of PP5 tend to plateau or even fall slightly after 36 weeks. PP5 falls rapidly after delivery; Obiekwe *et al.* (1980a) noted a half-life of 5–39 minutes and Nisbet *et al.* (1981) recorded 5–14 minutes. There is likely to be a multicompartmental distribution of PP5 as the subsequent half-life component is much longer, some PP5 still being detectable 7 days after delivery. The compartmental distribution of PP5 was studied by Grudzinskas *et al.* (1979a). They found the distribution to be much like that of hPL and concluded that PP5 too was secreted selectively into the maternal compartment. The diurnal and the day-to-day variation in the serum concentration of PP5 was studied by Obiekwe *et al.* (1979b) and by Nisbet *et al.* (1981). Neither found a consistent diurnal variation, but the day-to-day variation was large, the coefficient of variation being 5.1–15.1% in the 11 subjects studied by Obiekwe *et al.* (1979b) and 5.5–26.9% in the 9 subjects studied by Nisbet *et al.* (1981).

E. PP5 in Abnormal Pregnancy

Although Nisbet *et al.* (1981) found a significant, albeit weak, correlation between PP5 concentration and placental weight ($r = 0.29, p < 0.05$), this correlation did not extend to fetal birthweight and Obiekwe *et al.* (1980b) in a study on an unselected population of 400 patients concluded that PP5 assays were "unpromising" as a test for intrauterine growth retardation. Salem *et al.* (1981a) did a screening test in early pregnancy at 16 weeks. They compared the value of PP5, hPL, and SP_1 and came to the conclusion that there was significant association between low SP_1 levels and fetal growth retardation, even at this early stage, but confirmed that there was no correlation between PP5 and fetal growth retardation. On the other hand, they found a significant elevation of PP5 in association with premature labor. This is an important observation. Prematurity is the major cause of fetal loss and any clinical test which predicts this with reasonable accuracy would be very valuable. Salem *et al.* (1982) have also shown that PP5 levels are often elevated just before the clinical diagnosis of major abruption. The St. Bartholomew's group have also adduced evidence that PP5, like PAPP-A, is raised in preeclampsia and eclampsia (Lee *et al.*, 1981b). The same group have also examined PP5 levels in patients with untreated gestational trophoblastic tumors (Lee *et al.*, 1981a). They found that PP5 was detectable in all cases of hydatidiform mole, but in none of the patients with choriocarcinoma, and surmised that PP5 assays might be valuable in distinguishing between benign and malignant trophoblastic tumors.

F. The Function of PP5

Bohn and Winckler (1977) found that PP5 inhibited the proteolytic action of trypsin and of plasmin and suggested that it might *in vivo* function as a serine protease inhibitor. Obiekwe *et al.* (1979a) found that serum levels of PP5 were higher than in heparin plasma from the same subject, and later showed that this was due to the formation of a heparin–PP5 complex which could be split by addition of protamine sulfate (Salem *et al.*, 1980). Further work also showed the addition of protamine sulfate to pregnancy serum also caused an apparent increase in the level of PP5 (Salem *et al.*, 1981b). They surmised that PP5 may be capable of combining with endogenous heparin-like substances and this led them to investigate the role of PP5 in coagulation (Salem *et al.*, 1981c). They found evidence of interaction with thrombin and suggested that PP5 may be a naturally occurring anticoagulant factor, analogous to antithrombin III.

There are many curious similarities between PP5 and PAPP-A. Both are raised in preeclampsia, abruptio placentae, and premature labor. There is some evidence that both act as serine protease inhibitors. Both complex with heparin. Neither is affected by fetal growth retardation. If both have functions in pregnancy, they are likely to be related.

One further surprising finding which may bear upon the function of PP5 has to be recorded. Ranta *et al.* (1981) have shown lately that human seminal plasma contains a protein which shares physicochemical and immunological properties with PP5. This finding is very difficult to explain. If it is confirmed it casts doubt upon the putative placental role of PP5.

VI. Other Pregnancy-Associated Proteins

New proteins are being identified in placental extracts almost every day. It is likely that some of them will be of clinical interest but at the present time it is not possible to tell which they will be. Leading this field is the laboratory of Hans Bohn in Marburg, where human placentas are processed on a large scale and nearly 20 different proteins have been isolated and characterized. Many of them are proteins also found in other tissues. The ones which are found only in the placenta are of two kinds: proteins which are easily soluble in distilled water or buffers and insoluble proteins which require detergents or other agents to render them soluble. These are probably structural proteins of no particular interest in the context of the present discussion. The field has recently been reviewed (Bohn, 1972b, 1980) and the findings do not require repetition other than to point out that PP10 (Bohn and Kraus, 1979), PP11 (Bohn and Winckler, 1980), and PP15 (Bohn *et al.*, 1980) are the leading candidates, waiting in the wings.

The Russian pioneer in this field, Tatarinov, also continues to be active and two new placenta-specific α-globulins have recently been announced from his laboratory in Moscow (Tatarinov *et al.*, 1980). Two other interesting lines which do not fall strictly within the scope of this article are the surveys of placental proteins by means of immunofluorescent staining done by Faulk and his collaborators (Faulk and Johnson, 1977) and the isolation of antigens from preparations of the microvilli of the syncytiotrophoblast (Ogbimi and Johnson, 1980).

VII. Envoy

There is little to counter Gordon and Chard's despairing thesis that placental proteins have no function; that their concentration in the mother's blood is but a pale reflection of placental mass. That they are at most general indicators of fetal nutrition and growth and no one is better than another for this (Gordon and Chard, 1979). Certainly that hypothesis has as much force with respect to hPL and SP_1 as it ever had. hCG has always been a maverick. Its pregnancy curve bears no resemblance to that of the others and its luteotrophic function is probably real. PP5 and PAPP-A appear more and more different from the others. Their concentration is very doubtfully related to placental weight and they do not reflect fetal growth. They look more and more like essential agents in maternal adaptation to pregnancy, exercising a vital function somewhere where coagulation and immunology meet. If their concentration in the mother's blood has any bearing on that vital function, the answer is to hand. It lies in finding the feedback stimulus which controls their production. If they do anything in the mother there has to be a signal which tells them when to do it and how much to do. PP5 and PAPP-A have the potential for enlarging our understanding of the physiology of pregnancy. They may yet be "Charmed magic casements, opening on the foam of perilous seas in faery lands forlorn."

References

Ahmed, G., and Klopper, A. (1980). *Arch. Gynecol.* **230,** 95–108.
Ahmed, A. G., and Klopper, A. (1981a). *Arch. Gynecol.* **230,** 283–291.
Ahmed, A. G., and Klopper, A. (1981b). *Placenta* **2,** 223–232.
Ahmed, G., and Klopper, A. (1982). *Placenta* **3,** 211–216.
Ahmed, A., M., Toop, K., and Klopper, A. (1981). *Placenta* **2,** 45–52.
Anthony, F., Spencer, K., Mason, P., Masson, G., Price, C. P., and Wood, P. J. (1980a). *Clin. Chim. Acta* **105,** 287–295.
Anthony, F., Masson, G., and Wood, P. (1980b). *Br. J. Obstet. Gynaecol.* **87,** 496–500.
Azer, P. C., Braunstein, G. D., Van de Velde, R., Van de Velde, S., Kogan, R., and Engval, E. (1980). *J. Clin. Endocrinol. Metab.* **50,** 234–239.
Bischof, P. (1979). *Arch. Gynäkol.* **227,** 315–326.
Bischof, P. (1980). *In* "The Human Placenta: Proteins and Hormones" (A. Klopper, A. Genazzani, and P. G. Crosignani, eds.), pp. 47–55. Academic Press, New York.

Bischof, P. (1981). *Placenta* **2,** 29–34.
Bischof, P., Bruce, D.,Cunningham, P., and Klopper, A. (1979). *Clin. Chim. Acta* **95,** 243–247.
Bischof, P., Hughes, G., and Klopper, A. (1980). *Am. J. Obstet. Gynecol.* **138,** 494–499.
Bischof, P., Haenggeli, L., Sizonenko, M., Herrmann, W., and Sizonenko, P. (1981). *Biol. Reprod.* **24,** 1076–1081.
Bischof, P., DuBerg, S., and Schindler, A. (1982). *In* "Immunology of the Placental Proteins" (A. Klopper, ed), pp. 93–102. Saunders, Philadelphia, Pennsylvania.
Bohn, H. (1971). *Arch. Gynäkol.* **210,** 440–457.
Bohn, H. (1972a). **Arch. Gynäkol. 212,** 165–175.
Bohn, H. (1972b). *Blut.* **24,** 292–302.
Bohn, H. (1978). *Scand. J. Immunol.* **7,** 119–125.
Bohn, H. (1979a). In "Carcino-embryonic Proteins" (F. -G. Lehman, ed.). Elsevier, Amsterdam.
Bohn, H. (1979b). *In* "Placental Protcins" (A. Klopper and T. Chard, eds.), pp. 71–85. Springer-Verlag, Berlin and New York.
Bohn, H. (1980). *In* "The Human Placenta: Proteins and Hormones" (A. Klopper, A. Genazzani, and P. Crosignani, eds.), pp. 23–34. Academic Press, New York.
Bohn, H., and Kranz, T. (1973). *Arch. Gynäkol.* **215,** 63–71.
Bohn, H., and Kraus, W. (1977). *Arch. Gynäkol.* **223,** 33–39.
Bohn, H., and Kraus, W. (1979). *Arch. Gynäkol.* **227,** 125–134.
Bohn, H., and Ronneberger, H. (1973). *Arch. Gynäkol.* **215,** 277–281.
Bohn, H., and Sedlacek, H. (1975). *Arch. Gynäkol.* **220,** 105–121.
Bohn, H., and Weinmann, E. (1974). *Arch. Gynäkol.* **217,** 209–218.
Bohn, H., and Weinmann, E. (1976). *Arch. Gynäkol.* **221,** 305–312.
Bohn, H., and Winckler, W. (1977). *Arch. Gynäkol.* **223,** 179–186.
Bohn, H., and Winckler, W. (1980). *Arch Gynäkol.* **229,** 293–301.
Bohn, H., Johannsen, R., and Kraus, W. (1980). *Arch. Gynäkol.* **230,** 167–172.
Bruce, D., and Klopper, A. (1978). *Clin. Chim. Acta* **84,** 107–113.
Cerni, C., Tatra, G., and Bohn, H. (1977). *Arch. Gynäkol.* **223,** 1–7.
Chapman, M. G., and Jones, W. R. (1978). *Aust. N. Z. J. Obstet. Gynaecol.* **18,** 172–175.
Faulk, W. P., and Johnson, P. M. (1977). *Clin. Exp. Immunol.* **27,** 365–375.
Folkersen, J., Westergaard, J., Hindersson, P., and Teisner, B. (1979). *In* "Carcino-embryonic Proteins" (F. -G. Lehman, ed.), Vol. 2, pp. 503–508. Elsevier, Amsterdam.
Folkersen, J., Grudzinskas, J., Hindersson, P., Teisner, B., and Westergaard, J. (1981). *Am. J. Obstet. Gynecol.* **139,** 910–914.
Gall, S. A., and Halbert, S. P. (1972). *Int. Arch. Allergy Appl. Immunol.* **42,** 503–515.
Gordon, Y. B., and Chard, T. (1979). *In* "Placental Proteins" (A. Klopper and T. Chard, eds.), pp. 1–21. Springer-Verlag, Berlin and New York.
Gordon, Y. B., Grudzinskas, J. G., Lewis, J. D., Jeffery, D., and Letchworth, A. T. (1977a). *Br. J. Obstet. Gynaecol.* **84,** 642–647.
Gordon, Y., Grudzinskas, J., Jeffery, D., and Chard, T. (1977b). *Lancet* **1,** 331–333.
Gordon, Y., Lewis, J., Pendlebury, D., Leighton, M., and Gold, J. (1978). *Lancet* **1,** 1001–1003.
Grenner, G. (1978). *Fresenius Z. Anal. Chem.* **290,** 99.
Griffiths, B. W., and Godard, A. (1981). *J. Reprod. Immunol.* **3,** 117–129.
Grudzinskas, J. G., Gordon, Y. B., Jeffery, D., and Chard,T. (1977). *Lancet* **1,** 333–335.
Grudzinskas, J. G., Evans, D. G., Gordon, Y. B., Jeffrey, D., and Chard, T. (1978). *Obstet. Gynecol.* **52,** 43–45.
Grudzinskas, J. G., Menabawey, M., Wiley, B. A., Teisner, B., and Chard, T. (1979a). *Br. J. Obstet. Gynaecol.* **86,** 891–893.

Grudzinskas, J. G., Lenton, E. H., and Obiekwe, B. C. (1979b). *In* "Placental Proteins" (A. Klopper and T. Chard, eds.), pp. 119–131. Springer-Verlag, Berlin and New York.

Grudzinskas, G., Humphreys, J. D., Brudenell, M., and Chard, T. (1979c). *Br. J. Obstet. Gynaecol.* **86,** 978–980.

Grudzinskas, J. G., Charnock, M., Obiekwe, B., Gordon, Y. B., and Chard, T. (1979d). *Br. J. Obstet. Gynaecol.* **86,** 642–644.

Halbert, S. P. (1979). *In* "Placental Proteins" (A. Klopper and T. Chard, eds.), pp. VII-VIII. Springer-Verlag, Berlin and New York.

Halbert, S. P., and Lin, T. -M. (1979). *In* "Placental Proteins" (A. Klopper and T. Chard, eds.), pp. 89–104. Springer-Verlag, Berlin and New York.

Hau, J., Westergaard, J. G., Svendsen, P., Bach, A. and Teisner, B. (1980). *J. Reprod. Fertil.* **60,** 115–119.

Hau, J.,Westergaard, J. G., Svendsen, B., Teisner, B., Bach, A., and Pedersen, P. (1982). *In* "Immunology of the Placental Proteins" (A. Klopper, ed.), Saunders, Philadelphia Pennsylvania. In press.

Heikenheimo, M., Unnerus, H. A., Rantz, T., Jalanko, H., and Seppälä, M. (1978). *Obstet. Gynecol.* **52,** 276–279.

Higuchi, M.,Tokunaga, A., Haruna, N., Tukeuchi, Y. Ozaki, S.,Iwata, K., Takahashi,K., and Takeuchis, S. (1978). *Acta Obstet. Gynaecol. Jpn.* **30,** 323–329.

Hindersson, P., Folkersen, J., Westergaard, J. G., Teisner, B., and Svehag, S. E. (1979). *J. Reprod. Immunol.* **1,** 159–166.

Hindersson, P., Teisner, B., Folkersen, J., Grudzinskas, J. G., and Westergaard, J. G. (1981). *Placenta* **2,** 233–240.

Horne, C. H., Towler, C. M., Pugh-Humphreys, R. G., Thomson, A. W., and Bohn, H. (1976a). *Experientia* **32,** 1197–1199.

Horne, C. H., Reid, I. N., and Milne, G. D. (1976b). *Lancet* **1,** 279–282.

Horne, C. H., Bremner, R. D., Jandial, V., Glover, R. G., and Towler, C. M. (1979a). *In* "Placental Proteins" (A. Klopper and T. Chard, eds.), pp. 143–160. Springer-Verlag, Berlin and New York.

Horne, C. H., Pugh-Humphreys, R. G., and Bremner, R. (1979b). *In* "Carcino-embryonic Proteins" (F. -G. Lehman, ed.), Vol. 1, pp. 301–311. Elsevier, Amsterdam.

Hughes, G., Bischof, P., Wilson, G., Smith, R., and Klopper, A. (1980a). *Br. J. Obstet. Gynaecol.* **87,** 650–656.

Hughes, G., Bishcof, P., Wilson, G., and Klopper, A. (1980b). *Br. Med. J.* **1,** 671–673.

Jandial, V., Towler, C., Horne, C., and Abramovich, D. (1978). *Br. J. Obstet. Gynecol.* **85,** 832–836.

Jouppila, P., Seppälä, M., and Chard, T. (1980). *Lancet* **1,** 667–668.

Karg, N. J., Than, G., Arany, I., Szigetvari, I., and Csaba, I. (1978). *IRCS Med. Sci.* **6,** 74.

Klopper, A. (1980). *Excerpta Med. Int. Congr. Ser.* **512,** 1066–1071.

Klopper, A. (1981a). *In* "Current Status of EPH Gestosis" (A. Kurjak, E. Rippman, and V. Salovic, eds.), pp. 288–291. Excerpta Medica, Amsterdam.

Klopper, A. (1981b). *In* "Endocrinology of Pregnancy" (J.R. Givens, ed.), pp. 203–211. Year Book Medical Publ. Chicago, Illinois.

Klopper, A. (1982). *In* "Immunology of Placental Proteins" (A. Klopper, ed.), pp. 83–92. Saunders, Philadelphia, Pennsylvania.

Klopper, A., and Hughes, G. (1980). *In* "The Human Placenta: Proteins and Hormones" (A. Klopper, A. Genazzani, and P. G. Crosignani, eds.), pp. 17–22. Acadmeic Press, New York.

Klopper, A., Masson, G., and Wilson, G. (1977). *Br. J. Obstet. Gynaecol.* **84,** 648–655.

Klopper, A., Buchan, P., and Wilson,G. (1978). *Br. J. Obstet. Gynaecol.* **85,** 738–747.

Klopper, A., Smith, R., and Davidson, I. (1979). *In* "Placental Proteins" (A. Klopper and T. Chard, eds.). Springer-Verlag, Berlin and New York.

Koh, S. H., and Cauchi, M. (1981). *Eur. J. Obstet Gynecol. Reprod. Biol.* **11,** 215–219..

Lee, J. N., Grudzinskas, J. G., and Chard, T. (1979). *Br. J. Obstet. Gynaecol.* **86,** 888–890.

Lee, J. N., Salem, H. T., Al-Ani, A., Chard, T., Huang, S. C., Ouyang, P. C., Wei, P. Y., and Seppälä, M. (1981a). *Am. J. Obstet. Gynecol.* **139,** 702–704.

Lee, J. N., Salem, H. T., Huang, S. C., Ouyang, P. C., Seppälä, M., and Chard, T. (1981b). *Int. J. Obstet. Gynecol.* **19,** 65–67.

Lin, T.-M., and Halbert, S. P. (1975). *Int. Arch. Allergy Appl. Immunol.* **48,** 101–115.

Lin, T.-M., and Halbert, S. P. (1976). *Science* **193,** 1249–1252.

Lin, T.-M., and Halbert, S P. (1978). *Int. Arch. Allergy Appl. Immunol.* **56,** 207–223,

Lin, T.-M., Halbert, S. P., Kiefer, D., Spellacy, W. N., and Gall, S. (1974a). *Am. J. Obstet. Gynecol.* **118,** 223–236.

Lin, T.-M., Halbert, S. P., and Kiefer, D. (1974b). *Proc. Soc. Exp. Biol. Med.* **145,** 62–66.

Lin, T.-M., Halbert, S. P., Kiefer, D., and Spellacy, W. N. (1974c) *Int. Arch. Allergy* **47,** 35–53.

Lin, T.-M., Halbert, S. P., and Spellacy, W. (1974d). *J. Clin. Invest.* **54,** 576–581.

Lin, T.-M., Halbert, S. P., Spellacy, W. N., and Gall, S. (1976a). *Am. J. Obstet. Gynecol.* **124,** 382–387.

Lin, T.-M., Halbert, S. P., and Spellacy, W. N. (1976b). *Am. J. Obstet. Gynecol.* **125,** 17–24.

Lin, T.-M., Halbert, S. P., and Kiefer, D. (1976c). *J. Clin. Invest.* **57,** 466–472.

Lin, T.-M., Halbert, S. P., Spellacy, W. N., and Berne, B. H. (1977). *Am. J. Obstet. Gynecol.* **128,** 808–810.

Lin, T.-M., Halbert, S. P., and Keifer, D. (1978a). *Int. Arch. Allergy Appl. Immunol.* **57,** 294–303.

Lin, T.-M., Halbert, S. P., and Spellacy, W. N. (1978b). *Br. J. Obstet. Gynaecol.* **85,** 652–656.

McIntyre, J. A., Hsi, B., Faulk, W. P., Klopper, A., and Thomson, R. (1981). *Immunology* **44,** 577–583.

Mancini, G., Cabonara, A. O., and Heremans, J. P. (1965). *Immunochemistry* **2,** 235–254.

Masson, G., Klopper, A., and Wilson, G. (1977). *Obstet. Gynaecol.* **50,** 435–438.

Menabawey, M., Grudzinskas, J. G., and Chard, T. (1979). *Br. J. Obstet. Gynaecol.* **86,** 894–896.

Nisbet, A. D., Bremner, R. D., Herrot, R., Jandial, V., Horne, C. H., and Bohn, H. (1981). *Br. J. Obstet. Gynaecol.* **88,** 484–491.

Obiekwe, B., Pendlebury, P. J., Gordon, Y. B., Grudzinskas, J. G., Chard, T. and Bohn, H. (1979a). *Clin. Chim. Acta* **95,** 509–516.

Obiekwe, B. C., Grudzinskas, J. G., Gordon, Y. B., and Chard, T. (1979b). *Br. J. Obstet. Gynaecol.* **86,** 897–900.

Obiekwe, B. C., Grudzinskas, J. G., and Chard, T. (1980a). *In* "The Human Placenta: Proteins and Hormones" (A. Klopper, A. Genazzani, and P. G. Crosignani, eds.), pp. 129–136. Academic Press, New York.

Obiekwe, B. C., Grudzinskas, J. G., and Chard, T. (1980b). *Br. J. Obstet. Gynaecol.* **87,** 302–304.

Ogbimi, A. O., and Johnson, P. M. (1980). *J. Reprod. Immunol.* **1,** 127–140.

Pluta, M., Hardt, W., Schmidt-Gollwitzer, K., and Schmidt-Gollwitzer, M. (1979). *Arch. Gynecol.* **227,** 327–336.

Ranta, T., Siteri, J., Koistinen, R., Salem, H. T., Bohn, H., Koskimies, A., and Seppälä, M. (1981). *J. Clin. Endocrinol. Metab.* **53,** 1087–1089.

Rosen, S. W., Kaminska, J., Calvert, I., Ellmore, N., and Aaronson, S. (1980). *Am. J. Obstet. Gynecol.* **137,** 525–529.

Salem, H. T., Obiekwe, B. C., Al-Ani, A. T., Seppälä, M., and Chard, T. (1980). *Clin. Chim. Acta* **107,** 211–215.

Salem, H. T., Lee, J. N., Seppälä, M., Vaara, L., Aula, P., Al-Ani, A. T., and Chard, T. (1981a). *Brit. J. Obstet. Gynaecol.* **88**, 371–374.
Salem, H. T., Seppälä, M., Ranta, T., Bohn, H., and Chard, T. (1981b). *Br. J. Obstet. Gynaecol.* **88**, 367–370.
Salem, H. T., Seppälä, M., and Chard, T. (1981c). *Placenta* **2**, 205–210.
Salem, H. T., Westergaard, J. G., Hindersson, P., Seppälä, M., and Chard, T. (1982). *Br. J. Obstet. Gynaecol.* In press.
Schultz-Larsen, P. (1978). *Scand. J. Immunol.* **8**, 591–597.
Schultz-Larsen, P., and Hertz, J. (1978). *Eur. J. Obstet. Gynecol. Reprod. Biol.* **8**, 253–257.
Schultz-Larsen, P., Sizaret, P., Martel, N., and Hindersson, P. (1979a). *Clin. Chim. Acta* **95**, 347–351.
Schultz-Larsen, P., Lyngbye, J., Westergaard, J. G., and Teisner, B. (1979b). *Clin. Chim. Acta* **99**, 59–69.
Searle, F., Bagshawe, K., Dent, J., and Leake, B. (1978). *Scand. J. Immunol.* **8**, 587–590.
Searle, F., Leake, B. A., Bagshawe, K. D., and Dent, J. (1981). *Lancet* **1**, 579–581.
Sedlacek, H. H., Rehkopf, R., and Bohn, H. (1976). *Behring Inst. Mitt.* **59**, 81–91.
Seppälä, M., Ratanen, E., Jalanko, H., Lehtovirta, P., Stenman, U., and Engval, E. (1978). *J. Clin. Endocrinol.* **47**, 1216–1219.
Seppälä, M., Ronnberg, L., Ylostala, P., and Jouppila, P. (1979). *Fertil. Steril.* **32**, 608–609.
Seppälä, M., Venesmaa, P., and Ratanen, E. (1980). *Am. J. Obstet. Gynecol.* **136**, 189–193.
Siekmann, U., and Heilmann, L. (1979). *Z. Geburtshilfe Perinatol.* **183**, 351–358.
Sinosich, M. J., Teisner, B., Davey, M., and Grudzinskas, J. G. (1981). *Aust. N. Z. J. Med.* **11**, 429–433.
Smith, R., Klopper, A., Hughes, G., and Wilson, G. (1979a). *Br. J. Obstet. Gynaecol.* **86**, 119–123.
Smith, R., Bischof, P., Hughes, G., and Klopper, A. (1979b). *Br. J. Obstet. Gynaecol.* **86**, 882–887.
Smith, R., Cooper, W., and Thomson, M. (1980). *In* "The Human Placenta: Proteins and Hormones" (A. Klopper, A. Genazzani, and P. Crosignani, eds.), pp. 109–113. Academic Press, New York.
Smith, R., Thomson, M., and Cooper, W. (1981). *Placenta* **2**, 143–148.
Sørensen, S. (1978). *Acta Obstet. Gynecol. Scand.* **57**, 193–197.
Sørensen, S., Borggaard, B., and Rolff, L. (1977). *Scand. J. Clin. Lab. Invest.* **37**, 537–543.
Stevens, V. C., Bohn, H., and Powell, J. E. (1976). *Am. J. Obstet. Gynecol.* **124**, 51–54.
Stimson, W. H. (1980). *Clin. Exp. Immunol.* **40**, 157–160.
Sutcliffe, R. G., Kukulska, B. M., Nicholson, L. V., and Paterson, W. F. (1979). *In* "Placental Proteins" (A. Klopper and T. Chard, eds.), pp. 55–70. Springer-Verlag, Berlin and New York.
Sutcliffe, R. G., Kukulska-Langlands, B. M., Coggins, J. R., Hunter, J. B., and Gore, C. H. (1980a). *Biochem. J.* **191**, 779–809.
Sutcliffe, R. G., Hunter, J. B., Gibb, S., and MacLean, A. B.(1980b). *In* "The Human Placenta: Proteins and Hormones" (A. Klopper, A. Genazzani, and P. G. Crosignani, eds.), pp. 57–66. Academic Press, New York.
Sykes, A., and Chard, T. (1980). *Clin. Chem.* **26**, 1224–1226.
Tatarinov, Y. S. (1979). *In* "Carcino-embryonic Proteins" (F.-G. Lehamn, ed.), Vol. 1, pp. 313–319. Elsevier, Amsterdam.
Tatarinov, Y. S., and Masyukevich, V. N. (1970). *Bull. Exp. Biol. Med. USSR* **69**, 66–68.
Tatarinov, Y. S., Falaleeva, D. M., and Kalashnikov, V. V. (1976a). *Int. J. Cancer* **17**, 626–630.
Tatarinov, Y. S., Falaleeva, D. M., Kalashnikov, V. V., and Toloknov, B. O. (1976b). *Nature London* **260**, 263.

Tatarinov, Y. S., Kozljaeva, G. A., Petrunina, D. D., and Petrunina, Y. A. (1980). *In* "The Human Placenta: Proteins and Hormones" (A. Klopper, A. Genazzani, and P. Crosignani, eds.), pp. 35–46. Academic Press, New York.

Tatra, G. (1979). *Fortschr. Med.* **97**, 459–462.

Tatra, G., Breitenecker, G., and Gruber, W. (1974). *Arch. Gynäkol.* **217**, 383–390.

Tatra, G., Placheta, P., and Breitenecker, G. (1975). *Wien. Klin. Wochenschr.* **87**, 279–281.

Tatra, G., Tempfer, H., and Placheta, P. (1976). *Eur. J. Obstet. Gynecol. Reprod. Biol.* **6**, 53–57.

Tatra, G., Riss, P., and Bohn, H. (1979). *Z. Geburtshilfe. Perinatol.* **183**, 254–256.

Tatra, G., Polak, S., and Nasr, F. (1981a). *Geburtshilfe. Frauenheilkd.* **41**, 359–361.

Tatra, G., Polak, S., Nasr, F., and Dati, F. (1981b). *Arch. Gynäkol.* **230**, 293–297.

Teisner, B., Westergaard, J. G., Folkersen, J., Husby, S., and Svehag, S. E. (1978). *Am. J. Obstet. Gynecol.* **131**, 262–266.

Teisner, B., Folkersen, J., Hindersson, P., Jensenuis, J. C., and Westergaard, J. G. (1979a). *Scand. J. Immunol.* **9**, 409–417.

Teisner, B., Grudzinskas, J. G., Hindersson, P., Al-Ani, A. T., Westergaard, J G., and Chard, T. (1979b). *J. Immunol. Methods* **31**, 141–149.

Toop, K., and Klopper, A. (1981). *In* "Placenta: Receptors, Pathology and Toxicology" (R. K. Miller and H. Thiede, eds.), pp. 167–171. Saunders, Philadelphia, Pennsylvania.

Toop, K., and Klopper, A. (1982). *Br. J. Obstet. Gynaecol.* In Press.

Towler, C. M., Horne, C. H., Jandial, V., Campbell, D. M., and MacGillvray, I. (1976a). *Br. J. Obstet. Gynaecol.* **83**, 775–779.

Towler, C., Jandial, V., Horne, C., and Bohn, H. (1976b). *Br. J. Obstet. Gynaecol.* **83**, 386–374.

Towler, C. M., Horne, C. H., Jandial, V., and Chesworth, J. M. (1977a). *Br. J. Obstet. Gynaecol.* **84**, 580–584.

Towler, C., Horne, C., Jandial, V., Campbell, D., and MacGillivary, I. (1977b). *Br. J. Obstet. Gynaecol.* **84**, 258–263.

Towler, C. M., Glover, R. G., and Horne, C. H. (1978). *Clin. Chim. Acta* **87**, 289–296.

Viala, J., Bastide, J., Guibal, J., Oudghiri, T., and Donati, R. (1980). *J. Gynecol. Obstet. Biol. Reprod.* **9**, 419–424.

Wahlström, T., Teisner, B., and Folkersen, J. (1981). *Placenta* **2**, 253–258.

Weber, H., Heller, S., and Seulen, P. (1980). *Geburtshilfe Frauenheilkd.* **40**, 339–343.

Westergaard, J.,Teisner, B., Folkersen, J. Hindersson, P., Schultz-Larsen, P. and Svehag, S-E., (1979a). *Scand. J. Clin. Lab. Invest.* **39**, 351–359.

Westergaard, J. G., Folkersen, J., Hindersson, P., Svehag, S-E., and Teisner, B. (1979b). *In* "Carcino-embryonic Proteins" (F.-G. Lehman, ed.), Vol. 2, pp. 463–468. Elsevier, Amsterdam.

Westergaard, J. G., Folkersen, J., Hindersson, P., and Teisner, B. (1980). *In* "The Human Placenta: Proteins and Hormones" (A. Klopper, A. Genazzani, and P. G. Crosignani, eds.), pp. 121–128. Academic Press, New York.

Wood, P. J., Cockett, D., and Mason, P. (1978). *Clin. Chim. Acta* **90**, 87–91.

Wurz, H. (1979). *Arch. Gynäkol.* **227**, 1–6.

Wurz, H., Geiger, W., Künzig, H. J., Jabs-Lehmann, A., Bohn, H., and Lüben, G. (1981). *J. Perinatol. Med.* **9**, 67–78.

HUMAN PLACENTAL LACTOGEN

T. Chard

DEPARTMENTS OF REPRODUCTIVE PHYSIOLOGY AND OBSTETRICS AND GYNAECOLOGY
ST. BARTHOLOMEW'S HOSPITAL MEDICAL COLLEGE
LONDON, ENGLAND

I. Introduction 168
II. Nomenclature 168
III. Placental Lactogenic Hormones in Other Species 169
IV. Placental Lactogen and Other Placental Proteins 169
V. Synthesis 169
VI. Immunochemical Nature 172
VII. Biological Nature 173
VIII. Biological Functions 174
IX. Control Mechanisms 176
X. Metabolism and Clearance 177
XI. Levels in Different Biological Fluids 178
XII. Assay of hPL in Blood 179
XIII. Maternal Levels in Normal Pregnancy 179
XIV. Interpretation of Biochemical Tests of Fetoplacental Function 180
XV. Maternal Levels in Complications of Pregnancy 181
   A. Trophoblastic Tumors 181
   B. Threatened Abortion 182
   C. Low Birthweight Infants 182
   D. Preeclampsia and Hypertension 183
   E. Diabetes Mellitus 184
   F. Rhesus Isoimmunization 184
   G. Fetal Death 185
   H. Fetal Distress and Neonatal Asphyxia 185

Current Topics in
Experimental Endocrinology, Vol. 4

ISBN 0-12-153204-6

I. Miscellaneous Conditions 186
XVI. Clinical Use of hPL—Conclusions 186
References 187

I. Introduction

That the human placenta contains a substance having mammotrophic activity was first clearly shown by Ito and Higashi (1961). Subsequently, Josimovich and MacLaren (1962) demonstrated that the material was immunochemically similar to human pituitary growth hormone (hGH) and that it occurred in maternal peripheral serum, retroplacental serum, and placental extracts. These early investigations have now been fully confirmed and extended, and further studies have yielded a very full picture of the physiology and pathophysiology of the hormone. In addition, measurement of placental lactogen in the mother's blood during pregnancy has become one of the most universally accepted biochemical tests of placental function for studying the clinical well being of the fetus and placenta in current obstetric practice.

II. Nomenclature

There is much confusion over the nomenclature of the protein which in this article will be referred to as human placental lactogen or hPL. However, several other designations have been put forward, including human chorionic growth hormone-prolactin (hCGP) (Grumbach and Kaplan, 1964), purified placental protein (PPP) (Florini *et al.,* 1966), human chorionic somatomammotrophin (hCS) (Li *et al.,* 1968), and choriomammotrophin (IUPAC-IAB, 1975). The term hCS is widely used and has been promoted by Bewley and Li (1974) on the grounds that it provides a clear description of the relationship of this protein to other hormones. In addition, the term "chorionic" is more specific than "placental" and is commonly used for other placental hormones such as chorionic gonadotrophin and chorionic corticotrophin. However, many find the term chorionic somatomammotrophin to be inelegant and cumbersome and accordingly prefer the original name of placental lactogen. A new problem is the fact that the "specificity" to the placenta/chorion is now in considerable doubt: thus, human seminal plasma contains *high* levels of hPL and several other proteins previously considered to be specific to the placenta (Salem and Chard, unpublished observations).

III. Placental Lactogenic Hormones in Other Species

Similar lactogenic hormones have been found in the placenta of other species such as the goat (Buttle *et al.,* 1972), the Rhesus monkey (Walsh *et al.,* 1977), and the sheep (Handwerger *et al.,* 1977). The only notable exceptions among mammals appear to be the pig and the dog (Porter, 1980).

IV. Placental Lactogen and Other Placental Proteins

Placental lactogen is one of a large group of placental "specific" proteins (Table I), some of which seem to be unique as they have no obvious counterpart in the adult while others, such as hPL, are similar but not necessarily identical to adult products. The production of these materials, most of which have no obvious physiological function *in vivo,* is a major biological enigma (Gordon and Chard, 1979).

It is possible to classify the placental proteins into two groups. Group I consists of those materials which appear to have "hormonal" function (in the broadest sense of "action at a distance"); these include the hormone analogs and the enzymes. Group II consists of materials which seem to have local function in respect of the coagulation and complement systems; these include PP5 and PAPP-A.

V. Synthesis

As with other placental proteins hPL appears to be a product of the syncytiotrophoblast. The experimental evidence for this arises from immunohistochemical studies (Ikonicoff and Cedard, 1973). More recently the molecular biological approach has also been used to confirm the site of synthesis of hPL (McWilliams and Boime, 1980). Using labelled complementary DNA (^{3}H-cDNA) as a gene probe, it was shown that the bulk of the mRNA for hPL is in the syncytiotrophoblast. A similar approach has also been used on rat/human cell hybrids to show that the genes for both growth hormone and hPL are on the long arm of human chromosome 17 (George *et al.,* 1981).

The localization of the protein-synthesizing machinery within the trophoblast was studied by Burgos and Rodrigues (1966) who showed a clear differentiation between thick areas of the trophoblast cytoplasm which are rich in endoplasmic reticulum and microvilli and therefore appear to be specialized for protein synthesis, together with thin areas without microvilli which lie in proximity to fetal capillaries and appear to be specialized for the

Table I
Proteins Produced by the Human Placenta

Protein	Abbreviation
Human chorionic gonadotrophin	hCG
Human placental lactogen	hPL
Human chorionic somatomammotrophin	hCS
Human chorionic corticotrophin	hCCT
Human chorionic thyrotrophin-releasing hormone	hC-TRH
Human chorionic gonadotrophin releasing hormone	hC-LRH
Schwangerschafts-spezifiches glykoprotein 1	SP_1
Pregnancy-associated plasma protein A	PAPP-A
Pregnancy-associated plasma protein B	PAPP-B
Heat stable alkaline phosphatase	HSAP
Cystine aminopeptidase (oxytocinase)	CAP
Diamine oxidase (histaminase)	DO
Placental protein 5	PP5

transport of nutrients and waste products (Fig.1). The differentiation between these areas is of potential clinical significance because it is possible that a process which damages the critically important transfer area would leave the synthetic areas intact. However, most trophoblast pathology is secondary to factors such as occlusion of fetal capillaries in the chorionic villus or maternal decidual arterioles and it is likely in practice that all areas will be equally affected. The synthetic mechanisms of hPL in the trophoblast are

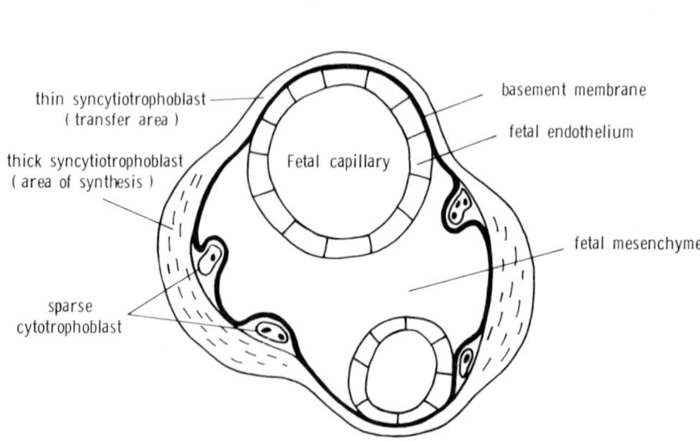

Fig. 1. Diagram of the structure of a chorionic villus of the human placenta. Note that separate areas of the trophoblast may be involved in synthesis and transfer.

similar to those of proteins in other tissues. Friesen and his co-workers (Friesen *et al.,* 1972; Suwa and Friesen, 1969a,b) examined the incorporation of ^{3}H-labeled amino acids by placental fragments *in vitro,* and showed that hPL accounts for a large proportion (up to 55% in some experiments) of the total labeled protein released into incubation medium. In the tissue itself the ratio of labeled hPL/labeled total protein was much lower (4%).The apparent molecular weight of labeled hPL released during the earlier stages of incubation was identical to that of authentic hPL; with more prolonged incubation a high molecular weight species appeared. In the tissue itself most of the hPL was of high molecular weight (> 100,000). The relationship between the high- and low-molecular-weight forms was not defined: their only common feature was the fact that both reacted with an antiserum to hPL. The specific activity of labeled hPL was higher in the medium than the tissue, suggesting the existence of two pools in the latter site: one of rapid turnover, and a second, more stable variety.The conclusions of these experiments are summarized in Fig. 2.

Subsequent studies have shown that polysomes and messenger RNA from the placenta can direct the synthesis of hPL in cell-free systems (Boime and Boguslawski, 1974; Boime *et al.,* 1976, 1977; Cox *et al.,* 1976); synthesis by polysomes from term placenta is four times greater than that of first trimester polysomes. As the efficiency of the first trimester and term mRNA is similar in terms of amino acid incorporation, it would appear that the relative levels of hPL–mRNA are greater in the term placenta (Boime *et al.,* 1976). When free polysomes are used in a cell-free system a "prelactogen" of molecular weight 25,000 is produced; the extra protein or "precursor piece" is at the NH_2-terminus of the molecule and contains an abundance of leucine residues. In the presence of membrane fractions from endoplasmic reticulum, the "prelactogen" is converted to authentic hPL; it has been suggested that the precursor piece is a 25 amino acid sequence which plays a part in the formation of membrane-bound ribosomal complexes (Fig. 3).

The primary gene product appears to be pre-hPL with a molecular weight of 25,000, and it is likely that the high-molecular-weight precursor (> 100,000) detected by Suwa and Freisen (1961) represented a complex of

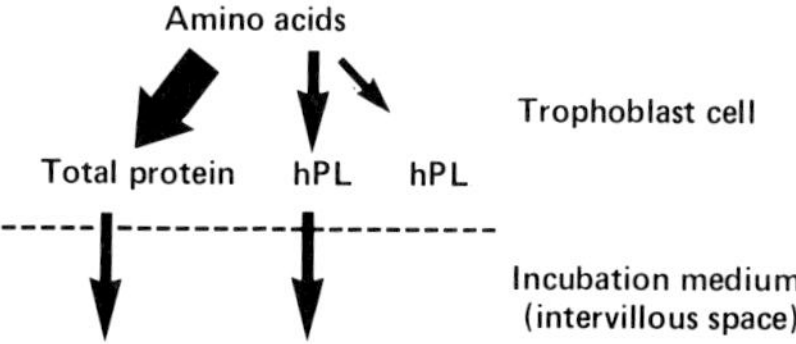

Fig. 2. Diagram of the conclusions reached by Suwa and Friesen on the synthesis and secretion of hPL by the human placenta *in vitro.*

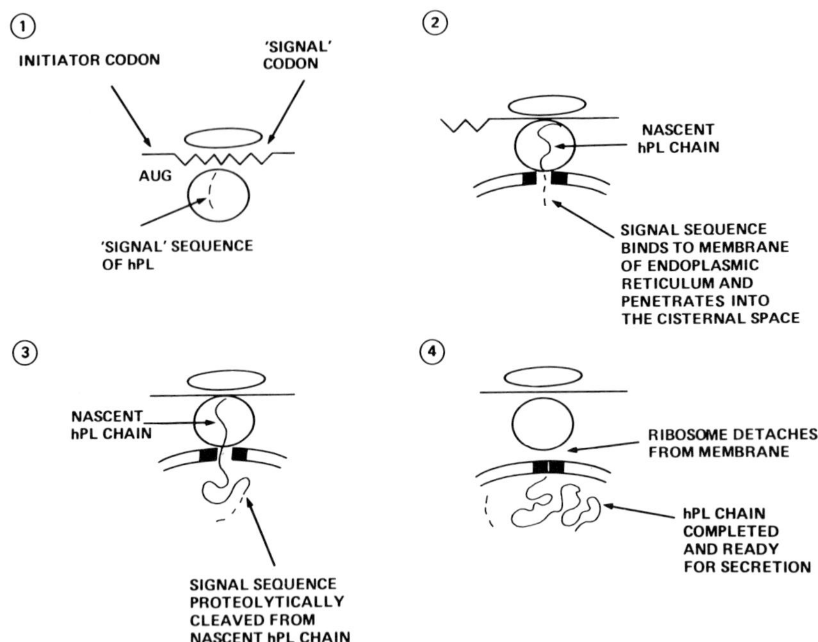

Fig. 3. A scheme for the synthesis and secretion of hPL by the trophoblast, based on the experimental findings described in the text and the "signal hypothesis" of protein secretion. (1) Synthesis of hPL is started by an initiator codon (AUG) on mRNA, together with two ribosome subunits. A unique sequence of codons, immediately to the right of the initiator codon, is translated into a unique sequence of amino acids on the N-terminus of the nascent hPL molecule. This is the so-called "signal sequence" or "precursor piece" which contains a high proportion of the hydrophobic amino acid leucine. (2) The signal sequence binds to a receptor on the membrane of the endoplasmic reticulum. This permits the nascent hPL chain to pass through the membrane into the cisterna. (3) The complete hPL chain enters the cisterna as it is translated by the ribosome (the ribosome remains bound to the membrane during this process). The signal piece is proteolytically cleaved from the nascent hPL chain. (4) The authentic hPL chain is completed and the ribsome dissociates from the membrane. This hypothesis explains why pre-hPL, i.e., with the signal sequence attached, is synthesized in cell-free systems containing only free polysomes, while authentic hPL is produced if a membrane fraction is included.

pre-hPL and membrane components or possibly a stable dimeric form of hPL (two hPL molecules joined by disulfide exchange links) (Schneider *et al.,* 1977).

VI. Immunochemical Nature

There have been several descriptions of the isolation and purification of hPL (Cohen *et al.,* 1964; Friesen,1965; Turtle *et al.,* 1966; Florini *et al.,*

1966). After extraction from placental tissue and chemical precipitation, final purification is achieved by combinations of gel filtration, ion-exchange chromatography, and electrophoresis.

Human placental lactogen is a polypeptide of MW 21,000 with a single chain of 191 amino acids and two intrachain disulfide bonds (Niall *et al.*, 1973). The amino acid composition is very similar to that of hGH, the main differences being in the number of methionine, histidine, and proline residues. The amino acid sequence of the two hormones is identical at 163 of the 191 residues (86% sequence homology), and the disulfide bonds are located in homologous portions of each molecule. Most of the differences are near the NH_2-terminus, and of the observed substitutions only one requires more than a single base change in the triplet codon. The amino acid sequences of hPL and hGH are also similar to that of prolactin (13% sequence homology with hPL, 16% with hGH), though prolactin has 198 amino acids and three intrachain disulfide bonds (Shome and Parlow, 1977).

Studies with recombined fragments generated by limited plasmin digestion and reduction of hPL and hGH have shown that most of the immunological and biological properties of these hormones are associated with the NH_2-terminal 1–134 amino acids (Russell *et al.*, 1981b). Cleavage of the hPL molecule at residue 86 (tryptophan) completely destroys the immunological and biological activity (Russell *et al.*, 1981a).

It is likely that hPL, hGH, and prolactin originated from a shorter primordial peptide of 25–30 amino acids. At an early stage a structural divergence produced two evolutionary lines: one with primarily lactogenic activity, and the other with somatotrophic activity. At a later stage individual species showed further divergence within these lines thus yielding the differences between, for instance, the structure of sheep and human pituitary growth hormone and prolactin. Finally divergences occurred within species leading to the existence of separate pituitary and placental proteins. These concepts are illustrated diagrammatically in Fig. 4.

VII. Biological Nature

A multiplicity of biological activities has been proposed for hPL including growth promotion, lactogenesis, an effect on carbohydrate and lipid metabolism, stimulation of the corpus luteum, erythropoiesis, inhibition of fibrinolysis, and immunosuppression. Although it is chemically similar to hGH, hPL has only weak somatotrophic activity equivalent to 0.1–1% of that of the pituitary protein. The extent of the lactogenic activity of hPL has been disputed. Early reports suggested that its potency was some 75% that of sheep prolactin (Josimovich and Brande, 1964). However, later studies

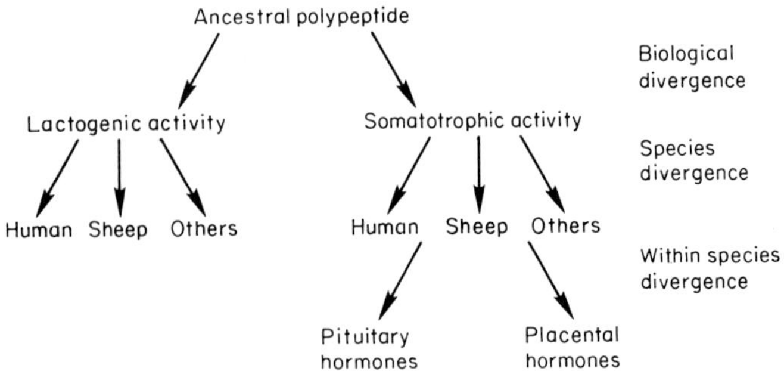

Fig. 4. Diagrammatic representation of the evolutionary divergence of the lactogenic and somatotrophic hormones (modified from Bewley and Li, 1974). It should be noted that the divergence between pituitary and placental forms seems to be universal, since it has been found in all species so far examined.

showed much lower activity (Friesen, 1965; Florini *et al.*, 1966) (1–4 U/mg in the pigeon crop-sac assay). The potency in the rabbit intraductal assay is greater than that in the pigeon crop-sac assay; a similar discrepancy has been observed with human growth hormone. Studies using intact animals have yielded estimates ranging from 20 to 100% of that of prolactin (Handwerger and Sherwood, 1974). Thus, the apparent lactogenic activity of hPL is highly dependent on the purity of the material examined, on the type of assay, and on the animal species used for the assay. It is difficult and perhaps impossible to assign an exact potency.

In rodents hPL has luteotrophic activity, and may influence placental progesterone secretion, particularly the interconversion of progesterone and the biologically inactive 20α-dihydroprogesterone (Josimovich and Archer, 1977). Administration of hPL in animals leads to a rise in blood sugar and impairment of carbohydrate tolerance (Burt *et al.*, 1966; Handwerger *et al.*, 1976); this may be due to increased peripheral resistance to insulin action, though in hypophysectomized rats hPL can cause an increase in insulin release *in vitro* from islet cells (Martin and Friesen, 1969).

In mice hPL stimulates erythropoietin secretion and thus the incorporation of iron into red blood cells (Jepson and Friesen, 1968). Both hPL and hCG can suppress phytohemagglutinin-induced lymphocyte transformation and may play a part in the immune survival of a pregnancy (Contractor and Davies, 1973).

VIII. Biological Functions

It is essential to distinguish between activity and function. A biological molecule may have a specific effect in an experimental system but this does not necessarily mean that it is responsible for the same effect in normal physiology. The distinction is especially notable with the biologically active placental proteins: none has been clearly identified as essential for any physiological event, and it has even been suggested that the placental proteins have no biological function but rather are waste products of the general activities of the placenta as an independent organism (Gordon and Chard,1979).

An important function of hPL in normal gestation could be the preparation of the breast for lactation. But there are several other potential candidates for this function, including placental estrogens and progesterone and maternal pituitary prolactin all of which are elevated concomitantly. Administration of hPL to nonpregnant subjects in amounts sufficient to yield blood levels comparable to those in mid-gestation does not induce lactation (Josimovich *et al.,* 1974). In addition lactation can be induced by appropriate breast stimulation even in subjects who have never been pregnant.

Similar reservations exist as to the possible role of hPL in carbohydrate and lipid metabolism. It is well recognized that pregnancy constitutes a diabetogenic stress, and impairment of carbohydrate tolerance with elevated levels of circulating insulin and free fatty acids are normal findings. It would be attractive to hypothesize that the pregnant woman tends to retain glucose within her circulation where it is available for transport across the placenta to the developing fetus, and especially to the fetal brain for which glucose is the essential and only energy source. This possibility is supported by several experimental observations. Administration of hPL to nonpregnant subjects leads to impaired carbohydrate tolerance and increased levels of insulin (Beck and Daughaday, 1967; Kalkhoff *et al.,* 1969), and plasma free fatty acids (Riggi *et al.,* 1966). Blood levels of hPL decrease following intravenous administration of glucose (Burt *et al.,* 1970; Spellacy *et al.,* 1971; Pavlou *et al.,* 1973) (Fig. 5). Pavlou and his colleagues showed that the change is small and inconsistent, and might also be attributed to trivial mechanisms such as the osmotic expansion of plasma volume which results from injection of a hypertonic solution; no response has been claimed after oral administration of glucose (Pavlou *et al.,* 1973). In the sheep maternal hyperglycemia produces no change in placental lactogen (oPL) levels in fetus or ewe (Brinsmead *et al.,* 1981). Others have shown increases of blood hPL levels during insulin-induced hypoglycemia (Spellacy *et al.,* 1971) and prolonged starvation (Tyson *et al.,* 1971; Kim and Felig,1971; Brinsmead *et al.,* 1981), but the changes are small when compared with those of pituitary growth hormone under similar circumstances. The case that hPL plays a major role in carbohydrate metabolism in pregnancy is not strong and equally good candidates would be the placental steroid hormones (estrogens and progesterone) which at levels much lower than those in late pregnancy (e.g., in

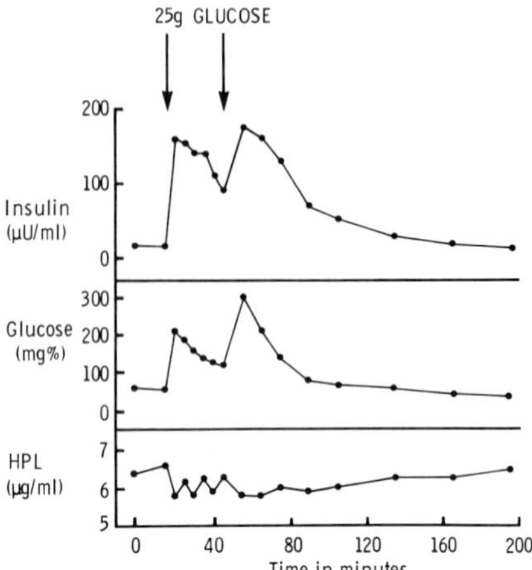

Fig. 5. Plasma levels of insulin, glucose, and hPL in 10 subjects following iv injection of glucose.

subjects on oral contraceptive agents) can produce all the changes characteristic of a prediabetic state.

It would also be attractive to speculate that hPL via its somatotrophic effect is an important growth-promoting factor for the fetus. But this possibility is ruled out by two observations: the somatotrophic activity of hPL is extremely low (1% or less) compared with that of pituitary growth hormone; and the levels of hPL in the fetal circulation are 1000-fold less than those in the mother.

IX. Control Mechanisms

As with other placental hormones there is little evidence for the existence of control mechanisms such as exist for comparable products of the adult. Though a variety of natural and synthetic agents have been examined as possible releasing or inhibiting factors, the doses examined are always pharmacological and the results are unlikely to reflect physiological events (Table II).

A hypothesis has been proposed (Chard, 1976) (Fig. 6) which suggests that the potential for placental protein production is a function of the total mass of the trophoblast; that the rate of release depends on the concentration of the protein in maternal blood in the intervillous space; and that this concentration, in turn, depends on the rate of blood flow in the intervillous space. Thus hPL will diffuse from the trophoblast cell down a concentration gra-

Table II
Effects of Various Pharmacological Agents on hPL Production by the Placenta

Agent	Observation	Author
Arginine	Rise in maternal hPL levels after intravenous injection	Prieto *et al.* (1976)
Arginine/ornithine	Rise in ovine maternal hPL levels after intravenous injection	Handwerger *et al.* (1978) Handwerger *et al.* (1981)
Cyclic AMP/theophylline	No effect on hPL secretion by placental explants *in vitro*	Handwerger *et al.* (1973)
Dopamine	Enhanced hPL secretion by placental explants *in vitro*	Macaron *et al.* (1978)
$PGF_{2\alpha}$	Progressive fall in maternal hPL levels after intraamniotic injection	Ward *et al.* (1977)
Pimozide	Decreased hPL secretion by placental explants *in vitro*	Macaron *et al.* (1978)
Somatostatin	No effect on hPL secretion by placental explants *in vitro*	Belleville *et al.* (1972)
TRH	Rise in maternal hPL levels after intravenous injection. No effect on hPL secretion by placental explants *in vitro*	Hershman *et al.* (1973)

dient; the faster the rate of blood flow the more rapid is the removal of hPL and hence the steeper the gradient. This hypothesis is fully compatible with all present evidence and has the important implication that the rate of hPL production and the circulating levels in the mother should be closely related to uteroplacental blood flow. In addition, it may explain why products which depend on both fetus and placenta, such as estriol, and products of the placenta alone, such as hPL, often show a concomitant decrease in pathological states.

X. Metabolism and Clearance

The half-life of hPL in the mother, as estimated by the rate of disappearance after delivery of the placenta, is 10–20 minutes (Spellacy *et al.*, 1966; Pavlou *et al.*, 1972). As with other biological molecules the disappearance is biphasic with an initial rapid fall (yielding the half-life stated above) followed by a period of less rapid decrease. The differences in half-lives between individual subjects cannot be explained by observational error alone (Pavlou *et al.*, 1972). Each subject has her own characteristic half-life and this can be attributed to differences in the mode of delivery and the physiological state of the patient.

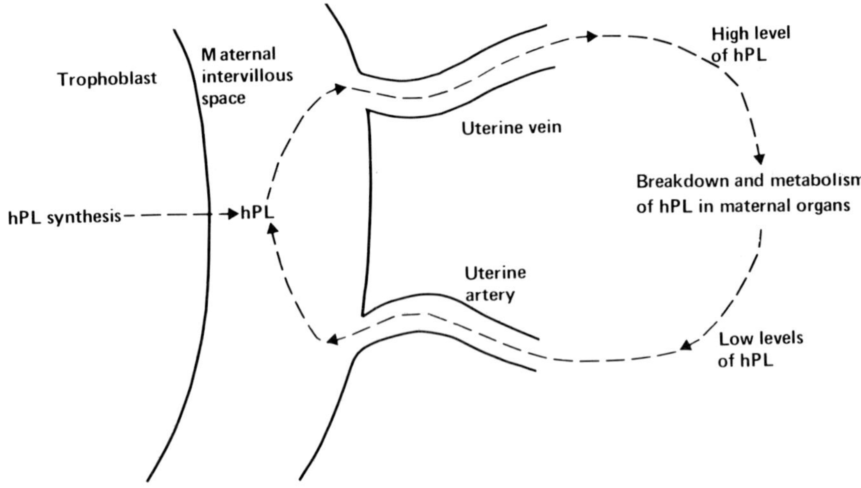

Fig. 6. Diagram to show how uteroplacental blood flow may control the rate of synthesis of hPL by the trophoblast.

The rate of synthesis of hPL has been estimated at 1–12 g/day (Beck *et al.*, 1965; Kaplan *et al.*, 1968). This is much greater than that of any other protein hormone, an interesting observation in the light of the dispute as to whether hPL has any function.

Maternal levels of hPL show no nyctohemeral rhythm (Beck *et al.*, 1965; Samaan *et al.*, 1966; Pavlou *et al.*, 1972; Lindberg and Nilsson, 1973a). However, the variation over a 24-hour period is greater than that which can be attributed to the assay itself (Pavlou *et al.*, 1972). Thus a single sample taken from an individual will not be representative of all samples taken from the individual, and the diagnostic significance of hPL levels is increased if serial levels are examined. The factors responsible for the variation are unknown. Posture has no effect (Ylikorkala *et al.*, 1973), nor does strenuous physical exercise (Lindberg and Nilsson, 1973a; Pavlou *et al.*, 1973). There is no change following the infusion of amino acids or ingestion of a protein meal (Tyson *et al.*, 1971). Some have claimed that there are wide fluctuations in levels during normal labor (e.g., Cramer *et al.*, 1971) but this has not been confirmed in other studies (Gillard *et al.*, 1973).

XI. Levels in Different Biological Fluids

The concentration of hPL in fetal blood is 100-fold less than that in the mother (Kaplan and Grumbach, 1965; Crosignani *et al.*, 1972). This differential is common to all specific proteins of the human placenta and is probably due to the fact that the trophoblast is in direct contact with the maternal circulation, whereas it is separated from the fetal circulation by a basement membrane and the fetal capillary endothelium.

The levels of hPL in amniotic fluid are 10-fold less than those in the mother (Niven *et al.*, 1974). Only small amounts of hPL are excreted in maternal urine (0.5 mg/day against a production rate of 1 g/day), a finding which is not surprising for a protein of this molecular weight.

XII. Assay of hPL in Blood

The majority of studies on hPL have been carried out using radioimmunoassay (see Chard, 1979), though other types of immunological assay have been developed, in particular enzymoimmunoassay (EIA) (Dittman *et al.*, 1979), and fluoroimmunoassay (FIA) (Chard and Sykes, 1979; Viinika *et al.*, 1981). Both EIA and, more especially, FIA are very promising techniques for the future.

One recent problem of hPL assays has been the apparent disappearance of purified hormone from the commercial market place. This vitiates one of the clinical advantages of the assay, namely, ready availability of materials at low cost.

XIII. Maternal Levels in Normal Pregnancy

Placental lactogen can be detected in maternal blood soon after implantation; thereafter the levels rise progressively to reach a plateau after the thirty-fifth week. This increase follows a sigmoid curve which characterizes all specific placental proteins and which closely parallels the growth of the placenta both in weight and in DNA content. The levels do not change at the onset of labor, and the absolute levels are not related to the time of onset of labor (Gillard *et al.*, 1973).

The normal range of hPL levels in the later part of pregnancy is shown in Fig. 7. In common with most other biochemical parameters the variation around the mean shows a skewed distribution (Chard, 1976); the range of variation is greater above the mean than below it. Thus a better approximation to the true mean and standard deviations is obtained after logarithmic transformation of the data. An alternative approach is the use of nonparametric statistics in which the results are expressed as medians and centiles. Appropriate analysis of the normal range is essential to the definition of cut-off points between normality and abnormality. The total spread of

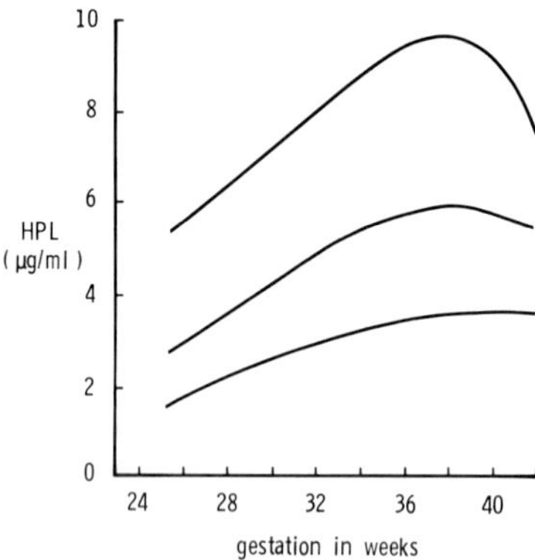

Fig. 7. The normal range of circulating hPL levels in the mother from the twentieth to forty-second weeks of gestation (200 subjects). The mean ± 2 standard deviations are shown. The distribution is skewed, the variation above the mean being greater than below it.

hPL values in normal pregnancies (coefficient of variation 36%) is less than that of circulating estrogens (Klopper *et al.,* 1977). As a generalization, the material showing the lowest coefficient of variation should be the best clinical test (Chard, 1976).

XIV. Interpretation of Biochemical Tests of Fetoplacental Function

The literature on the clinical use of biochemical tests of placental function is often confusing and contradictory. One group will claim a test is of great value, and another will disparage the procedure. Furthermore, it is often asked whether any such test is of any value when set against the strict criterion of whether it contributes to a decrease in perinatal mortality and morbidity. However, certain principles can be expressed about the interpretation of these tests (see also Chard, 1976):

1. A test is of no value unless an appropriate normal range is available. This should usually be based on results from at least 50 subjects at each week of gestation, and "normality" should be clearly defined.
2. The normal range should be submitted to the correct statistical evaluation. A Gaussian distribution is unusual and results should usually be analyzed after logarithmic transformation or in nonparametric form.
3. It is essential for an individual laboratory or group of laboratories to establish its own normal range. Differences in methodology can make the use of a published normal range misleading.

4. Ranges should be established for clinically defined abnormalities according to whether or not they are associated with fetal risk. Thus, it is of little value to know that the levels of a given material are generally low in preeclampsia: the obstetrician needs to know which case of preeclampsia is at greatest risk.

5. There is no such thing as a perfect test. All tests show a degree of overlap between normality and abnormality, with a "gray-zone" between. Results should be interpreted as a risk, not a certainty.

6. Serial levels are always of greater value than a single level. It is usually believed that this is because a trend may be apparent, i.e., a fall in a high-risk case. But far more important is the fact that serial levels give greater confidence to the observed relation between an individual subject and the population of which that subject is part (Fig. 8).

7. Placental products can be classified into two groups based on their biological properties (see Section IV): within any one group clinical measurement of the different products will give virtually identical results (Table III).

XV. Maternal Levels in Complications of Pregnancy

A. *Trophoblastic Tumors*

Trophoblastic tumors produce hPL but in smaller amounts than in normal pregnancy (Samaan *et al.*, 1966; Saxena *et al.*, 1968; Goldstein, 1971). The maternal levels appear to be related to tumor differentiation; the greater the

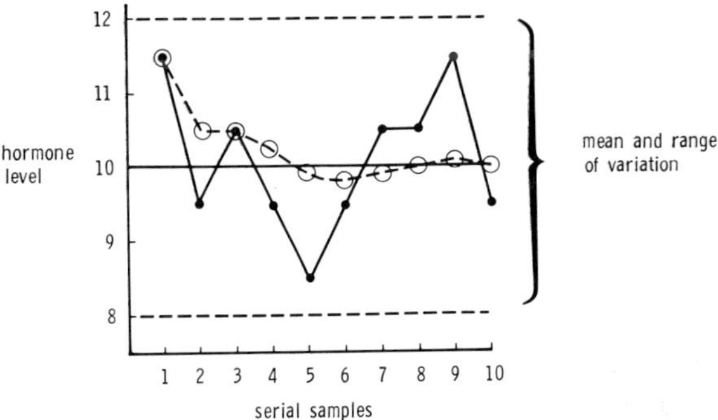

Fig. 8. Diagram to show the value of serial as opposed to single samples. The hormone has an overall day-to-day variation of ± 20% and serial samples (●—●) fluctuate within these limits. Calculation of the cumulative mean (○—○) shows that this becomes stable when five or more serial results are available, thus providing a very accurate estimate of the true situation in an individual patient.

Table III
A New Classification of Placental Products[a]

	Group I	Group II
Examples	Enzymes, steroids, hCG, hPL, SP_1	PP5, PAPP-A
Functions	Hormonal[b]	Local (Immune and coagulation systems)
Pathology	Fetal pathology (growth retardation, acute fetal distress)[c]	Placental pathology (placental abruption, premature labor, pre-eclampsia[d]

[a]The pathological changes refer to late pregnancy; in early pregnancy measurement of all fetoplacental products appears to give virtually identical results.
[b]Hormonal is used here in the broad sense of action at a distance.
[c]Group I compounds reflect fetal well being independently of other complications.
[d]Group II compounds reflect specific events which may lead to fetal risk, but which are associated with a normal fetus at their onset.

degree of malignancy, the lower the hPL value in relation to hCG (Saxena *et al.*, 1968; Goldstein, 1971). In some cases with active disease, hPL may disappear from the circulation while hCG remains detectable (Saxena *et al.*, 1968).

B. Threatened Abortion

The outcome for the fetus is uncertain in many cases of vaginal bleeding in early gestation. It is generally agreed that low maternal hPL levels after the eighth to tenth week indicate that the outcome is likely to be unsatisfactory, and thus provide a valuable guide to prognosis in this condition (Genazzani *et al.*, 1969; Niven *et al.*, 1972; Gartside and Tindall, 1975; Biswas *et al.*, 1980) (Fig. 9). This applies whether or not a sonogram is also abnormal (Vorster *et al.*, 1977). Low levels, and especially serial low levels after the tenth week indicate evacuation of the uterus without further delay unless there are contraindicating factors such as advanced maternal age or infertility.

C. Low Birthweight Infants

Placental lactogen levels are correlated with the weight of the placenta (Sciarra *et al.*, 1968; Cramer *et al.*, 1971; Lindberg and Nilsson, 1973a) and of the fetus (Letchworth *et al.*, 1971; Lindberg and Nilsson, 1973a; Boyce *et al.*, 1975). The latter relationship is secondary to that between the weight of the placenta and fetus, and there is disagreement as to whether hPL levels are an efficient guide to fetal growth and the prediction of delivery weight in an

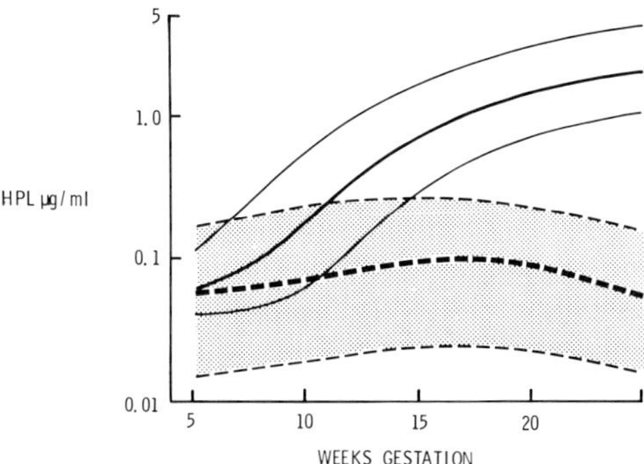

Fig. 9. Plasma hPL levels in 141 subjects who aborted on first admission (dashed lines and hatched area). The mean and range of normal subjects is also shown (solid lines).

individual patient. However, low levels have been described in association with severe intrauterine growth retardation (Lindberg and Nilsson, 1973b; Hensleigh *et al.,* 1977), particularly in cases of maternal hypertension (Granat *et al.,* 1977). The sensitivity of the test is around 40% (Morrison *et al.,* 1980). It has been suggested that hPL levels in IUGR became significantly lower than normal only after 33 weeks gestation (Daikoku *et al.,* 1979.) However, with other placental proteins, and possibly hPL it has been shown that low levels in *mid-trimester* may also be predictive of this complication (Salem *et al.,* 1981). Increased levels occur in twin pregnancies (Garoff and Seppälä, 1973), but because of the lack of a normal range for this condition clinical interpretation is difficult.

D. Preeclampsia and Hypertension

Spellacy and colleagues (1971) described a "fetal danger zone" for subjects with hypertension: levels less than 4 μg/ml after the thirtieth week indicated a fetal mortality of 24%. The levels are generally lower in multigravidae than in primigravidae (Letchworth and Chard, 1972a; Spellacy *et al.,* 1974), and it has been suggested that the greatest risk and lowest levels are associated with chronic vascular disease. Many workers have confirmed the association between low hPL levels and fetal outcome in hypertensive pregnancies (Keller *et al.,* 1971; Lindberg and Nilsson, 1973b; Christensen *et al.,* 1974). Kelly *et al.* (1975) showed a 75% fetal risk (growth retardation or perinatal asphyxia) for patients developing hypertension after the twenty-eighth week and having low hPL levels.

Some confusion in the literature on the precise clinical value of hPL levels in preeclampsia can be attributed to two factors. First, the condition itself is very heterogeneous and often not clearly defined. Second, it is very common for authors not to distinguish between preeclampsia per se, and the fetal risk arising from the preeclampsia.

E. Diabetes Mellitus

Diabetes mellitus is associated with a large placenta and it is therefore not surprising that hPL is generally elevated in this condition (Selenkow *et al.*, 1969; Cohen *et al.*, 1973; Ursell *et al.*, 1973; Soler *et al.*, 1975; Hertogh *et al.*, 1976) (Fig. 10). The levels are reduced in cases in which fetal outcome is unsatisfactory (Fig. 11). Thus, hPL levels in a diabetic pregnancy must be interpreted in relation to the elevated range for a "normal diabetic" pregnancy; whereas a level of 4 μg/ml is a useful dividing line for the diagnosis of abnormality under most circumstances, in patients with diabetes the critical level is 5 μg/ml.

Conflicting results in the literature on hPL levels in diabetes can be attributed to a number of factors, including the definition of the severity of the condition, the failure to appreciate that abnormality should be judged in relation to the general elevation of levels in this condition, and the fact that perinatal death may occur due to metabolic dysfunction in the absence of notable placental deficiency. A more recent problem is the fact that most diabetic pregnancies are so well controlled that they are, for all clinical and biochemical purposes, effectively normal.

F. Rhesus Isoimmunization

Placental lactogen levels are generally increased in this condition. The levels are most elevated in cases in which the child is severely affected (Lind-

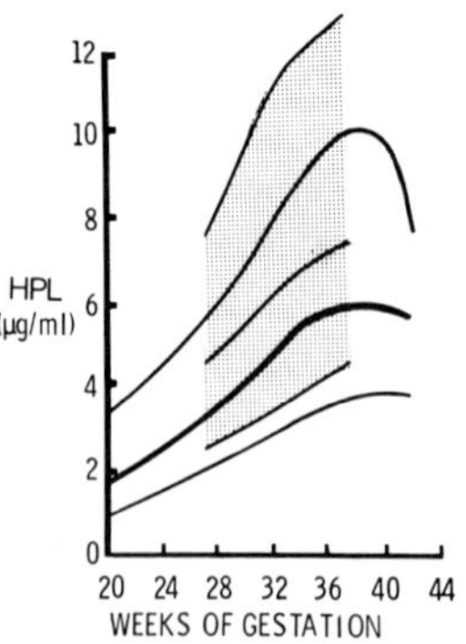

Fig. 10. hPL levels in pregnancies complicated by diabetes mellitus in which there was no evidence of placental dysfunction.

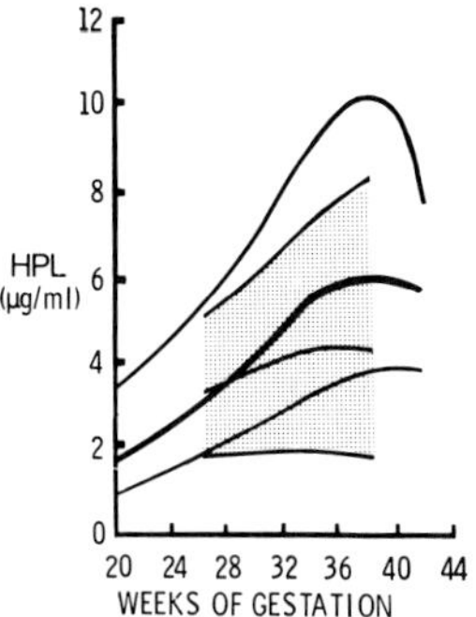

Fig. 11. hPL levels in pregnancies complicated by diabetes mellitus in which there was evidence of placental dysfunction. The normal range is shown by solid lines.

berg and Nilsson, 1973b; Ward *et al.,* 1974) (Fig. 12). Prior to the twenty-sixth week, a value greater than two standard deviations above the normal mean indicates a 90% likelihood that the case will be severe. Similar elevations are seen in amniotic fluid hPL (Niven *et al.,* 1974). The test has been advocated as an additional diagnostic aid at a stage when other parameters, such as liquor bilirubin, may be unhelpful.

G. Fetal Death

Placental lactogen levels often fall before fetal death occurs (Ward *et al.,* 1973). This is compatible with the fact that in many stillbirths the cause is placental insufficiency, rather than a primary defect in the fetus itself.

H. Fetal Distress and Neonatal Asphyxia

In some 12% of pregnancies with no obvious clinical abnormalities in the antenatal period, fetal complications occur either during labor or at the time

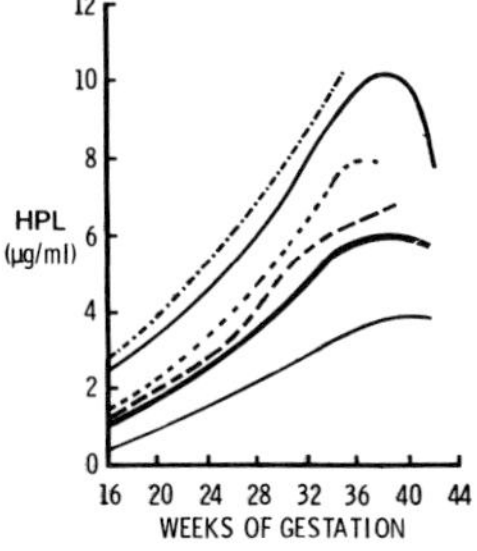

Fig. 12. Mean hPL levels in pregnancies complicated by rhesus isoimmunization (---, mildly affected cases, -----, moderately affected cases; -·-·-·-, severely affected cases).

of delivery. Some of these cases can be predicted by serial estimations of hPL (Letchworth and Chard, 1972b; England *et al.*, 1974); a patient who is otherwise normal and who has three or more levels below 4 μg/ml in the last 6 weeks of pregnancy has a 71% risk of fetal complications. Comparable observations have been made in a mixed group of "at risk" pregnancies, including patients with a clinical suspicion of fetal growth retardation, hypertension, preeclampsia, antepartum hemorrhage, and chronic renal disease (Edwards *et al.*, 1976).

There has been some argument as to whether hPL determinations can predict fetal distress in labor, when the latter complication is analyzed separately from IUGR. A recent study has shown an association between abnormal hPL levels and an abnormal result of an oxytocin challenge test (OCT) (Spellacy *et al.*, 1979).

I. Miscellaneous Conditions

Maternal blood hPL levels are generally lower in smokers than in nonsmokers (Moser *et al.*, 1974; Boyce *et al.*, 1975; Spellacy *et al.*, 1977). This is attributable to the associated growth retardation rather than to the smoking itself (Lee *et al.*, 1980). hPL levels are lower in mothers exposed to continuous aircraft noise (Ando and Hattori, 1977).

Several authors have described cases with an apparent absence of hPL in otherwise uneventful pregnancies (Gaede *et al.*, 1978; Nielsen *et al.*, 1979; Borody and Carlton, 1981). A similar condition has been reported with the new placental protein, SP_1 (Grudzinskas *et al.*, 1979) and both situations are probably similar to the rare sulfatase deficiency which leads to very low levels of estriol. The defects appear to be isolated because other placental products have invariably proved normal in these cases (Chard, unpublished observations).

The possible clinical importance of circulating antibodies to placental lactogen in the mother was observed many years ago (Gusdon *et al.*, 1970; Yamini *et al.*, 1972). A recent study has suggested that low hPL levels may be associated with the presence of a binding substance in maternal serum (Heal and Gluck, 1980).

XVI. Clinical Use of hPL—Conclusions

Two factors serve to explain the present widespread acceptance and use of hPL as a placental function test. First, the method of measurement is simple, reliable, and widely available. Second, and largely as a result of this, there is an extensive literature on its clinical applications so that interpretation is also relatively straightforward. In routine clinical practice the use of hPL or estriol (blood or urine) determinations should provide as much information as is likely to be achieved from the use of group I materials, and the combination of the two may be superior to either alone. Furthermore, it should be emphasized that negative information can often be as valuable as positive information: a value in the upper part of the normal range suggests almost regardless of the clinical situation that the fetus is at low risk.

The final question that may be asked is "is placental function testing worthwhile?" What is the value of an hPL result in relation to other features recorded as part of antenatal care, and can the information lead to a significant improvement in outcome? The first question has been answered in recent studies from Gordon *et al.* (1978) and Grudzinskas *et al.* (1981). Using a "relative risk factor" we demonstrated that low hPL levels, observed as part of a routine screening program on an entire obstetric population, were as effective a predictor of poor fetal outcome as the occurrence of severe preeclampsia, low maternal weight at 32 weeks, and heavy smoking by the mother. All of these parameters were superior to many other factors which are generally considered to be of great value in antenatal diagnosis. The second question has been answered in a pioneering study by Spellacy *et al.* (1975). Placental lactogen measurements were carried out on a large population of "at risk" patients; the subjects were divided into two randomized groups, one in which the results were reported to the obstetrician and the other in which they were not. In the first group the perinatal death rate was 3.4% while in the second it was 15%, a clear indication of the real practical value of these determinations. Since a substantial proportion of perinatal mortality and morbidity cannot be identified by existing clinical procedures, this constitutes a good argument for routine application of hPL measurement or a comparable determination in all pregnancies.

References

Ando, Y., and Hattori, H. (1977). *Br. J. Obstet. Gynaecol.* **84,** 115–118.

Beck, P., and Daughaday, W. H. (1967). *J. Clin. Invest.* **46,** 103–110.

Beck, P., Parker, M. L., and Daughaday, W. H. (1965). *J. Clin. Endocrinol. Metab.* **25,** 2457–1467.

Belleville, F., Absennes, A., Nabet, P., and Paysany, P. (1972). *C. R. Soc. Biol. (Paris)* **162,** 1030.

Bewley, T. A., and Li, C. H. (1974). *In* "Lactogenic Hormones, Fetal Nutrition, and Lactation" (J. B. Josimovich, ed.), p. 19. Wiley, New York.

Birken, S., Smith, D. L., Canfield, R. E., and Boime, I. (1977). *Biochem. Biophys. Res. Commun.* **74,** 106–112.

Biswas, S., Murrey, M., Buffoe, G., Graves, L., Jelowitz, J., and Dewhurst, J. (1980). *J. Obstet. Gynaecol.* **1,** 75–77.

Blobel, G., and Dobberstein, G. (1975). *J. Cell. Biol.* **67,** 835–851.

Boime, I., and Boguslawski, S. (1974). *Proc. Natl. Acad. Sci. U. S. A.* **71,** 1322–1325.
Boime, I., McWilliams, D., Szcesena, E., and Camel, M. (1976). *J. Biol. Chem.* **251,** 820–825.
Boime, I., Szcesena, E., and Smith, D. (1977). *Eur. J. Biochem.* **73,** 515–530.
Borody, I. B., and Carlton, M. A. (1981). *Br. J. Obstet. Gynaecol.* **88,** 447–449.
Boyce, A., Schwartz, D., Hubert, C., Cedard, L., and Dreyfus, J. (1975). *Br. J. Obstet. Gynaecol.* **82,** 964–967.
Brinsmead, M. W., Bancroft, B. J., Thorbrun, G. D., and Waters, M. J. (1981). *J. Endocrinol.* **90,** 337–343.
Burgos, M. H., and Rodriguez, E. M. (1966). *Am. J. Obstet. Gynecol.* **96,** 342–356.
Burt, R. L., Leake, N. H., and Pruitt, A. B. (1966). *Am. J. Obstet. Gynecol.* **95,** 579–585.
Burt, R. L., Leake, N. H., and Rhyne, A. L. (1970). *Obstet. Gynecol.* **36,** 233–237.
Buttle, H. L., Forsyth, I. A., and Knaggs, G. S. (1972). *J. Endocrinol.* **53,** 483–491.
Chard, T. (1976). *In* "Plasma Hormone Assays in Evaluation of Fetal Wellbeing" (A. Klopper, ed.), pp. 1–9. Churchill, London.
Chard, T. (1979). *In* "Hormones in Blood" (C. H. Gray and V. H. T. James, eds.), pp. 333–409. Academic Press, New York.
Chard, T. (1981). *In* "Hormones in Normal and Abnormal Human Tissues" (K. Fotherby and S. B. Pal, eds.), pp. 409–427. De Gruyter, Berlin.
Chard, T., and Sykes, A. (1979). *Clin. Chem.* **25,** 973–975.
Christensen, A., Frayshov. D., and Fylling, P. (1974). *Acta Endocrinol. Copenhagen* **77,** 344–355.
Cohen, H., Grumbach, M. M., and Kaplan, S. L. (1964). *Proc. Soc. Exp. Biol. Med.* **117,** 438–441.
Cohen, M., Haour, F., Dumont, M., and Bertrand, J. (1973). *Am. J. Obstet. Gynecol.* **115,** 202–210.
Contractor, S. F., and Davies, H. (1973). *Nature (London)* **243,** 284–285.
Cox, G. S., Weintraub, B. D., Rosen, S. W., and Maxwell, E. S. (1976). *J. Biol. Chem.* **251,** 1723–1728.
Cramer, D. W., Beck, P., and Makowski, E. L. (1971). *Am. J. Obstet. Gynecol.* **109,** 649–655.
Crosignani, P. G., Nencioni, T., and Brambati, B. (1972). *J. Obstet. Gynaecol. Br. Common W.* **79,** 122–126.
Daikoku, N. H., Tyson, J. E., Graf, C., Scott, R., Smith, B., Johnson, J. W. C., and King, I. M. (1979). *Am. J. Obstet. Gynecol.* **135,** 516–520.
Dittmar, D., Monji, N., Cid, A., Malkus, A., and Castro, A. (1979). *Clin. Chem.* **25,** 227–229.
Edwards, R. P., Diver, M. J., Davis, J. C., and Hipkin, L. J. (1976). *Br. J. Obstet. Gynaecol.* **83,** 229–237.
England, P., Lorrimer, D., Fergusson, J. C., Moffatt, A., and Kelly, A. (1974). *Lancet* **1,** 5–7.
Florini, J. R., Tonelli, G., Breuer, C. B., Coppola, J., Ringler, I., and Bell, P. H. (1966). *Endocrinology* **79,** 692–708.
Friesen, H. (1965). *Endocrinology* **76,** 369–381.
Friesen, H., Belanger, C., Guyda, H., and Hwang, P. (1972). *In* "Lactogenic Hormones" (G. E. W. Wolstenholme and J. Knight, eds.), pp. 83–103. Churchill, London.
Gaede, P., Trolle, D., and Pedersen, H. (1978). *Acta Obstet. Gynecol. Scand.* **57,** 203–209.
Garoff, L., and Seppälä, M. (1973). *J. Obstet. Gynaecol. Br. Common W.* **80,** 695–700.
Gartside, M. W., and Tindall, V. R. (1975). *Br. J. Obstet. Gynaecol.* **82,** 303–309.
Genazzani, A. R., Aubert, M. L., Casoli, M., Fioretti, P., and Felber, J.-P. (1969). *Lancet* **2,** 1385–1387.
George, D. L., Phillips, J. A., Francke, U., and Seeburg, P. H. (1981). Hum. Genet. **57,** 138–141.
Gillard, M., Letchworth, A. T., and Chard, T. (1973). *Obstet. Gynecol.* **41,** 774–775.
Goldstein, D. P. (1971). *Am. J. Obstet. Gynecol.* **110,** 583–587.

Gordon, Y. B., and Chard, T. (1979). *In* "Human Placental Proteins" (A. Klopper and T. Chard, eds.), pp. 1–21. Springer-Verlag, Berlin and New York.

Gordon, Y. B., Lewis, J. D., Pendlebury, D. J., Leighton, M., and Gold, J. (1978). *Lancet* **1**, 1001–1003.

Granat, M., Sharf, M., Diengott, D., Spindel, A., Kahana, L., and Elrad, H. (1977). *Am. J. Obstet. Gynecol.* **129**, 647–654.

Grudzinskas, J. G., Gordon, Y. B., Humphreys, J. D., Brudenell, M., and Chard, T. (1979). *Br. J. Obstet. Gynaecol.* **86**, 978.

Grudzinskas, J. G., Gordon, Y. B., Wadsworth, J., Menabawey, M., and Chard, T. (1981). *Aust. N. Z. J. Obst. Gynaecol.* **21**, 103–105.

Grumbach, M. M., and Kaplan, S. L. (1964). *Trans. N. Y. Acad. Sci.* **27**, 167–188.

Gusdon, J. J., Leake, N. H., and Burt, R. L. (1970). *Am J. Obstet. Gynecol.* **108**, 1056–1062.

Handwerger, S., Barret, J. Tyrey, L, and Schonberg, D. (1973). *J. Clin. Endocrinol. Metab.* **36**, 1268–1270.

Handwerger, S., Fellows, R E., Crenshaw, M. C., Hurley, T., Barrett, J. and Maurer, W. F. (1976). *J. Endocrinol.* **69**, 133–137.

Handwerger, S., Crenshaw, C., Maurer, W. F., Barrett, J. M., Hurley, T. W., Golander, A., and Fellows, R. E. (1977). *J. Endocrinol.* **72**, 27–34.

Handwerger, S., Crenshaw, M. C., Lansing, A., Golander, A., Hurley, T. W. and Fellows R. E. (1978). *Endocrinology* **103**, 1752–1758.

Handwerger, S., Grandis, A., Barry, S., and Crenshaw, M. C. (1981). *J. Endocrinol.* **88**, 283–288.

Heal, A. B., and Gluck, J. (1980). *Am. J. Obstet. Gynecol.* **137**, 975–977.

Hensleigh, P. A., Cheaton, S. G., and Spellacy, W. N. (1977). *Am. J. Obstet. Gynecol.* **129**, 675–678.

Hershman, J. M., Kojima, A., and Friesen, H. G. (1973). *J. Clin. Endocrinol. Metab.* **36**, 497–501.

Hertogh, R., de, Thomas, K., Hoet, J. J., and Vanderheyden, I. (1976). *Diabetologia* **12**, 455–461.

Ikonicoff, L. K., de, and Cedard, L. (1973). *Am. J. Obstet. Gynecol.* **116**, 1124–1132.

Ito, Y., and Higashi, K. (1961). *Endocrinology Jpn.* **8**, 279–287.

IUPAC-IUB Commission on Biochemical Nomenclature (1975). *Eur. J. Biochem.* **55**, 485–486.

Jepson, J. H., and Friesen, H. G. (1968). *Br. J. Haematol.* **15**, 465–471.

Josimovich, J. B. (1966). *Endocrinology* **78**, 707–714.

Josimovich, J. B., and Archer, D. F. (1977). *Am. J. Obstet. Gynecol.* **129**, 777–780.

Josimovich, J. B., and Brande, B. L. (1964). *Trans. N. Y. Acad. Sci.* **27**, 161–166.

Josimovich, J. B., and MacLaren, J. A. (1962). *Endocrinology* **71**, 209–211.

Josimovich, J. B., Stock, R. J., and Tobon, H. (1974). *In* "Fetal Nutrition and Lactation" (J. B. Josimovich, ed.), pp. 335–50. Wiley, New York.

Kalkhoff, R. K., Richardson, B. L., and Beck, P. (1969). *Diabetes* **18**, 153–163.

Kaplan, S. L., and Grumbach, M. M. (1965). *J. Clin. Endocrinol. Metab.* **25**, 1370–1374.

Kaplan, S. L., Gurpide, E., Sciarra, J. J., and Grumbach, M. M. (1968). *J. Clin. Endocrinol. Metab.* **28**, 1450–1460.

Keller, P. J., Baertschi, U., Bader, P., Gerber, C., Schmid, J., Solterman, R., and Kopper, E. (1971). *Lancet* **2**, 729–730.

Kelly, A. M., England, P., Lorrimer, J. D., Fergusson, J. C., and Govan, A. D. T.(1975). *Br. J. Obstet. Gyanecol.* **82**, 272–275.

Kim, Y. J., and Felig, P. (1971). *J. Clin. Endocrinol. Metab.* **32**, 864–867.

Klopper, A., and Chard, T., eds. (1979). "Placental Proteins." Springer-Verlag, Berlin and New York.

Klopper, A., Masson, G., and Wilson, G. (1977). *Br. J. Obstet. Gynaecol.* **84**, 648–655.

Lee, J. N., Grudzinskas, J. G., and Chard, T. (1980). *J. Obstet. Gynecol.* **1**, 87–89.
Letchworth, A. T.,and Chard, T. (1972a). *J. Obstet. Gynaecol. Br. Common W.* **79**, 680.
Letchworth, A. T., and Chard, T. (1972b). *Lancet* **2**, 704–706.
Letchworth, A. T., Boardman, R., Bristow, C., Landon, J., and Chard, T., (1971). *J. Obstet. Gynaecol. Br. Common W.* **78**, 542–548.
Li, C. H., Grumbach, M. M., Kaplan, S. L., Josimovich, J. B., Friesen, H., and Catt, K. J. (1968). *Experientia* **24**, 1288.
Lindberg, B. S., and Nilsson, B. A. (1973a). *J. Obstet. Gynaecol. Br. Common. W.* **80**, 619–626.
Lindberg, B. S., and Nilsson, B. A. (1973b). *J. Obstet. Gynaecol. Br. Common W.* **80**, 1046–1053.
Lolis, D., Konstantinidis, K., Paparangelou, G., and Kaskarelis, D. (1977). *Am. J. Obstet. Gynecol.* **128**, 724–726.
Macaron, C., Famuyima, O., and Singh, S. P. (1978). *J. Clin. Endocrinol. Metab.* **47**, 168–170.
McWilliams, D., and N. Boime, I. (1980). *Endocrinology* **107**, 761–765.
Martin, J. M., and Friesen, H. (1969). *Endocrinology* **84**, 619–621.
Morrison, I., Green, P., and Oomen, B. (1980). *Am. J. Obstet. Gynecol.* **135**, 1055–1060.
Moser, R. J., Hollingsworth, D. R., Carlson, J. W., and Lamotte, L. (1974). *Am. J. Obstet. Gynecol.* **120**, 1080–1086.
Niall, H. D., Hogan, M. L., Tregear, G. W., Segre, G. V., Hwang, P., and Friesen, H. G. (1973). *Recent Prog. Horm. Res.* **29**, 387–398.
Nielsen, P. V., Pedersen, H., and Kampmann, E. (1979). *Am. J. Obstet. Gynecol.* **135**, 322–326.
Niven, P. A. R., Landon, J., and Chard, T. (1972). *Br. Med. J.* **3**, 799–801.
Niven, P. A. R., Ward, R. H. T., and Chard, T. (1974). *J. Obstet. Gynaecol. Br. Common W.* **81**, 988–990.
Pavlou, C., Chard, T., and Letchworth, A. T. (1972). *J. Obstet. Gynaecol. Br. Common W.* **79**, 629–634.
Pavlou, C., Chard, T., Landon, J., and Letchworth, A. T. (1973). *Eur. J. Obstet. Gynecol. Reprod. Biol.* **3**, 45–49.
Porter, D. G. (1980). *Placenta* **1**, 259–274.
Prieto, J. C., Cifuentes, I., and Serrano-Rios, M. (1976). *Obstet. Gynecol.* **48**, 297.
Riggi, S. J., Boshart, C. R., Bell, P. H., and Ringler, I. (1966). *Endocrinology* **79**, 709–715.
Russell, J., Katzhendler, J., Kowalski, K., Schneider, A. B., and Sherwood, L. M. (1981a). *J. Biol. Chem.* **256**, 304–307.
Russell, J., Sherwood, L. M., Kowalski, K., and Schneider, A. B. (1981b). *J. Biol. Chem.* **256**, 296–300.
Salem, H. T., Lee, J. N., Seppälä, M., Vaara, L., Aula, P., Al-Ani, A. T. M., and Chard,T. (1981). *Br. J. Obstet. Gynaecol.* **88**, 371–374.
Saxena, B. N., Goldstein, D. P., Emerson, K., and Selenkow, H. A. (1968). *Am. J. Obstet. Gynecol.* **103**, 115–121.
Saxena, B. N., Emerson, K., and Selenkow, H. A. (1969). *New Engl. J. Med.* **281**, 225–231.
Schneider, A. B., Kowalski, K., Buckman, G., and Sherwood, L. M. (1977). *Biochim. Bio Phys. Acta* **493**, 69–77.
Sciarra, J. J., Sherwood, L. M., Varma, A. A., and Lundberg, W. B. (1968). *Am. J. Obstet. Gynecol.* **101**, 413–421.
Selenkow, H. A., Varma, K., Younger, D., White, P., and Emerson, K. (1969). *Diabetes* **20**, 696–706.
Shome, B., and Parlow, A. F. (1977). *J. Clin. Endocrinol. Metab.* **45**, 1112–1115.
Soler, N. G., Nicholson, H. O., and Malins, J. M. (1975). *Lancet* **2**, 54–57.

Spellacy, W. N. (1972). *In* "Lactogenic Hormones" (G. E. W. Wolstenholme and J. Knight, eds.), p. 223. Churchill, London.

Spellacy, W. N., Buhi, W. C., Schram, J. D., Birk, S. A., and McCreary, S. A. (1971). *Obstet. Gynecol.* **96**, 1164.

Spellacy, W. N., Buhi, W. C., Birk, S. A., and McCreary, S. A. (1974). *Am. J. Obstet. Gynecol.* **120**, 214–223.

Spellacy, W. N., Buhi, W. C., and Birk, S. A. (1975). *Am. J. Obstet. Gynecol.* **121**, 835–843.

Spellacy, W. N., Buhi, W. C., and Birk, S. A.(1977). *Am. J. Obstet. Gynecol.* **127**, 232–234.

Spellacy, W. N., Cruz, A. C., Kalra, P. S., Kellner, K. R., Quinlan, R. W. Buhi, W. C., and Birk, S. A. (1979). *Am. J. Obstet. Gynecol.* **135**, 917–921.

Suwa, S., and Friesen, H. (1969a). *Endocrinology* **85**, 1028–1036.

Suwa, S., and Friesen, H. (1969b). *Endocrinology* **85**, 1037–1045.

Turtle, J. R., Beck, B., and Daughaday, W. H. (1966). *Endocrinology* **79**, 197.

Tyson, J. E., Austin, K. L, and Farinholt, J. W. (1971). *Am. J. Obstet. Gynecol.* **109**, 1080.

Ursell, W., Brudenell, J., and Chard, T. (1973). *Br. Med. J.* **2**, 80–82.

Viinikka, L., Landon, J., and Pourfarzaneh, M. (1981). *Clin. Chim. Acta* (in press).

Vorster, C. S., Pannall, P. R., and Slabber, C. F. (1977). *Am. J. Obstet. Gynecol.* **128**, 879–880.

Walsh, S. W., Wolf, R. C., Meyer, R. K., Aubert, M. L. and Friesen, H. (1977). *Endocrinology* **100**, 851–855.

Ward, H., Rochman, H., Varnavides, L. A., and Whyley, G. A. (1973). *Am. J. Obstet. Gynecol.* **116**, 1105–1113.

Ward, R. H. T., Letchworth, A. T., Niven, P. A. R., and Chard, T. (1974). *Br. Med. J.* **1**, 347–349.

Ward, R. H. T., Whyley, G. A., Fairweather, D. V. I., Allen, E. I., and Chard, T. (1977). *Br. J. Obstet. Gynaecol.* **84**, 363.

Yamini, G., Chard, T., and Blake, M. E. (1972). *J. Endocrinol.* **55**, 29,

Ylikorkala, O., Haapalahti, J., and Jarvinen, P. A. (1973). *J. Obstet. Gynaecol. Br. Common. W.* **80**, 546.

ESTROGEN AND PROGESTRONE PRODUCTION IN HUMAN PREGNANCY

Robert E. Oakey

DIVISION OF STEROID ENDOCRINOLOGY
DEPARTMENT OF CHEMICAL PATHOLOGY
SCHOOL OF MEDICINE
UNIVERSITY OF LEEDS
LEEDS, ENGLAND

I. Introduction ... 194
II. Nomenclature ... 194
III. Biosynthesis of Estrogens ... 196
IV. Control of Estrogen Production ... 197
  A. Effects of Alterations in the Supply of Precursors ... 198
  B. Effects of Alterations in Activities of Placental Enzymes ... 208
V. Estrogens in Plasma in Relation to the Onset of Labor ... 211
VI. Biosynthesis of Progesterone ... 213
VII. Control of Progesterone Production ... 215
  A. Effects of Alterations in the Supply of Precursors ... 215
  B. Effects of Alterations in the Activities of Placental Enzymes ... 216
  C. Effects of Polypeptides of Placental or Pituitary Origin ... 217
VIII. Progesterone in Plasma in Relation to the Onset of Labor ... 218
IX. Conclusions ... 219
  References ... 223

Current Topics in Experimental Endocrinology, Vol. 4

ISBN 0-12-153204-6

I. Introduction

The daily excretion of the urinary metabolites of estrogen and progesterone increases as gestation proceeds (Fig. 1), reflecting increased production of each hormone, although this itself is technically difficult to measure with accuracy. The purpose of this article is to assess current understanding of how these increases in the production of estrogen and progesterone are brought about. Attention will be focused on the last two trimesters, when ovarian contributions are small enough to be neglected.

The opportunity for experimental endocrinology in human pregnancy is severely restricted by ethical considerations. The fetal circulation proper is inaccessible. Samples from the scalp or cord become available only during or after the stressful process of delivery which diminishes any value the samples may have as reflecting the status of the undisturbed fetus, particularly when steroids secreted by the fetal adrenal gland are being considered. Consequently, information regarding the resting fetus is sparse, in marked contrast to that obtained by the application of elegant surgical procedures to pregnant farm animals and lower primates. In view of the proper limitations imposed, evidence has had to be gathered from pregnancies complicated by failure of the development of particular fetal organs (e.g., anencephaly) or of specific enzymes (e.g., steroid sulfatase, steroid hydroxylases). Another valuable source of information has been pregnancies in which, for therapeutic or diagnostic reasons, the patient has received steroid or pituitary hormones. Finally experiments *in vitro* with adrenal and placental tissue and their exposure to various agents thought likely to affect steroid synthesis have yielded important information.

The biosynthesis of estrogen and its regulation will be considered separately from that of progesterone. The concentrations of these hormones in peripheral plasma which are achieved near term by these processes will be described, particularly in relation to changes which precede parturition. Finally, a personal interpretation of these changes will be presented.

I. Nomenclature

Steroids are referred to by trivial names; systematic names are listed below.

Androstenedione, 4-androstene-3,17-dione

Cortisol, 11β,17α,21-trihydroxy-4-pregnene-3,20-dione

Dehydroepiandrosterone (DHA), 3β-hydroxy-5-androsten-17-one

Dehydroepiandrosterone sulfate (DHAS), 3β-hydroxy-5-androsten-17-one 3β-yl sulfate

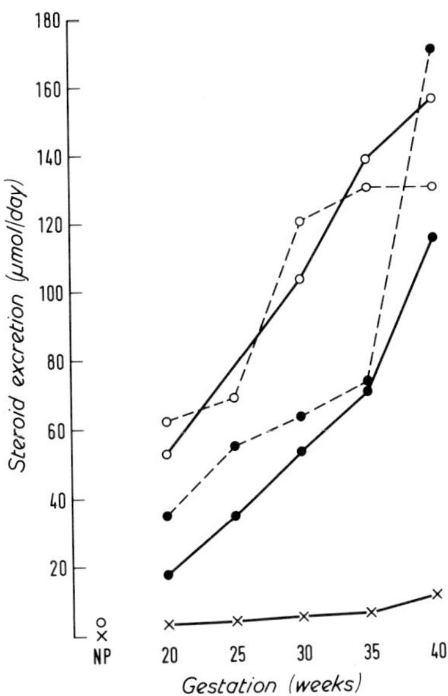

Fig. 1 Urinary excretion (μmole/day) of pregnanediol (○), estrone + estradiol (×), and estriol (●) in nonpregnant (NP) and in the last half of human pregnancy. Solid lines are mean values for estrogens from Brown (1956) and for pregnanediol from Klopper and Billewicz (1963). Broken lines join values for a single patient studied in our laboratory.

Dexamethasone, 9α-fluoro-16α-methyl-11β,17α,21-trihydroxy-1,4-pregnadiene-3,20-dione

20α-Dihydroprogesterone, 20α-hydroxy-4-pregnen-3-one

Estradiol, 1,3,5,(10)-estratriene-3,17β-diol

Estriol, 1,3,5(10)-estratriene-3,16α,17β-triol

Estrone, 3-hydroxy-1,3,5(10)-estratrien-17-one

16α-Hydroxyandrostenedione, 16α-hydroxy-4-androstene-3,17-dione

19-Hydroxyandrostenedione, 19-hydroxy-4-androstene-3,17-dione

16α-Hydroxy dehydroepiandrosterone (16α-OH-DHA), 3β,16α-dihydroxy-5-androsten-17-one

16α-Hydroxydehydroepiandrosterone sulfate (16α-OH-DHAS), 3β,16α-dihydroxy-5-androsten-17-one 3β-yl sulfate

16α-Hydroxyestrone, 3,16α-dihydroxy-1,3,5(10)-estratrien-17-one

17α-Hydroxypregnenolone, 3β,17α-dihydroxy-5-pregnen-20-one

16α-Hydroxytestosterone, 16α,17β-dihydroxy-4-androsten-3-one

β-Methasone, 9α-fluoro-16β-methyl-11β,17α,21-trihydroxy-1,4-pregnadiene-3,20-dione

Pregnanediol, 5β-pregnane-3α,20α-diol

Pregnenolone, 3β-hydroxy-5-pregnen-20-one
Pregnenolone sulfate, 3β-hydroxy-5-pregnen-20-one 3β-yl sulfate
Progesterone, 4-pregnene-3,20-dione
Testosterone, 17β-hydroxy-4-androsten-3-one.

III. Biosynthesis of Estrogens

The pathways by which the three classical estrogens (estrone, estradiol, and estriol) are produced were established from studies of the conversion of radioactive precursors in the fetus, placenta, and mother, alone or in combination, and from measurement of the concentration of precursors in cord and maternal blood in normal and pathological pregnancies. The contributions of Diczfalusy, Simmer, Colas, Frandsen, and their colleagues have been reviewed (e.g., Diczfalusy, 1969; Oakey, 1970a) and details will not be described again here. Any pathway proposed must take into account (1) the inability of the placenta to use C_{21} steroids for estrogen synthesis (thereby breaking the biosynthetic chain $C_{27} \rightarrow C_{21} \rightarrow C_{19} \rightarrow C_{18}$ found in adrenals and gonads) and (2) the dominance of estriol production. This compound, in a conjugated form, comprises about 40% of urinary estrogens in nonpregnant women (~ 150 nmole/day), but accounts for 90% of the estrogens excreted near term (~ 150 μmole/day).

The consensus reached (Fig. 2) is that the fetal adrenal, and, in particular the fetal zone (Seron-Ferre *et al.*, 1978b), synthesizes dehydroepiandrosterone sulfate (DHAS), from acetate or blood-borne cholesterol. This DHAS is the precursor of almost all of the estrogen eventually secreted by the placenta. A large proportion of secreted DHAS is hydroxylated at C-16α by the fetal liver before uptake by the placenta. Insertion of the hydroxyl into the C_{19} steroid in this particular position provides the distinctive precursor (16α-hydroxydehydroepiandrosterone sulfate, 16α-OH-DHAS) for estriol. Another portion of secreted DHAS reaches the placenta unchanged. Here both these steroid sulfates (DHAS and 16α-OH-DHAS) are first converted into the corresponding unconjugated steroids (DHA and 16α-OH-DHA) by steroid sulfatases. The unconjugated steroids are next transformed to the corresponding -4-en-3-oxo steroids by means of the 3β-hydroxysteroid dehydrogenase-isomerase complex. Another enzyme complex, aromatase, acts to convert the A-ring of the -4-en-3-oxo steroids into an aromatic ring, while 17β-hydroxysteroid dehydrogenase ensures reduction at C-17, so that a mixture of estrone and estradiol (from DHAS) and estriol (from 16α-OH-DHAS) is secreted by the placenta. Some hydroxylation of estrone at C-16α takes place in the fetal and maternal liver and also gives rise to estriol. Hydroxylation of estrone in this way is the dominant pathway of estriol

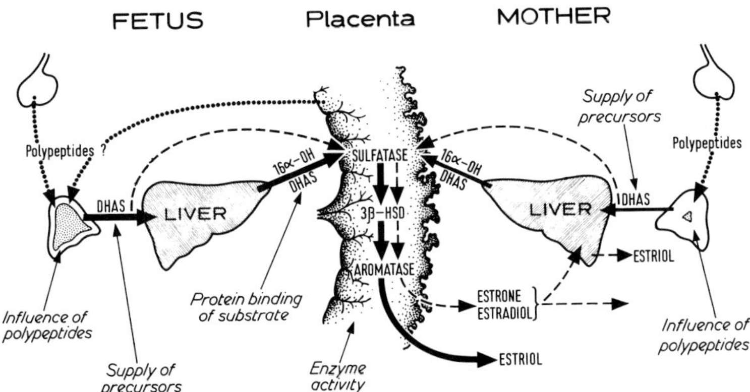

Fig. 2 Representation of the pathways of estrogen biosynthesis in late pregnancy. Possible points of control, as discussed in the text, are in italic. DHAS, Dehydroepiandrosterone sulfate; 16α-OH-DHAS, 16α-hydroxydehydroepiandrosterone sulfate; 3β-HSD, 3β-hydroxysteroid dehydrogenase-isomerase.

biosynthesis in nonpregnant women. This process is overshadowed in late pregnancy by that involving hydroxylation of the neutral steroid precursor before aromatization.

DHAS and 16α-OH-DHAS are present in maternal circulation and can be converted in the placenta to estrone–estradiol and estriol, respectively, but precursors presented from the maternal circulation appear to be poorly utilized. For example, when the fetus is anencephalic the daily excretion near term of estrone–estradiol is reduced by 70% (Michie, 1966) although the mean concentration of DHAS in maternal plasma remains unchanged (normal pregnancy, 1.6 μmole/liter; anencephalic fetus, 1.8 μmole/liter; Tulchinsky *et al.,* 1977). There is a significant fall in the concentration of this precursor in umbilical cord blood in this condition (normal fetus, 5.1 μmole/liter; anencephalic fetus, 0.2 μmole/liter). Measurements of the concentration of 16α-OH-DHAS [the direct precursor of estriol, the excretion of which is reduced by 90% when the fetus is anencephalic (Frandsen and Stakeman, 1961)] in maternal plasma in pregnancies with an anencephalic fetus have not been made with sufficient sensitivity to illustrate the differences. Relevant mean plasma concentrations in normal pregnancies are maternal, 0.6 μmole/liter; umbilical artery, 10.5 μmole/liter; umbilical vein, 8.9 μmole/liter (Laatikainen *et al.,* 1980).

IV. Control of Estrogen Production

The pathway of biosynthesis (Fig. 2) offers several points at which control of production could be exercised. These include (1) alterations in the provision of precursors and (2) variations in placental enzyme activity. Investigations of both possibilities will be considered in turn.

A. *Effects of Alterations in the Supply of Precursors*

1. From the Fetus

The associaton between subnormal concentrations of DHAS and 16α-OH-DHAS and subnormal estrogen excretion in pregnancies complicated by anencephaly has already been discussed (Section III). Subnormal production of these precursors would also be expected in primary hypoplasia of the fetal adrenal glands. Measurements have not been reported, but estrogen excretion is low (Roberts and Cawdry, 1970; Fliegner *et al.*, 1972; Laverty *et al.*, 1973). Congenital adrenal hyperplasia lies at the opposite end, from anencephaly, of the spectrum of abnormalities of the fetal adrenal gland. In those forms, e.g., 21- or 11β-hydroxylase deficiency, associated with excessive androgen production an increase in maternal estrogen excretion might be expected. An initial report was encouraging (Cathro *et al.*, 1969) but the association is not obligatory (Nichols and Gibson, 1969). The reason for this is not clear but may relate to the different zones of the fetal adrenal gland being affected by the enzyme deficiencies to different degrees.

Only exceptionally has it been possible to present precursors of estrogen to the placenta from the fetal side. Michie (1966) noted increases in the excretion of conjugated estrone, estradiol, and estriol on the day following intraamniotic injection of DHAS (250 mg) to four women near term pregnant with an anencephalic fetus. Eighty-six to 94% of the increase was due to estriol indicating involvement of the fetus. Confirmation was provided by Maeyama *et al.* (1976), who found that intraamniotic injection of DHAS (200 mg) into two women with an anencephalic fetus was followed by an additional excretion of estrogen of 30–40 μmole during the next 2 days representing about 5% of precursor. Again 70–85% of the increase was estriol. Thus in these abnormal pregnancies, in which a diminished precursor supply has been demonstrated (Tulchinsky *et al.*, 1977), the placentas retain the capacity to convert precursors to estrogen. Better yields of estrogen were found during investigations of normal pregnancies (Crystle *et al.*, 1973). In these patients intraamniotic injection of saline–ethanol vehicle caused a fall in estrogen excretion during the following 3 days. Injection of 100, 150, or 200 mg DHAS was followed by increases in estrogen excretion of 30–120 μmole. Hausknecht and Mandelman (1969) used a dose of 200 mg DHAS and found increases in estriol excretion of 37–60 μmole (equivalent to 5–9% of substrate) on the following day. This evidence demonstrates that the human placenta is not saturated with precursors presented from the fetal side and has the capacity to increase estrogen production if additional supplies of precursors are provided by the fetus.

Changes in estrogen production are also evident, transiently in the peripheral circulation (Crystle *et al.*, 1973). When DHAS was given intraamniotically the concentration of unconjugated estradiol in maternal serum increased markedly within 2 hours and remained elevated for 48 hours. Conjugated estriol showed a response provided more than 100 mg DHAS had been given. Interestingly, direct injection of DHAS (25–50 mg in an oily vehicle) into the fetal thigh muscle at 36–41 weeks of gestation failed to evoke changes in the concentration of unconjugated estrone or estradiol or conjugated estriol in maternal plasma within 2 hours of injection (Gamissans *et al.*, 1977). Presumably the oily vehicle and the intramuscular injection prevented an uptake of precursor rapid enough for metabolites to be detected in 2 hours.

16α-OH-DHAS has not been tested as a precursor in this way. It would be challenging to our hypothesis to compare the response obtained with this material with that established with DHAS. Estriol concentrations and excretion should increase while those of estrone and estradiol should be unchanged.

2. From the Mother

There are a number of reports of pregnancies in adrenalectomized women (Charles *et al.*, 1970; Maeyama *et al.*, 1975) which, by comparison with normal women, might be expected to illustrate the contribution to estrogen production of precursors from the maternal adrenal. Inevitably such patients receive corticosteroid therapy, which may exert, indirectly, a suppressive effect on the fetal pituitary–adrenal axis. This invalidates the interpretation of any unusually low estrogen excretion observed as due entirely to lack of precursors from the maternal adrenal.

Alterations in the supply of estrogen precursors from the maternal side of the placenta have received much more attention than have manipulations involving the fetus. Most commonly DHAS or DHA has been injected iv or taken by mouth with the intention of assessing increases in the concentration of estrogens in plasma as an index of placental function (Lauritzen, 1967; Strecker *et al.*, 1978) or of their clearances from blood to predict subsequent development of preeclampsia (Gant *et al.*, 1976). Although neither of these tests has been widely adopted, valuable information was collected during their development.

Formal investigation of the behaviour of infused DHAS has been carried out by Buster *et al.* (1974), Belisle *et al.* (1977), and Madden *et al.* (1976), while Belisle *et al.* (1980) studied DHA. The half-life of DHAS in plasma, measured within the first 8 hours following an injection of DHAS (2.5 mg/kg body wt in 5 minutes) at about 18 weeks of gestation was found to be about 2.9 hours whether the fetus was alive or not (Buster *et al.,* 1974). When measurements were made within 12 hours after delivery the half-life had increased to 4.8 hours. Similar measurements near term and after delivery (Belisle *et al.,* 1977) gave half-lives of 2.4 and 3 hours, respectively, whereas in nonpregnant women the half-life is 8–11 hours (Baulieu *et al.,* 1965). The increased clearance rate in pregnancy is therefore independent of the fetus and persists for some time after delivery of the placenta. The two important organs for the clearance of DHAS appear to be the placenta (presumably involving hydrolysis and aromatization) and the liver where hydroxylation at C-16α to form 16α-OH-DHAS is quantitatively important (Madden *et al.,* 1976). This pathway appears to be inducible by estrogens (Gurpide *et al.,* 1973), and probably accounts for the persistance of the high clearance rate of DHAS in the puerperium. Androstenedione and testosterone lie on the pathway of placental estrogen biosynthesis intermediate between DHAS and estrone–estradiol. Short-lived changes in the concentration of both these androgens in peripheral plasma have been recognized within 1 hour following injection of DHAS (50 mg iv, Klopper *et al.,* 1976; Ylikorkala *et al.,* 1980), but others (Belisle *et al.,* 1977) were unable to detect these intermediates.

Estrogen concentrations in maternal plasma respond promptly to infusion or iv injection of DHAS. Unconjugated estrone and estradiol concentrations increase within 1 hour, usually by a factor of 4 (Belisle *et al.,* 1977; Ylikorkala *et al.,* 1980; Kauppila and Ylikorkala, 1980; Buster *et al.,* 1974; Axelsson *et al.,* 1978); the estrone response is smaller and occurs more slowly (Fraser *et al.,* 1976). There was no change in the concentration of unconjugated estriol (Belisle *et al.,* 1977; Buster *et al.,* 1974; Fraser *et al.,* 1976) or of conjugated estriol (Ylikorkala *et al.,* 1980) within 5 hours of injection. This lack of immediate response after DHAS to the mother reflects the pathway of biosynthesis and the transfer constants (ρ values) reported by Madden *et al.* (1978). For example 29% of DHAS in the maternal plasma is converted to estradiol and 36% to 16α-OH-DHAS. Only 17% of this is converted to estriol. Conjugation of any estriol formed also delays the appearance of this metabolite in the plasma. The independence from fetal participation of the conversion of injected DHAS to estrone–estradiol is demonstrated by the dramatic increase in plasma estradiol after injection of DHAS (50–100 mg iv) to women 2–11 days following fetal death (Fraser *et al.,* 1976; Korda *et al.,* 1975). Evidence like this implies that the procedure could be seriously misleading if used as an index of fetal condition. Increased urinary estrogen excretion has also been reported. Scommegna *et al.* (1968) reported modest increases in estriol excretion (13–50 μmole/day in five normal patients at 34–38 weeks of gestation) following DHAS (200 mg, iv). Urinary estrone and estradiol were not measured.

3. Indirectly

Supplies of endogenous precursors might be expected to be altered by treatment which stimulated or suppressed the secretion of precursors from the fetal or maternal adrenal gland. Examples are available for consideration.

a. Challenge with Adrenocorticotrophin (ACTH). Several papers record the effects upon urinary estrogen excretion, of injection of ACTH (usually 25–40 IU ACTH-Zn) to the mother. Dassler (1966) found a clear increase in urinary estriol and a smaller one for estrone and estradiol the day following injection. Similar responses were found by Maeyama and Nakagawa (1970). These authors also established, by measurement of 17-hydroxycorticosteroid excretion, that some degree of adrenal stimulation had been achieved. Maeyama *et al.* (1969), like Dassler (1966), showed that there was no response after fetal death, and, in addition, in two pregnancies where the fetus was anencephalic. The results, particularly the greater response of estriol compared to that of estrone–estradiol and the lack of response after fetal death or anencephaly, imply that the fetal adrenal is participating in the responses found, through ACTH crossing the placenta. However, studies of a pregnant woman with Nelson's syndrome (inappropriate raised secretion of ACTH after adrenalectomy) indicated that endogenous ACTH does not cross the placenta (Allen *et al.,* 1973). Consequently, the interpretation of these findings, implying a regulation of the fetal adrenal by maternal ACTH remains unsatisfactory. Moreover, ACTH injected into the mother should also produce extra DHAS from the maternal gland and therefore a greater response of estrone–estradiol would be expected than was found. Scommegna *et al.* (1968), Dickey and Thompson (1969), and Jeffery *et al.* (1970) did not find consistent responses to ACTH injected into the mother. Concomitant excretion of 17-hydroxycorticosteroids, where measured, did not suggest that adrenal tissue had been adequately stimulated.

Probably the most detailed and well-designed studies of the effect of ACTH injected into the mother on estrogen precursors and products were reported by Simmer *et al.* (1974, 1975). The concentrations of cortisol, 16α-OH-DHAS, DHAS, 16α-OH-DHA, DHA, and unconjugated estrone, estradiol, and estriol were measured in plasma from the cord vein, cord artery, and a maternal peripheral vein of 17 patients who were delivered by elective cesarean section at term. Seven of these patients received ACTH (40 IU) 4–6.5 hours before delivery. Comparison of the results from control and ACTH-treated subjects indicated that ACTH had little effect on maternal 16α-OH-DHAS, DHAS, 16α-OH-DHA, DHA, estrone, estradiol, or estriol concentrations in these circumstances. Nor were there alterations in the concentrations of DHA, DHAS, estrone, or estradiol in the cord artery and vein plasma. The mean concentrations of 16α-OH-DHAS and estriol were reduced significantly in umbilical artery and vein plasma, while that of 16α-OH-DHA was reduced in the cord artery. Associated with these changes were significant increases in mean concentrations of cortisol and non-protein-bound cortisol but not of ACTH, in fetal and maternal plasma. Thus excess cortisol generated by the ACTH crosses the placenta and suppresses the supply of 16α-hydroxy-C_{19} steroid sulfates through effects on the fetal pituitary–adrenal axis. Intraamniotic injection of ACTH was given by Jorgensen and Lebech (1971) and rather small responses of increased estrogen and 17-oxosteroid excretion were achieved. Injection of ACTH into the mother (two patients) resulted in increases of 17-oxogenic steroid excretion, but not of estrogen. Following direct injection of ACTH (40 iu) into the fetus at mid gestation Arai *et al.* (1972) found the mean daily estrogen excretion increased 20–74% (n = 4) of which 84–94% was estriol, implicating a fetal response. In contrast, Burd *et al.* (1970) found no response to this dose of ACTH at term, even when endogenous steroid secretion was suppressed by dexamethasone (6 mg/day).

b. Challenge with Metyrapone. This drug interferes with cortisol synthesis. It is used to test the integrity of the pituitary–adrenal axis and to assess the potential of pituitary tissue to respond to diminished concentrations of cortisol in plasma with an increased secretion of ACTH. For this reason it has been used to examine whether there are changes in estrogen production in response to increased quantities of precursor, consequent upon raised secretion of ACTH. A prompt response in urinary estrogen excretion was seen in each of three normal subjects treated with 750 mg of metyrapone every 4 hours for 24 hours (Scommegna *et al.*, 1968). Fifteen patients were tested by Dickey and Thompson (1969) of whom five showed a clear response in urinary 17-oxosteroid excretion demonstrating sufficient drug had been given to stimulate extra ACTH secretion. These five patients all showed an increased excretion of urinary estriol. Independently, Oakey and Heys (1970) compared the response of six women with an intact fetus and three women with an anencephalic fetus to this standard dose. Changes in 17-oxogenic steroid excretion demonstrated that increased adrenal steroid production was provoked in all patients. Each woman with an intact fetus showed increased estrogen excretion (mean excretion before treatment was 100 μmole/day; maximum after treatment was 170 μmole/day) whereas no response in estrogen excretion was observed in women pregnant with an anencephalic fetus. These results imply that metyrapone acts, presumably through ACTH secreted by the fetal pituitary, to stimulate production of precursors from the fetal adrenal. Significant uptake of precursor from the maternal adrenal can be discounted in view of the results in pregnancies with an anencephalic fetus. These results imply also that a negative feedback system exists in the fetus with cortisol controlling the secretion of pituitary corticotrophins.

c. Challenge with Glucocorticosteroids. Information on the effects of glucocorticosteroids on estrogen excretion arose from casual observations on women receiving these steroids for diseases coexisting with their pregnancy, e.g., arthritis, asthma, inflammatory conditions. More recently responses to acute high dose treatment has been investigated in patients receiving β-methasone therapy in premature labor.

Early reports merely noted the association between maternal corticosteroid therapy and estrogen excretion inappropriate to the condition of the baby at birth. However, Brown *et al.* (1968) challenged patients with cortisol (100 mg on 2 consecutive days) and noted that mean estriol excretion fell by 40%, estrone by 50%, and estradiol by 50% of pretreatment values. A higher dose of glucocorticosteroid (dexamethasone 6 mg/day for 10 days) caused even greater suppression of estrogen excretion (Warren and Cheatum, 1967). In quantitative terms the effect on estriol was the greatest, implying suppression of the supply of precursors from the fetus. The response appears to be dose-related. Of 17 women who received 10–160 mg of cortisol (or equivalent) daily, after 34 weeks of gestation, those who delivered surviving infants of adequate birth weight showed normal estrogen excretion unless the dose exceeded 75 mg/day (Oakey, 1970b). Direct evidence that corticosteroids suppress estrogen production through reducing the supply of precursors from the fetus is due to Simmer and his colleagues (Simmer *et al.,* 1966, 1974, 1975). These workers compared the concentrations of DHAS, 16α-OH-DHAS, and unconjugated estrone, estradiol, and estriol in plasma from a maternal peripheral vein, cord artery, and cord vein in 16 patients undergoing elective cesarean section at term, 6 of whom received cortisol hemisuccinate (50 mg, 10, 6, and 2 hours before delivery). Under these circumstances the mean concentrations of each estrogen and their precursors were substantially diminished in the patients receiving corticosteroids.

Very high doses of glucocorticosteroids suppress production for several days after stopping treatment. For example, 3 days after ceasing cortisol therapy (100 mg/day for 2 days) estriol excretion was almost back to pretreatment values (Brown *et al.,* 1968). Five days after stopping dexamethasone (6 mg/day for 10 days) total estrogen excretion was close to normal (Warren and Cheatum, 1967). When even higher daily doses were given (12 mg dexamethasone for 3 days) urinary estrogen excretion did not return to pretreatment values for 3 weeks (Ohrlander *et al.,* 1975). Long-term suppressive effects were also noted in plasma estrone and estradiol concentrations which were still depressed up to 6 days after ceasing treatment, the longest sampling time tested (Ohrlander *et al.*, 1977). Despite these suppressive effects on androgen secretion few, if any, of the infants show evidence of adrenal suppression, possibly due to different effects of pituitary hormones on the fetal and definitive zones of the fetal adrenal.

Some authors, considering that cortisol from the maternal circulation might exert an indirect regulatory action on the fetal adrenal gland, have sought relationships between unconjugated estrogen and cortisol concentrations in maternal plasma. Patrick *et al.* (1979) noted that the lowest concentrations of estriol (found at 10.00 hours) were preceded by the highest concentrations of cortisol which occurred at 08.00 hours. The lowest concentrations of cortisol (24.00–02.00) were at times when estriol concentration was highest. A similar illustration of negative feedback control has been demonstrated by Reck *et al.* (1978) who found that a fall in the concentration of unconjugated estriol, from 125 to 41 nmole/liter, occurred in association with an increase in cortisol concentration from 1.1 up to 3.9 μmole/liter brought about by infusion of ACTH. It should be noted that the final concentration of cortisol reached is much in excess of normal (1.5 μmole/liter, Reck *et al.*, 1979) so that the physiological importance of these observations is rather limited. Other direct, rather than inverse, relationships were found between the times of maximum and minimal concentrations of estrone or estradiol and cortisol (Patrick *et al.*, 1979; Reck *et al.*, 1979) implying that these estrogens were derived from precursors from the maternal adrenal which were secreted in synchrony with cortisol.

d. Through Protein Binding of Substrate. The avidity and extent of substrate binding to plasma proteins may also modify the rate of estrogen production. In the reversible ligand–protein interaction the concentrations of free and bound substrate depend on the association constant and the concentrations of protein and ligand. Only non-protein-bound ligand is readily available for entry into cells, but uptake of this from the blood will provoke dissociation of bound ligand. Protein binding will delay metabolism to an extent depending on the transit time through the placenta and half-time of dissociation of the ligand–protein complex. Studies relating the dissociation of cortisol from its binding protein to its metabolism by liver have been reported (Paterson, 1973) but there has been no comparison of the dissociation of testosterone in relation to uptake by the placenta. Experiments *in vitro* involving sex hormone binding globulin (SHBG), which binds testosterone with high affinity $K_a = 8 \times 10^8$ liters/mole, but has little affinity for androstenedione, DHA, or DHAS, have been reported. The rate of conversion of testosterone to estradiol by placental microsome preparations was inhibited by preincubation of the substrate with SHBG (Mowszowciz *et al.*, 1970). Physiological concentrations of albumin also inhibited the conversion, although its affinity for testosterone is weak (K_a = 3.6 × 10^4 liters/mole). The albumin effect was not reversible on denaturing the albumin, so it may be nonspecific. Similar experiments (Hampl and Starka, 1973) demonstrated that the inhibition by SHBG could be reversed by addition of excess estradiol, presumably through displacement of substrate from the protein. The authors incubated [^{3}H]testosterone, SHBG, and estradiol in concentrations designed to mimic those of the fetal or maternal blood. Higher conversions of substrate were recorded under fetal conditions (68% substrate used) than under maternal conditions (0.2% substrate used). This was also reflected in the mass of substrate converted. However, testosterone must be considered a minor substrate, compared with the androgen sulfates. DHAS is bound with weak affinity (K_a = 1 × 10^5 liters/mole) to albumin. Until the rate of dissociation is measured and compared with the transit time through the placenta, no proper assessment of the role of substrate binding in the regulation of estrogen synthesis can be made.

4. Indirectly *in Vitro:* Challenges with Polypeptides of Placental or Pituitary Origin

Because of the difficulties inherent in sampling the human fetal compartment and of isolating it from the placenta, many experiments have been carried out *in vitro* to assess the response of the fetal adrenal toward possible trophic agents. Relatively short-term exposures—a few hours to a few days—have been given; changes in steroid production have been used to assess the response. The time scale *in vivo* is much longer and the response may involve effects on tissue growth, rather than only on steroid biosynthesis, although in adrenal tissue these effects appear to be closely associated (Roos, 1974). Inevitably most experiments have used tissue collected at termination of pregnancies of less than 24 weeks of gestation. Extrapolation of the results obtained to the circumstances at term is hardly justifiable particularly with tissue which grows through gestation. The results quoted below should therefore be considered with this reservation in mind. Early reports (Bloch and Benirschke, 1959, 1962) showed that the incorporation of [^{14}C]acetate into [^{14}C]DHA by adrenal tissue obtained at 15 and 17 weeks of gestation increased 40–100% above control values on addition of 0.1–0.2 iu ACTH/100 mg tissue. ACTH and hCG were found to increase the quantity of [^{14}C]DHA formed from [^{14}C]cholesterol or [^{14}C]pregnenolone by slices of human fetal adrenals obtained at 12–25 weeks of gestation (Lehmann and Lauritzen, 1975). A similar approach was used by Isherwood and Oakey (1976) but with emphasis on the incorportion of [^{14}C]acetate into [^{14}C] DHAS. ACTH (12.5–50 iu/100 mg tissue) stimulated the incorporation of precursor by 8–65 times, relative to the controls. Even more substantial was the effect of human growth hormone (hGH, 25 μg/100 mg tissue); incorporation was 130 times that of control levels. Chorionic somatomammotrophin (placental lactogen, 200 μg/100 mg tissue) increased the yield of [^{14}C]DHAS 22-fold.

More recent work has involved measurement of steroids produced from endogenous precursors, rather the estimation of the incorporation of labeled substrates into products. The use of tissue and cell culture techniques has also been applied to the problem. Kahri *et al.* (1976) drew attention to differences in behavior during culture between cells of the fetal zone (which were rapidly lost from the cultures) and cells of the definitive zone (which proliferated). Consequently cells kept in culture for 6 days or more may be quite unrepresentative of the original tissue source. Despite this Kahri *et al.* (1976) demonstrated increased secretion (16–160 times control) of DHAS in response to ACTH (0.1 IU/ml/day) during the seventh to twelfth days of culture. Explants of fetal adrenal still respond to ACTH in the early days of culture (Carr *et al.*, 1980a). Omission of ACTH from the culture medium in this early phase led to a decline in daily production of DHAS and to an exaggerated response when ACTH was eventually added. Apparently cell surface receptors for ACTH appear to maintain their sensitivity to ACTH for at least 6 days. Cell culture was also used by Branchaud *et al.* (1978) to assess the response of fetal adrenal cells to ACTH, α-MSH, and CLIP. These latter two polypeptides were selected because Silman *et al.* (1976) had proposed they were the dominant pituitary hormones of fetal life and were replaced by hACTH only before parturition, although some doubt has been cast on their identification of α-MSH (Tilders *et al.*, 1981). α-MSH, at concentrations about $10^{-6} M$, was equipotent with ACTH (2×10^{-8}–2×10^{-9} *M*) at stimulating production of DHAS. CLIP was without effect.

Exposure of tissue slices to a stream of buffer which can bring stimulants/inhibitors to the tissue and carries away products (superfusion) has also been used. The response of fetal zone tissue to ACTH was reported by Seron-Ferre *et al.* (1978b). Incorporation of ACTH into the buffer at a concentration of $5 \times 10^{-5} M$ provoked a twofold increase in DHAS production within 1 hour. The definitive zone showed little response to ACTH when assessed by assay of DHAS. In a different experimental design, Seron-Ferre *et al.* (1978a) showed that fetal zone tissue exposed to hCG (250 μg/liter) for 6 hours produced significantly more DHAS than corresponding tissue not exposed to hCG. These and other peptides were tested by Brown *et al.* (1981). ACTH (2×10^{-7}–4×10^{-9} *M*), hCG (1.5–15 IU/ml), hGH (2–4 × 10^{-8} *M*), and α-MSH (1–6 × 10^{-8} *M*) appeared equally active in stimulating DHAS in this preparation. Metenkephalin (2×10^{-6} *M*) and β-LPH (1 × 10^{-7} – 5×10^{-8} *M*) were almost as active while ovine prolactin (2–4.5 × 10^{-7} *M*) was weaker. CLIP (2×10^{-7} *M*) was without effect.

The effect of extracts of fetal pituitaries rather than of individual polypeptides has also been assessed. Seron-Ferrc *et al.* (1978b) found a response from fetal zone tissue in only one of three experiments while Goodyer *et al.* (1977) found a positive response to all five adrenal samples tested in tissue culture.

These experiments have established that a number of polypeptide hormones of pituitary or chorionic origin possess the ability to stimulate secretion of DHAS *in vitro*. The effect does not appear to be nonspecific since steroid production from bovine adrenal tissue was unresponsive to gonadotrophins, albumin, or dextran (Brown *et al.*, 1981). However, the variety of materials giving responses and the multiplicity of peptides which may be secreted by the pituitary gland suggest that this approach has little further to offer in terms of identifying the polypeptide essential for adrenal stimulation. There may not be, of course, a single polypeptide responsible, but rather a number of hormones acting synergistically or sequentially. Future experiments might examine extracts of pituitary tissue or of fetal blood as corticotrophins and use specific antisera to neutralize the effects of individual components.

In the most recent experiments to investigate control of steroid production by the fetal adrenal gland, cell culture techniques have been used to assess the response of these fetal adrenal cells to polypeptides. During preparation for culture, the cells of necessity are exposed to collagenase and trypsin, which might be thought to modify cell surface characteristics. Despite this treatment, cells prepared in this way show the typical retraction on exposure to ACTH (Simonian and Gill, 1981). Nevertheless, intracellular features characteristic of fresh fetal zone or definitive zone cells disappear during culture for 6 days (Fujieda *et al.*, 1981a). After this period in culture, the two types of cell appear indistinguishable, an observation recorded earlier (Kahri *et al.*, 1976). Dispersed cells in culture produce little steroid unless ACTH is incorporated in the medium (Fujieda *et al.*, 1981b). Responses in the production of DHA and cortisol can be detected within 2 hours of addition of ACTH, but usually cultures were maintained for several days before the response was assessed. Fujieda *et al.* (1981a) reported that both fetal and definitive zone cells secreted both DHA and cortisol in culture, and considered that specialization of steroid production within the two zones was not supported by their results. The conclusions were based on assay of DHA rather than of DHAS. The cells were exquisitely sensitive to ACTH. When culture was maintained for 6 days, ACTH in a concentration of 10^{-12} *M* clearly stimulated production of DHA and cortisol. Other polypeptides, for example hCG (650 IU/liter), hGH (10^{-9} *M*), hPRL (10^{-9} *M*), α-MSH (10^{-12} *M*), CLIP (10^{-7} *M*), or β-LPH (10^{-11} *M*) failed to provoke the response in the output of DHA or cortisol under these conditions (Fujeida *et al.*, 1981c).

Using similar techniques, Simonian and Gill (1981) also demonstrated the response of monolayers of cells to ACTH (10^{-9} *M*). Fetal zone cells examined within the first 24 hours of culture secreted more DHAS, relative to cortisol, than was secreted by definitive zone cells. However, during culture for 4 or 5 days, the ratio of secreted DHAS to cortisol fell, an observation also made by Fujieda *et al.* (1981c). This was interpreted as due to induction of 3β-hydroxysteroid dehydrogenase-isomerase by ACTH. This evidence again calls into question the proposal that specialization exists in the two zones in regard to the nature of the steroid output. However, exposure of cells in monolayer culture to polypeptides may evoke responses different from those obtained when the cell is incorporated into the tissues of an organ. The differences in results obtained from the cell culture and the tissue slice approaches may be due to the distinct differences in preparation techniques used and in the duration of exposure. Which approach provides the more accurate reflection of the physiological response remains to be determined.

The system for delivery of substrate to the adrenal gland may play a significant role in regulating steroid secretion. Like the adult adrenal gland, the fetal adrenal gland can use cholesterol or acetate in the blood as substrate (Telegdy *et al.,* 1970a; Archer *et al.,* 1971). Cholesterol held in the low-density lipoprotein fraction of serum is the preferred substrate, at least in tissue cultured in the presence of ACTH (Carr *et al.,* 1980b). Under these circumstances *de novo* synthesis of cholesterol from acetate by the tissue is also stimulated (Carr *et al.,* 1980c).

B. Effects of Alterations in Activities of Placental Enzymes

1. In Association with Complications of Pregnancy

Estrogen production could be controlled by regulation of enzyme activities in the placenta. This idea was attractive because complications of pregnancy, such as high blood pressure, which were believed to alter placental blood flow and diminish placental growth, were often associated with lower than normal estrogen excretion. Results have been inconsistent. Laumas *et al.* (1968) and Rahman *et al.* (1975) measured the conversions of 19-hydroxyandrostenedione, androstenedione, and testosterone to estrone and estradiol by microsomes from a standard mass of placenta. Mean conversions by placentas from pregnancies complicated by toxemia were significantly lower than those from uncomplicated pregnancies. This finding was confirmed with DHA, DHAS, and androstenedione as substrates. However, initial reaction rates were not measured, although saturation of enzymes with substrate was apparent. Independently, Lehmann *et al.* (1973) showed that the mean conversion of DHA or androstenedione to estrogen was lower with preparations of placentas from toxemic pregnancies than from normal. This is so if their values reported after 5-minute incubations are considered as initial rates, but only four normal tissues were studied. In contrast, yields from experiments with 15 normal placentas were in a range similar to those from pregnancies complicated by diabetes (*n* = 6) or retarded fetal growth (*n* = 11) (Sybulski, 1969). In a large study based on measurement of initial reaction rates, Townsley *et al.* (1973) found no differences in aromatase and sulfatase activities in placentas from 22 normal and 44 abnormal pregnancies. This research must weigh heavily in assessing the balance of the evidence. Inhibition of 3β-hydroxysteroid dehydrogenase-isomerase *in vitro* with cyanoketone abolished the conversion of DHA to estrone and estradiol, emphasizing the importance of this enzyme in estrogen biosynthesis (Yates and Oakey, 1972). It seems unlikely therefore that placental enzyme activities, as measured *in vitro,* play an important role in regulating the level of estrogen production. This is particularly so in view of the evidence quoted earlier regarding the effects of an enhanced supply of precursor.

There is one notable exception to the conclusion that the level of enzyme activities in the placenta plays little part directly in regulating estrogen production.This is the condition known as steroid sulfatase deficiency which is an example of an inherited enzyme deficiency rather than an illustration of a physiological control mechanism. In this condition the fetus inherits, in an X-linked recessive mode, the inability to express steroid sulfatase activity (France and Liggins, 1969). The deficiency is apparent in skin cells, and presumably throughout the body tissues of the affected (male) subjects (Shapiro *et al.,* 1978). The placenta, a product of conception, also fails to express steroid sulfatase activity. Because of its involvement in estrogen biosynthesis and the relatively large quantities of tissue available, interest has focused on enzyme activity in this tissue.

The test which establishes the condition is the failure of preparations of the placenta to hydrolyze DHAS *in vitro* while showing ability for estrogen synthesis from DHA. This test is only carried out after birth but experience with injection of precursors in pregnancies subsequently demonstrated to lack steroid sulfatase *in vitro* is informative. For example, France (1980) compared the urinary excretion of estrone, estradiol, and estriol before and after DHA (100 mg) and DHAS (100 mg) to two patients on different occasions. The excretion of each estrogen increased noticeably after DHA but not after DHAS. Bedin *et al.* (1980) reported that the mean urinary estrogen excretion, estimated by fluorimetry without separation into individual estrogens, was 10.5 ± 5.1 (SD) μmole/24 hours before DHAS and 11.3 ± 5.2 μmole/24 hours afterward (*n* = 9). In contrast when three of these patients were given DHA (100 mg) estrogen excretion increased from 3.4 to 15.5, 12.7 to 20.5, and 9.4 to 18.0 μmole/24 hours, respectively. Lack of estrogen response is also seen after intraamniotic instillation of DHAS in affected pregnancies (Tabei and Heinrichs, 1976).

Similar evidence of the role of placental steroid sulfatase is shown if plasma estrogen concentrations are measured within 6 hours after injection of DHAS (Bedin *et al.,* 1980). In seven cases the mean estradiol concentration was 8.38 ± 5.9 (SD) nmole/liter before injection of DHAS and 10.1 ± 6.5 nmole/liter afterward. This response should be compared with the corresponding values of 20.7 ± 13.0 and 87.6 ± 35.2 nmole/liter in normal pregnancy.

The relative activities of placental steroid sulfatase activity *in vitro* in sulfatase deficiency and in normal pregnancy (Marton and Oakey, 1980) were (pmole/mg protein/minute) boiled tissue, 124 ± 92 (mean ± SD, n = 6); affected tissue, 194 ± 147 (n = 9); normal tissue, 2940 ± 184 (n = 7). Other enzymes in the chain required for estrogen biosynthesis appear to show somewhat depressed activity *in vitro* (France and Liggins, 1969; France *et al.,* 1973; Osathanondh *et al.,* 1976; Marton and Oakey,1980; Oakey *et al.,* 1974). This may be due to the effect of freezing and thawing the tissue (Marton and Oakey, 1980) which affects 3β-hydroxysteroid dehydrogenase-isomerase of sulfatase-deficient placentas more than that of normal placentas. This abnormality in turn may be related to deficiencies in membrane composition (McNaught and France, 1980; McKee *et al.,* 1981).

2. Through Inhibition by Steroids

Despite the lack of regulation of estrogen synthesis by placental enzyme activity there is evidence to suggest that these enzymes do not act in an uncontrolled environment. Townsley *et al.* (1970) noticed that steroid sulfatase activity was rate limiting for estrogen synthesis *in vivo,* but not *in vitro* with washed placental microsomes. These authors found that steroid sulfatase was susceptible to inhibition *in vitro* by progesterone, pregnenolone sulfate, 20α-dihydroprogesterone, pregnenolone, estradiol, and DHA in the concentrations encountered in cord blood. This effect was not observed when cultured choriocarcinoma cells were studied (Schut and Townsley, 1977). 3β-Hydroxysteroid dehydrogenase-isomerase activity, an essential link in the conversion of DHA to androstenedione, is also amenable to inhibition from endogenous steroids at concentrations found in maternal plasma (Townsley, 1975). There are also reports (Story *et al.,* 1974; Schut and Townsley, 1977) that estrogen production *in vitro* from DHA, androstenedione, and DHAS is enhanced by addition of cyclic adenosine monophosphate and its derivatives. The physiological importance of this observation has not been assessed.

3. Through Chorionic Gonadotrophin

In view of the relatively large quantities of hCG synthesized by the placenta, even in late pregnancy, some workers have questioned whether this hormone has any effect on estrogen biosynthesis at the level of the placental enzymes. The results have been inconsistent. Varangot *et al.* (1965) measured the influence of hCG (20,000 IU) on aromatase activity during *in vitro* perfusion of placentas and found a significant effect of this polypeptide on the conversion of 16α-hydroxytestosterone or 16α-hydroxyandrostenedione to estriol. An effect of luteinizing hormone (LH) on aromatase activity was also reported (Cedard *et al.*, 1968). Others, admittedly using different conditions, failed to confirm these findings. In particular, Macome *et al.* (1972) were unable to detect differences in the conversion of [^{14}C]androstenedione to radioactive estrone and estradiol due to addition of hCG (350 IU), 300 units of anti-hCG, or both, to preparations of human placentas.

V. Estrogens in Plasma in Relation to the Onset of Labor

The pathways of estrogen biosynthesis outlined earlier, together with appropriate production of DHAS and DHA from the fetal and maternal adrenal glands, lead to production of increasing quantities of estrone, estradiol, and estriol as gestation progresses. These processes are reflected in increasing quantities of unconjugated estrogen in maternal blood. The estrogens are released from the placenta in an unconjugated form, but a high proportion is rapidly converted into conjugated forms by addition of β-glucuronic acid or sulfuric acid residues. These are without estrogenic activity and may be considered as inactivated material proceeding toward elimination. The overall pattern of estrogen concentrations in the last few weeks of gestation takes the form shown in Table I. In the umbilical vein plasma the relative concentrations are estriol > estrone> estradiol; concen-

Table I

Concentrations of Estrone, Estradiol, and Estriol in the Umbilical Circulation at Delivery[a]

Number of patients and mode of delivery[b]	Estrone		Estradiol		Estriol		Reference
	UA	UV	UA	UV	UA	UV	
n = 5; sp.	27.7	57.7	7.0	18.9	316	543	Antonipillai and Murphy (1977)
n = 14; c.s.	16.3	36.3	8.5	16.8	350	508	Antonipillai and Murphy (1977)
n = 5; c.s.	21.9	40.7	10.0	23.7	116	235	Tulchinsky (1973)
n = 6; sp.	9.2	30.3	6.6	28.5	67	336	Shutt *et al.* (1974)
n = 5; c.s.	5.2	44.4	5.2	24.4	77	267	Shutt *et al.* (1974)
n = 10; c.s.	61.9	83.7	54.6	58.9	382	466	Simmer *et al.* (1974)

[a]Values are means from the several works cited and the units are nmole/liter.
[b]sp., Spontaneous delivery; c.s., cesarean section; UA, umbilical artery; UV, umbilical vein.

Table II

Concentrations of Estrone, Estradiol, and Estriol in Maternal Peripheral Plasma during the Last 10 weeks of Gestation[a]

Estrone			Estradiol			Estriol			
30 weeks	35 weeks	40 weeks	30 weeks	35 weeks	40 weeks	30 weeks	35 weeks	40 weeks	Reference
18.1	16.7	27.7	40.7	54.4	74.0	17.5	26.0	51.9	Lindberg *et al.* (1974)
19.2	29.6	26.6	56.2	57.4	64.0	22.1	41.4	51.5	De Hertogh *et al.* (1975)
22.2	27.4	27.4	38.6	51.8	59.3	24.5	28.0	47.4	Tulchinsky *et al.* (1972)
25.9	44.4	—	51.5	95.3	—	10.5	21.0	—	Loriaux *et al.* (1972)
						21.0	35.0	66.6	Katagiri *et al.* (1976)

[a]Values are means from the various works cited and the units are nmole/liter.

trations in the umbilical arterial plasma are in the same relative proportions. The relative concentrations in maternal peripheral plasma (Table II) are quite different since estradiol > estriol > estrone. The concentration of each estrogen increases as gestation progresses.

It must be assumed that the biochemical events of estrogen synthesis and removal are organized to achieve this pattern. It has been argued that a yet to be defined concentration of, or exposure to, estrogen is required to bring about normal parturition. However, there are sufficient examples to suggest that the onset of labor and parturition in the human, as in other species, has many components, not all of which are absolute requirements e.g., Knight and O'Connor (1977). Thus labor may be delayed in spite of relatively high estrogen titers in blood, or may occur even when estrogen concentrations are low. Csapo (1969) has argued that the relative concentration of estrogen and progesterone is an important factor. Progesterone inhibits and estrogen permits uterine contractions. Therefore labor may commence when progesterone concentrations fall, or estrogen concentrations rise, or when both these occur. In this section some of the experimental findings that have been collected on this topic in relation to estrogens will be considered.

A clear indication of sharply rising concentrations of unconjugated estradiol in maternal plasma before onset of labor was reported by Turnbull *et al.* (1974) in a study of 33 selected primigravid patients. Mean values began to increase 5 weeks before the onset of labor and rose steadily. In the final week the mean concentration (67 nmole/liter) was almost twice that 5 weeks earlier. An increase was found in all patients but large ones in only 13, so that these changes may have been overemphasized (Flint, 1978). Mathur *et al.* (1980) could not confirm these findings in a study of 25–30 women with uncomplicated pregnancy. Mean estradiol concentration was maximal 2–3 weeks before the onset of labor and was significant lower at labor.

No consistent changes in estradiol or estriol concentrations were found in the last 3 weeks of gestation by Shaaban and Klopper (1973). On the other hand, Chew and Ratnam (1976) reported a steady rise in mean estradiol concentrations in 32 women, which increased from 83 nmole/liter at 35 weeks of gestation to 120 nmole/liter at term. Increasing estriol concentrations were observed in 3 out of 5 normal women (as judged from 10-day rolling mean values) commencing 16–40 days before the onset of labor (Boroditsky *et al.*, 1978). Changes in estradiol concentrations in these patients were less clear, showing a steady rise in only two. An interest in estriol was also recorded by Buster *et al.* (1976) and by Sakakini *et al.* (1977) who detected a surge in mean estriol concentration from 39 nmole/liter at 35 weeks of gestation to 56 nmole/liter at 37 weeks. Mean values before and after this discontinuity increased only slowly. An independent investigation failed to substantiate this surge in estriol (Penney, 1980) but time trend analysis of estriol concentrations in 42 patients enabled prediction of gestational age at delivery to within 2 weeks (Buster *et al.*, 1980). In another approach, the concentrations of estradiol from the twenty-sixth week of gestation onward in normal pregnancy and in pregnancies complicated by prematurity of no known cause were compared (Cousins *et al.*, 1977). If estradiol plays some special role in the etiology of premature delivery higher concentrations would be expected in this condition. However lower values, in general, were found. There does not seem consistent evidence for any abrupt changes in plasma estrogen titer related to the onset of delivery. The findings will be discussed later in the article.

Measurements usually assess all of the unconjugated estrogen in plasma, but only the portion of this which is not bound to protein is readily available to evoke a biological response. This fraction is more difficult to measure. The proportion of estriol in maternal peripheral plasma which is not protein bound appears to be unchanged (approx 17%) in the luteal phase, early pregnancy, and at term (Tulchinsky, 1973). Consequently the concentration of nonprotein-bound estriol parallels that of total unconjugated estriol. In contrast, the proportion of estradiol which is not bound to protein falls between early pregnancy (1.2%) and term (0.7%) so that the concentration of non-protein-bound estradiol bears no simple relationship to total unconjugated estradiol (Tulchinsky, 1973). Perhaps more detailed investigation of changes in the non-protein-bound portions of estrogen in relation to the onset of labor would be revealing.

VI. Biosynthesis of Progesterone

The most striking feature of progesterone biosynthesis is its independence from estrogen synthesis. In the gonads, for example, estrogen arises from further metabolism of the C_{21} steroids pregnenolone and progesterone, which in turn arise from cholesterol. These steroids are linked in a chain:

$$C_{27} \rightarrow C_{21} \rightarrow C_{19} \rightarrow C_{18}$$

The placenta however has no ability to carry out the reactions necessary for $C_{21} \rightarrow C_{19}$. The enzymes concerned with introduction of the C-17 hydroxyl group and subsequent C-17 → C-20 cleavage are inactive. Perfusion of placentas *in situ* with [^{14}C]progesterone, [^{3}H]pregnenolone, or [^{3}H]17α-hydroxy pregnenolone failed to show conversion to C_{19} or C_{18} steroids yet conversion of [^{14}C]androstenedione to [^{14}C]estrone took place (Jaffe *et al.*, 1965; Pion *et al.*, 1965). Occasionally minor conversions have been reported (Little and Shaw, 1961; Telegdy *et al.*, 1970b, 1973). Ovarian tissue will convert all these substrates to estrogens (Ryan and Smith, 1965).

Further evidence of the independence of estrogen and progesterone synthesis can be found in the measurements reported by Cassmer (1959). Pregnanediol excretion (used as an index of progesterone production) was hardly disturbed by ligation of the umbilical cord during second trimester abortions; estrogen excretion was immediately disrupted. Similarly, plasma progesterone may show little change after fetal death, whereas estrogen excretion is very sensitive (Coyle *et al.*, 1962; Lurie *et al.*, 1966).

The source of progesterone appears to be cholesterol present in fetal and maternal plasma (Fig. 3). This conclusion was drawn from one of the first metabolic experiments with isotopically labeled steroids. Bloch (1945) administered [^{2}H]cholesterol to a pregnant woman and was able to isolate [^{2}H]pregnanediol (a metabolite of progesterone) from the urine. Twenty-

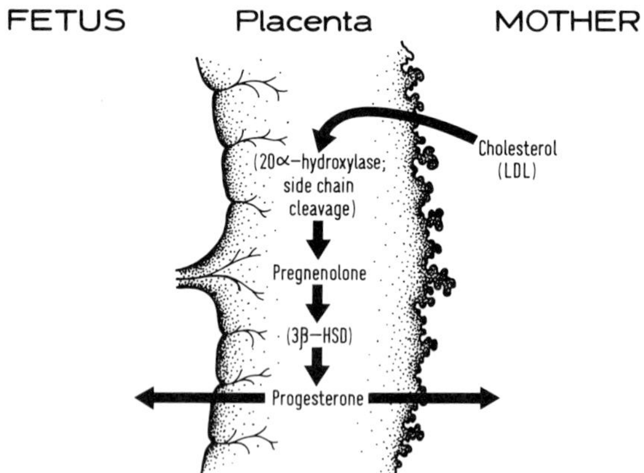

Fig. 3 Representation of the pathways of progesterone biosynthesis in late pregnancy. LDL, low-density lipoprotein; 3β-HDS, 3β-hydroxysteroid dehydrogenase-isomerase.

five years later this was put on a quantitative basis by Hellig *et al.* (1970) who injected two pregnant women near term with [^{3}H]cholesterol. Subsequent analysis of the specific activities of pregnanediol in the urine, free cholesterol in plasma, and progesterone in the placenta showed that cholesterol in maternal plasma was the source of more than 80% of placental progesterone. Perfusion *in vitro* of the intact fetus and placenta (Telegdy *et al.*, 1970b; 1973) indicated that cholesterol, not acetate, was the favored precursor.

By term progesterone production is estimated to be some 250 mg/day (Pearlman, 1957; Lin *et al.*, 1972) contrasting with 20 mg/day in the luteal phase. This increasing production in gestation is reflected in increasing concentrations in maternal peripheral blood (Table III) and in increasing daily excretion of pregnanediol glucuronide, the major urinary metabolite (Fig. 1). The concentration of progesterone in umbilical vein plasma exceeds that in the arterial plasma indicating secretion of progesterone to the fetus, and concentration in maternal peripheral plasma is less than that in umbilical vein plasma. Zander (1961) estimated that half the progesterone secreted near term passed to the fetus.

VII. Control of Progesterone Production

The points in the biosynthetic pathway at which progesterone production might be regulated are (1) supply of precursor; (2) variations in placental enzyme activity; and (3) influence of pituitary and/or placental polypeptides (Fig. 3).

A. Effects of Alterations in the Supply of Precursors

Cholesterol in maternal plasma is the most important precursor of pro-

Table III

Concentrations of Progesterone in Plasma from a Maternal Peripheral Vein during the last 10 weeks of Pregancy and from the Umbilical Artery and Vein[a]

Number of patients and mode of delivery	30 weeks	35 weeks	40 weeks	Umbilical artery	Umbilical vein	Reference
Not stated	382	510	573	—	—	Tulchinsky *et al.* (1972)
32, uncomplicated	318	414	510	—	—	Parker *et al.* (1979)
10, elective section	—	—	—	1012	1440	Tulchinsky and Okada (1975)
16, not stated	—	—	—	1203	2156	Effer *et al.* (1973)

[a]Values are means taken from the authors cited and units are nmole/liter.

gesterone in human pregnancy. An abundant supply is available, since the mean concentration of total cholesterol in maternal plasma (n = 111) was 5.7 mmole/liter (Spellacy *et al.*, 1974). No experiments on the effect of altering plasma cholesterol levels have been reported. Administration of pregnenolone sulfate (100–200 mg iv) to five pregnant women near term was without consistent effect on progesterone production, as assessed by urinary pregnanediol excretion (Chattoraj *et al.*, 1970). Apparently pregnenolone sulfate is not easily introduced into the chain of enzymes concerned. In perfusion *in situ* pregnenolone sulfate can serve as a precursor of progesterone (Palmer *et al.*, 1966).

Studies on placental cells in culture have shown that low-density lipoprotein in the serum acts as a carrier for cholesterol to enter the trophoblast cell (Winkel *et al.*, 1980). In culture, low-density lipoprotein (concentration 200 μg protein/ml) doubled progesterone production during 72 hours, compared to that occurring in the presence of lipoprotein-poor serum. High-density lipoprotein was less efficient but both lipoprotein fractions exert similar effects when present in amounts which provide equivalent cholesterol concentrations. In addition, low-density lipoprotein inhibits the rate of conversion of acetate to cholesterol in this system thus suppressing any *de novo* synthesis of cholesterol, an effect opposite to that reported for adrenal tissue (Carr *et al.*, 1980c). These effects are evident *in vitro* but may be difficult to recognize *in vivo*.

B. *Effects of Alterations in the Activities of Placental Enzymes*

The enzymes concerned in the conversion of cholesterol are (1) 20α-hydroxylase; (2) side chain cleavage complex, and (3) 3β-hydroxy steroid dehydrogenase-isomerase. Manipulations involving the first and the last enzymes have been carried out (Fig. 3).

1. 20α-Hydroxylase

This enzyme is involved in the first step in removal of the C_6 fragment of the side chain. Aminoglutethimide inhibits C-20 hydroxylation (Kahnt and Neher, 1966; Cash *et al.*, 1967) and its effect on steroid biosynthesis in human pregnancy has been examined. McIntosh *et al.* (1974) measured the plasma concentrations of steroid hormones in women in the first two trimesters who received aminoglutethimide. After a single dose plasma progesterone concentrations fell and remained depressed for 8–12 hours. Continued daily administration resulted in prolonged depression of plasma progesterone levels. The magnitude of the decrease was said to be proportional to dose and inversely related to the gestation period. Such manipulations cannot be carried out in continuing pregnancies where interruption of progesterone synthesis may threaten their stability. These measurements provide some indication of the reliance of progesterone production on cholesterol as substrate.

2. 3β-Hydroxy Steroid Dehydrogenase-Isomerase Activity

This enzyme complex is concerned with the conversion of pregnenolone to progesterone in the placenta. Studies have suggested that some degree of regulation of this enzyme activity is exerted by other steroids present in fetal and placental blood. Wiener and Allen (1967) reported that this enzyme was inhibited by 20α-dihydroprogesterone with an apparent $K_i = 2 \times 10^6$ *M*, similar to the concentration of this steroid in peripheral blood. Townsley (1975), using DHA as substrate, also noted inhibition of this enzyme by androstenedione and progesterone. These reports have now to be considered in the light of more recent evidence from Blomquist *et al.* (1978) and Gibb (1979) who found K_m for this enzyme to be 40×10^{-9} *M*, substantially lower than reported earlier. These findings raise some doubt on the interpretation of those studies in which micromolar concentrations of inhibitor were used. The important differences between the two sets of investigations was the use of β-mercaptoethanol to protect sulfhydryl groups in the later studies.

C. Effects of Polypeptides of Placental and Pituitary Origin

The placenta is the source of large quantities of a gonadotrophin (hCG) which can enhance progesterone production by the corpus luteum (Hanson *et al.*, 1971) at the time of implantation and for a few weeks afterward. Macome *et al.* (1972) examined the effect of hCG on progesterone biosynthesis in minces and homogenates of human term placentae. Neither addition of hCG (300 IU) nor of an antiserum to hCG (to inhibit endogenous activity) had any effect on the conversion of [^{14}C]cholesterol to [^{14}C]progesterone, implying that placental progesterone production is independent of hCG. A similar conclusion was reached by Runnebaum *et al.* (1972) who were unable to detect a change in the peripheral concentration of progesterone during or after infusion of hCG (5000–20000 IU over 2 hours) into all pregnant women at 31–39 weeks of gestation. The converse of this finding has been reported, i.e., that progesterone (17–70 μmole/liter) added to incubations of washed placental villi suppressed the production of hCG (measured by radioimmunoassay of the β-subunit). The concentrations used were many times higher than those encountered in plasma but equivalent to those recorded in tissue. Pregnenolone and 20α-dihydroprogesterone showed this suppressive effect, but cortisol, testosterone, 5α-dihydrotestosterone, and estriol did not (Wilson *et al.*, 1980).

Evidence for effects of pituitary corticotrophins on progesterone synthesis has been sought either by direct injection of ACTH or by studying the effect of suppression of pituitary activity. Administration of ACTH (40 IU, im) to 17 patients 1.5–9.5 hours before delivery or cortisol (150 mg) 10, 6, and 2 hours before delivery to six patients failed to alter the concentration of progesterone in maternal or cord plasma at elective cesarean section compared with that of similar, untreated patients (Tulchinsky and Okada, 1975). Larger doses of cortisol (1 g, repeated after 8 hours) appeared to decrease mean progesterone concentrations relative to those of untreated patients (Elsner *et al.,* 1979). This effect may be due to increased clearance of progesterone associated with its displacement from cortisol binding globulin by these high doses of cortisol. β-Methasone, which does not bind to cortisol binding globulin, given for 3 days at 12 mg/day, did not alter progesterone concentrations in maternal plasma during, or in the 5 days following treatment (Ohrlander *et al.,* 1977).

VIII. Progesterone in Plasma in Relation to the Onset of Labor

Others have argued (see Section V) that changes in the relative concentrations of progesterone and estradiol precede the onset of labor. Excellent evidence exists for a fall in progesterone concentrations at this time in the sheep. In humans a consensus has not been achieved. Csapo *et al.* (1971) collected samples from 12 pregnant women during the last 7 weeks of their pregnancies. Progesterone estimations were carried out independently in three laboratories. Mean ($\pm$ SE) maximum values 540 $\pm$ 19 nmole/liter (n = 26) were found 2–3 weeks before delivery, while the mean value at the start of contractions was 463 $\pm$ 35 nmole/liter. In 10 out of 12 individuals maximum progesterone concentrations preceded the onset of labor by more than 1 week. Supporting evidence was provided by Turnbull *et al.* (1974) who studied 33 obstetrically normal, primigravid women. Maximum mean progesterone levels (495 $\pm$ 2.2 nmole/liter) was found 5 weeks before the onset of labor. Other workers have been unable to confirm such changes. Tulchinsky *et al.* (1972) found no significant changes in the ratio of the concentrations of progesterone and estradiol as labor approached. Mathur *et al.* (1980) found mean plasma progesterone concentrations in 25 patients were unchanged from 4 weeks before labor and neither Llauro *et al.* (1968) nor Boroditsky *et al.* (1978) were able to find significant falls in maternal progesterone levels before delivery in studies of 13 and 5 subjects, respectively.

The concentration of non-protein-bound progesterone near term was reported to be 33.6 nmole/liter representing about 9% of total progesterone in plasma (Yannone *et al.,* 1969) and a similar proportion of progesterone in plasma was not bound to protein at the eighth week of gestation. Tulchinsky and Okada (1975) found 5% of progesterone was not bound to protein at the thirteenth week and at term which represented a fourfold increase in the concentration of non-protein-bound progesterone. Others (Batra *et al.*, 1976) found increasing proportions of progesterone were not protein bound as pregnancy proceeded. This implied changes in the concentration of unbound progesterone from 9.5 nmole/liter at 24 weeks to 63 nmole/liter at term. Greenstein *et al.* (1977), using a column technique, reported that 2% of progesterone in peripheral plasma was not bound to protein at term compound with 2.5% during the second and third trimesters. No serial study of changes in the concentration of unbound progesterone in individual patients has been reported. This might clarify the conflicting evidence, and help define any changes which occur before the onset of labor.

IX. Conclusions

Probably the most significant feature of the pathways of biosynthesis of the estrogens and progesterone in human pregnancy is their independence from each other. This comes about because of the inability of the placenta to convert progesterone to C_{19} and C_{18} steroids. To a lesser extent the avidity of the placenta for androgens presented from the fetal side (following their exposure to 16α-hydroxylase in fetal liver) compared with those presented from the maternal side provides the opportunity for estriol synthesis at the expense of that of estrone and estradiol.

Investigation of the control of steroid hormone production in human pregnancy would be greatly aided if there was a clear recognition of the biological need for these hormones. Progesterone secretion is essential; there are no conditions known in which progesterone production is abnormally low yet the pregnancy continues. Neither is it possible to arrange surgically or biochemically to interrupt progesterone production near term without interruption of the pregnancy.

Estrogen production and the maintenance of estrogen concentrations normally found in the later part of gestation are not essential for the continuation of the pregnancy and for proper fetal development and growth. There appears to be a wide tolerance in the concentration of estradiol maintained in peripheral plasma before the timing of the onset of labor is disturbed. For example, in those women receiving chronic treatment with high doses of glucocorticosteroids for coexisting conditions, postmaturity is not a recognized association. Yet plasma estrogen concentrations are diminished. Disturbed gestation length is often a feature of anencephaly (Anderson *et al.*, 1969; Honnebier and Swaab, 1973) and plasma estradiol concentrations may be low at term. In pregnancies complicated by placental steroid sulfatase deficiency, postmaturity is sometimes, but not always, a feature. When it occurs here postmaturity is associated failure of cervical ripening and dilation. In Fig. 4 are shown the concentrations of estradiol achieved before and after glucocorticosteroids (Simmer *et al.*, 1974), in pregnancies with an anencephalic fetus (Cawood *et al.*, 1976), in three cases of pregnancy complicated by sulfatase deficiency where delivery was spontaneous before term (personal observation), and one similar case in which delivery could be achieved only by cesarean section (Oakey *et al.*, 1974). Estradiol concentrations only 20% of normal were compatible with spontaneous delivery; in the single illustration of delayed delivery the plasma estradiol concentration was only 6% the normal value. This may illustrate the extremely low concentrations of estradiol required to delay the onset of labor. Anecdotal material such as this can only be quoted in an effort to encourage the collection of samples from other abnormal pregnancies with a view to providing a more detailed and critical assessment of any associaton between estradiol concentrations and the onset of labor. Progesterone concentrations in the subjects illustrated in Fig. 4, where measured, did not decline to the same extent as did those of estradiol.

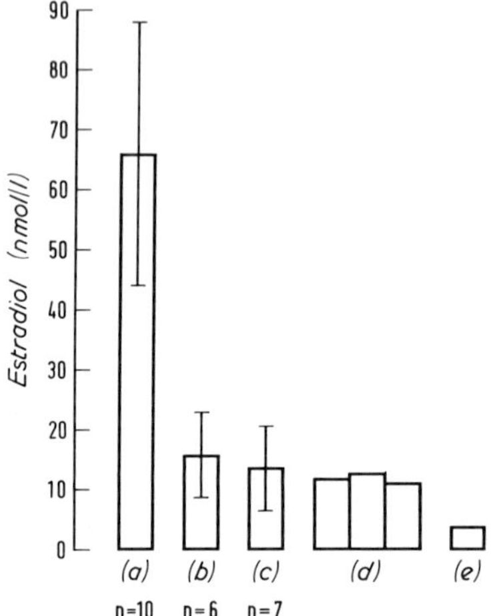

Fig. 4 Concentrations of estradiol (nmole/liter) in maternal plasma near term (a) in normal pregnancy (Simmer *et al.*, 1974); (b) in normal pregnancy after acute cortisol (150 mg) therapy (Simmer *et al.*, 1974); (c) in pregnancies with an anencephalic fetus (Cawood *et al.*, 1976); (d) in pregnancies complicated by steroid sulfatase deficiency but which ended with spontaneous delivery (personal observations); (e) in a pregnancy complicated by steroid sulfatase deficiency in which labor was delayed (Oakey *et al.*, 1974). Values shown for (a), (b), and (c) are means ± SD.

So far discussion of this point has considered only estradiol. Estriol was long regarded as having only weak uterotrophic action or even being an antiestrogen. Recent evidence (Clark *et al.,* 1977; Schiff *et al.,* 1980) requires that this view be reconsidered. Estriol, when presented continuously to the uterus, is equipotent with estradiol in promoting uterine growth at least in rats (Martucci and Fishman, 1977). The contributions of other C_{18} steroids often regarded as ineffective estrogens, for example, 16α-hydroxyestrone (Fishman and Martucci, 1980), may also require reevaluation. Consequently, the concentration of estriol in peripheral plasma, the production of which can be varied to a significant extent in a manner independently of that of estrone and estradiol, should now be given more attention than it has received in recent years. Earlier reports, based on analysis of urine, suggested a role for estriol in the timing of delivery. For example, relatively high estriol excretion at 30 weeks gestation was associated with earlier delivery (Klopper and Billewicz, 1963; Turnbull *et al.,* 1967). The changes in plasma estriol occurring 4 weeks before delivery described by Buster and his colleagues have been discussed in Section V. If estriol production and its plasma concentration are involved in the initiation of parturition the fetal liver must be brought into consideration. This again is responsible for insertion into the precursor of the 16α-hydroxyl group which distinguishes estriol. Assay techniques for estriol with the necessary sensitivity are available so the results of their application in selected conditions can be awaited with interest.

Although the biological reasons for the progressively increasing production of, and, in consequence, increasing plasma concentrations of estrone, estradiol, estriol, and progesterone are not at all clear, evidence has been reviewed in this article relating to the regulation of the production of these hormones.

The increasing production of progesterone is based on adequate supplies of cholesterol as precursor. Polypeptide hormones of placental or pituitary origin have not been shown to have inhibitory or stimulatory effects. There is likely to be some intracellular control, probably involving inhibition by steroid hormones. Consequently, progesterone production appears to be regulated only by placental size and availability and activity of the necessary enzymes.

The increasing production of estrogens represents a different problem. Since there is increased estrogen excretion when the supply of precursors is increased experimentally, it is generally supposed that rising estrogen production is dependent on the increasing supplies of precursor. It has not been demonstrated rigorously that precursor supply does increase during pregnancy. Indeed, comparison of concentrations of androgen sulfates in cord blood at mid-gestation (Huhtaniemi and Vihko, 1970) with values at term (Laatikainen *et al.,* 1980) implies that precursor concentrations do not increase appreciably, although the analytical methods used may not be strictly comparable and the fetuses were not undisturbed. If one accepts, with some reservations, that increased estrogen production is related to an increasing supply of precursors, the question then becomes "What factor(s) regulate the growth and steroid secretion of the fetal adrenal gland?" Observations in anencephaly and in patients receiving glucocorticosteroids or metapyrone emphasizes the importance of the fetal hypothalamus and pituitary glands in any mechanism. But can the corticotrophic factor(s) be identified?

The effects of potential corticotrophins have been assessed only over short time periods (relative to the duration of gestation) and only in terms of steroid secretion response (which may differ from the growth response). Given this restriction ACTH, α-MSH, β-LPH, hGH, prolactin, and metenkephalin, but not CLIP, must be considered. Additionally, placental factors hCG and hPL also affect androgen synthesis by the fetal adrenal gland and the placenta is recognized as a source of ACTH (Genazzani *et al.,* 1975; Rees *et al.,* 1975). From this evidence it is not possible to identify the corticotrophin. It must be recognized too that tests *in vitro* are usually carried out between about 12 and 20 weeks of gestation. It is quite possible that a different response would occur with more mature tissue. Different corticotrophins could operate at different periods of gestation. Considering the concentrations of possible corticotrophins in fetal blood, that of GH shows a maximum between the twentieth and twenty-ninth weeks (Kaplan *et al.,* 1972) whereas that of ACTH declines steadily throughout gestation (Winters *et al.,* 1974). This is contrary to expectations if ACTH is responsible for stimulating adrenal growth. Prolactin (which provokes a relatively poor response in terms of DHAS synthesis at 13–18 weeks of gestation) is present in increasing concentrations as gestation proceeds (Aubert *et al.,* 1975; Winters *et al.,* 1975). Thus prolactin exhibits more of the properties required of a trophic hormone for the fetal zone than does either hGH or ACTH. There is now indirect evidence (Cohen *et al.,* 1981) that synergism between hGH and prolactin may be responsible for the increase in secretion of adrenal androgens, of which DHAS is the most abundant, which occurs before puberty. A parallel might be drawn between this behavior and that of the fetal adrenal.

The relevance of ACTH cannot entirely be dismissed, since the evidence reviewed in Section IV indicates that manipulations which result in a raised, or in a decreased concentration of glucocorticosteroid in fetal plasma lead, respectively, to a lower or a higher production of estrogens, and, by implication to a lower or higher output of androgens from the fetal adrenal gland. This evidence implies the existence of a negative feedback system. In such a system the release of the factor which stimulates the production of the adrenal androgen DHAS is related inversely to the glucocorticosteroid titer of fetal plasma. The relationship between an adrenal steroid stimulating factor and glucocorticosteroids in adults is recognized to involve ACTH. Growth hormone and Prl, suggested as adrenal androgen stimulating factors for the fetus, are not known to be secreted in adults in response to diminished plasma concentrations of cortisol. The increased production of adrenal androgen stimulating factor in the fetus brought about by treatment with metyrapone may be considered to be an unphysiological imposition on the system. Such an argument cannot be used with justification to discount the inhibitory effects of high doses of glucocorticosteroids. This evidence demonstrates suppression of a normal regulatory effect of the adrenal androgen stimulatory factor. Thus, by analogy with studies in adults, ACTH is a strong candidate for the role of adrenal androgen stimulatory factor in the human fetus. Dispersal of all the evidence into a rational scheme is difficult, particularly since the mean concentration of ACTH in fetal plasma appears to be lower at term than in mid-gestation (Winters *et al.*, 1974). The values quoted were obtained on samples taken from the umbilical cord after termination or after normal delivery and might therefore be suspect as reflecting the status of the undisturbed fetus. No significant effects of the mode of delivery at term on ACTH concentration were found. If this evidence is confirmed then one might need to suggest that adrenal androgen production is more sensitive to ACTH later in gestation than earlier. Moreover, the mean concentration of ACTH in fetal plasma near term reported by these authors is about three times greater than that in samples collected from adults between 13.00 and 16.00 hours. The concentrations of ACTH in fetal plasma would therefore be high enough to respond to manipulation by glucocorticosteroid therapy in the ways described. It is worth pointing out also that, at least in the adult, the adrenal secretory product of interest here, DHAS, is not recognized as having a role in regulation of ACTH secretion. This appreciation of the data excludes a direct role for hGH or Prl as adrenal androgen stimulatory factors because of the involvement of a glucocorticosteroid-sensitive negative feedback. However, the evidence from studies *in vitro* is persuasive and involvement of these and other peptides cannot be discounted with confidence.

It must be concluded that, at present, sufficient information is not available to provide a satisfactory and consistent hypothesis for the regulation of adrenal androgen production in the fetus and, therefore, for much of the estrogen production in pregnancy.

References

Allen, J. P., Cook, D. M., Kendall, J. W., and McGilvra, R. (1973). *J. Clin. Endocrinol. Metab.* **37**, 230–234.

Anderson, A. B. M., Laurence, K. M., and Turnbull, A. C. (1969). *J. Obstet. Gynaecol. Br. Commonw.* **76,** 196–199.

Antonipillai, I., and Murphy, B. E. P. (1977). *Br. J. Obstet. Gynaecol.* **84,** 179–185.

Arai, Kuwabara, Y., and Okinaga, S. (1972). *Am. J. Obstet. Gynecol.* **113,** 316–322.

Archer, D. F., Mathur, R. S., Wiqvist, N. F., and Diczfalusy, E. (1971). *Acta Endocrinol. (Copenhagen)* **66,** 666–678.

Aubert, M. L., Grumbach, M. M., and Kaplan, S. L. (1975). *J. Clin. Invest.* **56,** 155–164.

Axelsson, O., Nilsson, B. A., and Johansson, E. D. B. (1978). *Acta Endocrinol. (Copenhagen)* **89,** 359–371.

Batra, S., Bengtsson, L. P., Grundsell, H., and Sjoberg, N. O. (1976). *J. Clin. Endocrinol. Metab.* **42,** 1041–1047.

Baulieu, E. E., Corpechot, C., Dray, F., Emiliozzi, R., Lebeau, M. C., Mauvais-Jarvis, P., and Robel, P. (1965). *Recent Prog. Horm. Res.* **21,** 411–500.

Bedin, M., Alsat, E., Tanguy, G., and Cedard, L. (1980). *Eur. J. Obstet. Gynaecol. Reprod. Biol.* **10,** 21–34.

Belisle, S., Osathanondh, R., and Tulchinsky, D. (1977). *J. Clin. Endocrinol. Metab.* **45,** 544–550.

Belisle, S., Schiff, I., and Tulchinsky, D. (1980). *J. Clin. Endocrinol. Metab.* **50,** 117–121.

Bloch, K. (1945). *J. Biol. Chem.* **157,** 661–666.

Bloch, E., and Benirschke, K. (1959). *J. Biol. Chem.* **234,** 1084–1088.

Bloch, E., and Benirschke, K. (1962). *In* "The Human Adrenal Cortex" (A. R. Currie, T. Symington, and J. K. Grant, eds.), pp. 589–595. Livingstone, Edinburgh.

Blomquist, C. H., Kotts, C. E., and Hakanson, E. Y. (1978). *J. Steroid Biochem.* **9,** 685–690.

Boroditsky, R. S., Reyes, F. I., Winter, J. S. D., and Faiman, C. (1978). *Obstet. Gynaecol.* **51,** 686–691.

Branchaud, C. T., Goodyer, C. G., Hall, C. St. G., Arato, S., Silman, R. E., and Giroud, C. J. P. (1978). *Steroids* **31,** 557–572.

Brown, J. B. (1956). *Lancet* **1,** 704–707.

Brown, J. B., Beischer, N. A., and Smith, M. A. (1968). *J. Obstet. Gynaecol. Br. Commonw.* **75,** 819–828.

Brown, T. J., Ginz, B., Milne, C. M., and Oakey, R. E. (1981). *J. Endocrinol.* **91,** 111–122.

Burd, L. I., Bieniarz, J., Nedoss, B. R., Charles, A. G., and Scommegna, A. (1970). *Obstet. Gynaecol.* **36,** 574–581.

Buster, J. E., Abraham, G., Kyle, W. F., and Marshall, J. R. (1974). *J. Clin. Endocrinol. Metab.* **38,** 1031–1037.

Buster, J. E., Sakakini, J., Killam, A. P., and Scragg, W. H. (1976). *Am. J. Obstet. Gynecol.* **125,** 672–676.

Buster, J. E., Freeman, A. G., Tataryn, I. V., and Hobel, C. J. (1980). *Obstet. Gynecol.* **56,** 743–747.

Carr, B. R., Parker, C. R., Milewich, L., Porter, J. C., Macdonald, P. C., and Simpson, E. R. (1980a). *Steroids* **36,** 563–574.

Carr, B. R., Parker, C. R., Milewich, L., Porter, J. C., Macdonald, P. C., and Simpson, E. R. (1980b). *Endocrinology* **106,** 1854–1860.

Carr, B. R., Macdonald, P. C., and Simpson, E. R. (1980c). *Endocrinology* **107,** 1000–1006.

Cash, R., Brough, A. J., Cohen, M. N. P., and Satoh, P. S. (1967). *J. Clin. Endocrinol. Metab.* **27,** 1239–1248.

Cassmer, O. (1959). *Acta Endocrinol. (Copenhagen) Suppl.* **45.**

Cathro, D. M., Bertrand, J., and Coyle, M. G. (1969). *Lancet* **1,** 732.

Cawood, M. L., Heys, R. F., and Oakey, (1976). *Clin. Endocrinol.* **5,** 341–347.

Cedard, L., Alsat, E., Ego, C., and Varangot, J. (1968). *Steroids* **11,** 179–186.

Charles, D., Harkness, R. A., Kenny, F. M., Menini, E., Ismail, A. A. A., Durkin, J. W., and Loraine, J. A. (1970). *Am. J. Obstet. Gynecol.* **106,** 66–74.

Chattoraj, S. C., Pinkus, J. L., and Charles, D. (1970). *Steroids* **16,** 523–537.

Chew, P. C. T., and Ratnam, S. S. (1976). *J. Endocrinol.* **71,** 267–268.

Clark, J. H., Pasko, Z., and Peck, E. J. (1977). *Endocrinology* **100,** 91–95.

Cohen, H. N., Wallace, A. M., Beastall, G. H., Fogelman, I., and Thompson, J. A. (1981). *Lancet* **1,** 689–692.

Cousins, L. M., Hobel, C. J., Chang, E. J., Okada, D. M., and Marshall, J. R. (1977). *Am. J. Obstet. Gynecol.* **127,** 612–615.

Coyle, M. G., Greig, M., and Walker, J. (1962). *Lancet.* **2,** 275–277.

Crystle, C. D., Dubin, N. H., Grannis, G. F., Stevens, V. C., and Townsley, J. D. (1973). *Obstet. Gynecol.* **42,** 718–724.

Csapo, A. (1969). *In* "Ciba Foundation Study Group No. 34" (G. E. Wolstenholme and J. Knight, eds.), pp. 4–55. Churchill, London.

Csapo, A. I., Knobil, E., van der Molen, H. J., and Wiest, W. G. (1971). *Am. J. Obstet. Gynecol.,* **110,** 630–632.

Dassler, C. G. (1966). *Acta Endocrinol. (Copenhagen)* **53,** 401–406.

De Hertogh, R., Thomas, K., Bietlot, Y., Vanderheyden, I., and Ferin, J. (1975). *J. Clin. Endocrinol. Metab.* **40,** 93–101.

Dickey, R. P., and Thompson, J. P. (1969). *J. Clin. Endocrinol. Metab.* **29,** 701–706.

Diczfalusy, E. (1969). *In* "The Foeto-Placental Unit" (A. Pecile and C. Finzi, eds.), pp. 65–109. Excerpta Medica, Amsterdam.

Effer, S. B., Gupta, K., and Younglai, E. V. (1973). *Am. J. Obstet. Gynecol.* **116,** 643–647.

Elsner, C. W., Buster, J. E., Preston, D. L., and Killam, A. P. (1979). *J. Clin. Endocrinol. Metab.* **49,** 30–33.

Fishman, J., and Martucci, C. (1980). *J. Clin. Endocrinol. Metab.* **51,** 611–615.

Fliegner, J. R. H., Schnidler, I., and Brown, J. B. (1972). *J. Obstet. Gynaecol. Br. Commonw.* **79,** 810–815.

Flint, A. P. F. (1978). *In* "Human Parturition" (M. J. N. C. Keirse, A. B. M. Anderson, and J. Bennebroek Gravenhorst, eds.), p. 87. Leiden Univ. Press, Leiden.

France, J. T. (1980). *In* "International Reviews of Perinatal Medicine" (E. M. Scarpelli and E. V. Cosmi, eds.), Vol. 4, pp. 248–272. Raven, New York.

France, J. T., and Liggins, G. C. (196). *J. Clin. Endocrinol. Metab.* **29,** 138–141.

France, J. T., Seddon, R. J., and Liggins, G. C. (1973). *J. Clin. Endocrinol. Metab.* **36,** 1–9.

Frandsen, V. A., and Stakeman, G. (1961). *Acta Endocrinol. (Copenhagen)* **38,** 383–381.

Fraser, I. S., Leask, R., Drife, J., Bacon, L., and Michie, E. (1976). *Obstet. Gynecol.* **47,** 152–158.

Fujieda, K., Faiman, C., Reyes, F. I., and Winter, J. S. D. (1981a). *J. Clin. Endocrinol. Metab.* **53,** 34–48.

Fujieda, K., Faiman, C., Reyes, R. I., Thliveris, J., and Winter, J. S. D. (1981b). *J. Clin. Endocrinol. Metab.* **53,** 401–405.

Fujieda, K., Faiman, C., Reyes, F. I., and Winter, J. S. D. (1981c). *J. Clin. Endocrinol. Metab.* **53,** 690–693.

Gamissans, O., Wilson, G. R., Cuyas, J., Davi, E., and Pujol-Amat, P. (1977). *Obstet. Gynecol.* **50,** 439–441.

Gant, N. F., Madden, J. D., Chand, S., Worley, R. J., Strong, J. D., and Macdonald, P. C. (1976). *Obstet. Gynecol.* **47,** 319–326.

Genazzani, A. R., Fraioli, F., Hurliman, J., Fioretti, P., and Felber, J. P. (1975). *Clin. Endocrinol.* **4,** 1–14.

Gibb, W. (1979). *Steroids* **33,** 459–466.

Goodyer, C. G., Hall, C. St. G., Branchaud, C., and Giroud, C. J. F. (1977). *Steroids* **29**, 407–416.
Greenstein, B. D., Puig-Duran, E., and Franklin, M. (1977). *Steroids* **30**, 331–341.
Gurpide, E., Giebenhain, M., Stolee, A., Notation, A., Dixon, R., and Blackard, C. E. (1973). *J. Clin. Endocrinol. Metab.* **37**, 867–872.
Hampl, R., and Starka, L. (1973). *Steroids Lipids Res.* **4**, 257–265.
Hanson, F. W., Powell, J. E., and Stevens, V. C. (1971). *J. Clin. Endocrinol. Metab.* **32**, 211–215.
Hausknecht, R. U., and Mandelman, N. (1969). *Am. J. Obstet. Gynecol.* **104**, 433–435.
Hellig, H., Gattereau, D., Lefebvre, Y., and Bolte, E. (1970). *J. Clin. Endocrinol. Metab.* **30**, 624–631.
Honnebier, W. J., and Swaab, D. F. (1973). *J. Obstet. Gynaecol. Br. Commonw.* **80**, 577–588.
Huhtaniemi, I., and Vihko, R. (1970). *Steroids* **16**, 197–205.
Isherwood, D. M., and Oakey, R. E. (1976). *J. Endocrinol.* **68**, 321–329.
Jaffe, R., Pion, R., Eriksson, G., Wiqvist, N., and Diczfalusy, E. (1965). *Acta Endocrinol. (Copenhagen)* **48**, 413–422.
Jeffery, J., Swapp, G., Wilson, G. R., and Fotherby, K. (1970). *J. Endocrinol.* **48**, 591–598.
Jorgensen, P. I., and Lebech, P. E. (1971). *J. Steroid Biochem.* **2**, 269–277.
Kahnt, F. W., and Neher, R. (1966). *Helv. Chim. Acta* **49**, 725–732.
Kahri, A. I., Huhtaniemi, I., and Salmenpera, M. (1976). *Endocrinology* **98**, 33–41.
Kaplan, S. L., Grumbach, M. M., and Shepard, T. H. (1972). *J. Clin. Invest.* **51**, 3080–3093.
Katagiri, H., Distler, W., Freeman, R. K., and Goebelsmann, U. (1976). *Am. J. Obstet. Gynecol.* **124**, 272–280.
Kauppila, A., and Ylikorkala, O. (1980). *Am. J. Obstet. Gynecol.* **138**, 271–272.
Klopper, A. I., and Billewicz, W. (1963). *J. Obstet. Gynaecol. Br. Commonw.* **70**, 1024–1033.
Klopper, A., Varela-Torres, R., and Jandial, V. (1976). *Br. J. Obstet. Gynaecol.* **83**, 478–483.
Knight, J., and O'Connor, M., eds. (1977). "The Fetus and Birth." Ciba Foundation Symp. No. 47. Elsevier, Amsterdam.
Korda, A. R., Challis, J. J., Anderson, A. B. M., and Turnbull, A. C. (1975). *Br. J. Obstet. Gynaecol.* **82**, 656–661.
Laatikainen, T., Pelkonen, J., Apter, D., and Ranta, T. (1980). *J. Clin. Endocrinol. Metab.* **50**, 489–494.
Laumas, K. R., Malkani, P. K., Koshti, G. S., and Hingorani, V. (1968). *Am. J. Obstet. Gynecol.* **101**, 1062–1067.
Lauritzen, C. (1967). *Acta Endocrinol. (Copenhagen) Suppl.* **119**, 188.
Laverty, C. R. A., Fortune, D. W., and Beischer, N. A. (1973). *Obstet. Gynecol.* **41**, 655–664.
Lehmann, W. D., and Lauritzen, C. (1975). *J. Perinat. Med.* **3**, 231–236.
Lehmann, W. D., Lauritzen, C., and Schumann, R. (1973). *Acta Endocrinol. (Copenhagen)* **73**, 771–789.
Lin, T. J., Lin, S. C., Erlenmeyer, F., Kline, I. T., Underwood, R., Billiar, R. B., and Little, B. (1972). *J. Clin. Endocrinol. Metab.* **34**, 287–297.
Lindberg, B. S., Johansson, E. D. B., and Nilsson, B. A. (1974). *Acta Obstet. Gynecol. Scand. Suppl.* **32**, 21–36.
Little, R. B., and Shaw, A. (1961). *Acta Endocrinol. (Copenhagen)* **36**, 455–461.
Llauro, J. L., Runnebaum, B., and Zander, J. (1981). *Am. J. Obstet. Gynecol.* **101**, 867–873.
Loriaux, D. L., Ruder, H. J., Knab, D. R., and Lipsett, M. (1972). *J. Clin. Endocrinol. Metab.* **35**, 887–891.
Lurie, A. O., Reid, D. E., and Villee, C. A. (1966). *Am. J. Obstet. Gynecol.* **96**, 670–675.
McIntosh, E. N., Holtrop, H. R., Alonso, C., and Salhanick, H. A. (1974). *Annu. Meet. Endocrine Soc., 56th* p. A145 (Abstr.).

McKee, J. W. A., Abeysekera, R., and France, J. T. (1981). *J. Steroid Biochem.* **14,** 195–198.
McNaught, R. W., and France, J. T.(1980). *J. Steroid Biochem.* **13,** 363–373.
Macome, J. C., Bischoff, K., Uma Bai, R., and Diczfalusy, E. (1972). *Steroids* **20,** 469–485.
Madden, J. D., Siiteri, P. K., Macdonald, P. C., and Gant, N. F. (1976). *Am. J. Obstet. Gynecol.* **125,** 915–920.
Madden, J. C., Gant, N. F., and Macdonald, P. C. (1978). *Am. J. Obstet. Gynecol.* **132,** 392–395.
Maeyama, M., and Nakagawa, T. (1970). *Steroids* **15,** 267–274.
Maeyama, M., Nakagawa, T., Tuchida, Y., and Matuoka, H. (1969). *Steroids* **13,** 59–67.
Maeyama, M., Mori, N., Miyakawa, I., and Higashi, S. (1975). *J. Endocrinol.* **64,** 389–390.
Maeyama, M., Ichimaru, S., Nakahara, K., Nakayama, M., and Miyakawa, I. (1976). *J. Endocrinol.* **71,** 305–313.
Marton, I., and Oakey, R. E. (1980). *J. Steroid Biochem.* **13,** 475–479.
Martucci, C., and Fishman, J. (1977). *Endocrinology* **101,** 1709–1715.
Mathur, R. S., Landgrebe, S., and Williamson, H. O. (1980). *Am. J. Obstet. Gynecol.* **136,** 25–27.
Michie, E. A. (1966). *Acta Endocrinol. (Cophenhagen)* **51,** 535–542.
Mowszowicz, I., Kahn, D., and Dray, F. (1970). *J. Clin. Endocrinol. Metab.* **31,** 584–586.
Nichols, J., and Gibson, G. G. (1969). *Lancet* **2,** 1068.
Oakey, R. E. (1970a). *Vitam. Horm.* **28,** 1–36.
Oakey, R. E. (1970b). *J. Obstet. Gynaecol. Br. Commonw.* **77,** 922–927.
Oakey, R. E., and Heys, R. F. (1970). *Acta Endocrinol. (Copenhagen)* **65,** 502–508.
Oakey, R. E., Cawood, M. L., and Macdonald, R. R. (1974). *Clin. Endocrinol.* **3,** 131–148.
Ohrlander, S. A. V., Gennser, G. M., and Grennert, L. (1975). *Am. J. Obstet. Gynecol.* **123,** 228–236.
Ohrlander, S., Gennser, G., Batra, S., and Lebech, P. (1977). *Obstet. Gynecol.* **49,** 148–153.
Osathanondh, R., Canick, J., Ryan, K. J., and Tulchinsky, D. (1976). *J. Clin. Endocrinol. Metab.* **43,** 208–214.
Palmer, R., Eriksson, G., Wiqvist, N., and Diczfalusy, E. (1966). *Acta Endocrinol. (Copenhagen)* **52,** 598–606.
Parker, C. R., Everett, R. B., Quirk, J. G., Whalley, P. J., and Gant, N. F. (1979). *Am. J. Obstet. Gynecol.* **135,** 778–782.
Paterson, J. Y. F. (1973). *J. Endocrinol.* **56,** 551–570.
Patrick, J., Challis, J., Natale, R., and Richardson, B. (1979). *Am. J. Obstet. Gynecol.* **135,** 791–798.
Pearlman, W. H. (1957). *Biochem. J.* **67,** 1–5.
Penney, L. L. (1980). *J. Steroid Biochem.* **13,** 1443–1447.
Pion, R., Jaffe, R., Eriksson, G., Wiqvist, N., and Diczfalusy, E. (1965). *Acta Endocrinol. (Copenhagen)* **48,** 234–248.
Rahman, S. A., Hingorani, V., and Laumas, K. R. (1975). *Clin. Endocrinol.* **4,** 333–341.
Reck, G., Nowostawskyji, H., and Breckwoldt, M. (1978). *Acta Endocrinol. (Copenhagen)* **87,** 820–827.
Reck, G., Noss, U., and Breckwoldt, M. (1979). *Acta Endocrinol. (Copenhagen)* **90,** 519–524.
Rees, L. H., Burke, C. W., Chard, T., Evans, S. W., and Letchworth, A. T. (1975). *Nature (London)* **254,** 620–622.
Roberts, G., and Cawdry, J. E.(1970). *J. Obstet. Gynaecol. Br. Commonw.* **77,** 654–656.
Roos, B. A. (1974). *Endocrinology* **94,** 685–690.
Runnebaum, B., Holzmann, K., von Munstermann, A. M., and Zander, J. (1972). *Acta Endocrinol. (Copenhagen)* **69,** 739–746.
Ryan, K. J., and Smith, O. W. (1965). *Recent Prog. Horm. Res.* **21,** 367–409.

Sakakini, J., Buster, J. E., and Killam, A. P. (1977). *Am. J. Obstet. Gynecol.* **127,** 452–454.
Schiff, I., Tulchinsky, D., Ryan, K. J., Kadner, S., and Levitz, M. (1980). *Am. J. Obstet. Gynecol.* **138,** 1137–1142.
Schut, H., and Townsley, J. D. (1977). *Acta Endocrinol. (Copenhagen)* **84,** 633–641.
Scommegna, A., Nedoss, B. R., and Chattoraj, S. C. (1968). *Obstet. Gynecol.* **31,** 526–533.
Seron-Ferre, M., Lawrence, C. C., and Jaffe, R. B. (1978a). *J. Clin. Endocrinol. Metab.* **46,** 834–837.
Seron-Ferre, M., Lawrence, C. C., Siiteri, P. K., and Jaffe, R. B. (1978b). *J. Clin. Endocrinol. Metab.* **47,** 603–609.
Shaaban, M. M., and Klopper, A. (1973). *J. Obstet. Gynaecol. Br. Commonw.* **80,** 210–217.
Shapiro, L. J., Weiss, R., Webster, D., and France, J. T. (1978). *Lancet* **1,** 70–72.
Shutt, D. A., Smith, I. D., and Shearman, R. P. (1974). *J. Endocrinol.* **60,** 333–341.
Silman, R. E., Chard, T., Lowry, P. J., Smith, I., and Young, I. M. (1976). *Nature (London)* **260,** 716–718.
Simmer, H. H., Digman, W. J., Easterling, W. E., Frankland, M. V., and Naftolin, F. (1966). *Steroids* **8,** 179–193.
Simmer, H. H., Tulchinsky, D., Gold, E., Frankland, M., Greipel, M., and Gold, A. S. (1974). *Am. J. Obstet. Gynecol.* **119,** 283–296
Simmer, H. H., Frankland, M., and Greipel, M. (1975). *Am. J. Obstet. Gynecol.* **121,** 646–652.
Simonian, M. H., and Gill, G. N. (1981). *Endocrinology* **108,** 1769–1779.
Spellacy, W. N., Ashbacher, L. V., Harris, G. K., and Buhi, W. C. (1974). *Obstet. Gynecol.* **44,** 661–665.
Story, M. T., Hussa, R. O., and Pattillo, R. A. (1974). *J. Clin. Endocrinol. Metab.* **39,** 877–881.
Strecker, J. R., Killus, C. M., Lauritzen, C., and Neumann, G. K. (1978). *Am. J. Obstet. Gynecol.* **131,** 239–249.
Sybulski, S. (1969). *Am. J. Obstet. Gynecol.* **105,** 1055–1062.
Tabei, T., and Heinrichs, W. L. (1976). *Am. J. Obstet. Gynecol.* **124,** 409–414.
Telegdy, E., Weeks, J. W., Archer, D. F., Wiqvist, N., and Diczfalusy, E. (1970a). *Acta Endocrinol. (Copenhagen)* **63** 119–133.
Telegdy, G., Weeks, J. W., Wiqvist, N., and Diczfalusy, E. (1970b). *Acta Endocrinol. (Copenhagen)* **63,** 105–118.
Telegdy, G., Robin, M., and Diczfalusy, E. (1973). *Acta Endocrinol. (Copenhagen)* **72,** 127–136.
Tilders, F. J. H., Parker, C. R., Barnea, A., and Porter, J. C. (1981). *J. Clin. Endocrinol. Metab.* **52,** 319–324.
Townsley, J. D. (1975). *Acta Endocrinol. (Copenhagen)* **79,** 740–748.
Townsley, J. D., Scheel, D. A., and Rubin, E. J. (1970). *J. Clin. Endocrinol. Metab.* **31,** 670–678.
Townsley, J. D., Rubin, E. J., and Crystle, D. C. (1973). *Am. J. Obstet. Gynecol.* **117,** 345–350.
Tulchinsky, D. (1973). *J. Clin. Endocrinol. Metab.* **36,** 1079–1087.
Tulchinsky, D., and Okada, D. M. (1975). *Am. J. Obstet. Gynecol.* **121,** 293–299.
Tulchinsky, D., Hoebel, C. H., Yeager, E., and Marshall, J. R. (1972). *Am. J. Obstet. Gynecol.* **112,** 1095–1100.
Tulchinsky, D. Osathanondh, R., Belisle, S., and Ryan, K. J. (1977). *J. Clin. Endocrinol. Metab.* **45,** 1100–1103.
Turnbull, A. C., Anderson, A. B. M., and Wilson, G. R. (1967). *Lancet* **2,** 627–629.
Turnbull, A. C., Patten, P. T., Flint, A. P. F., Keirse, M. J. N. C., Jeremy, J. Y., and Anderson, A. B. M. (1974). *Lancet* **1,** 101–104.
Varangot, J., Cedard, L., and Yannotti, S. (1965). *Am. J. Obstet. Gynecol.* **92,** 534–547.

Warren, J. C., and Cheatum, S. G. (1967). *J. Clin. Endocrinol. Metab.* **27**, 433–436.
Wiener, M.,and Allen, S. H. G. (1967). *Steroids* **9**, 567–582.
Wilson, E. A., Jawad, M. J., and Dickson, L. R. (1980). *Am. J. Obstet. Gynecol.* **138**, 708–713.
Winkel, C. A., Snyder, J. M., Macdonald, P. C., and Simpson, E. R. (1980). *Endocrinology* **106**, 1054–1060.
Winters, A. J., Oliver, C., Colston, C., Macdonald, P. C., and Porter, J. C. (1974). *J. Clin. Endocrinol. Metab.* **39**, 269–273.
Winters, A. J., Colston, C., Macdonald, P. C., and Porter, J. C. (1975). *J. Clin. Endocrinol. Metab.* **41**, 626–629.
Yannone, M. E., Mueller, J. R., and Osborn, R. H. (1969). *Steroids* **13**, 773–781.
Yates, J., and Oakey, R. E. (1972). *Steroids* **19**, 119–135.
Ylikorkala, O., Kauppila,A., Reinila, M., and Tuimala, R. (1980). *Clin. Endocrinol.* **12**, 261–267.
Zander, J. (1961). *In* "Ciba Foundation Study Group No. 9" (G. E. Wolstenholme and M. P. Cameron, eds.), pp. 32–39. Churchill, London.

THE ROLE OF OXYTOCIN IN PARTURITION

Anna-Riitta Fuchs

DEPARTMENT OF OBSTETRICS AND GYNECOLOGY
CORNELL UNIVERSITY MEDICAL COLLEGE
NEW YORK, NEW YORK

I. Introduction ... 231
II. Indirect Evidence of a Role for Oxytocin ... 233
A. Effects of Exogenous Oxytocin ... 233
B. Effects of Endogenous Oxytocin ... 234
C. Pituitary and Hypothalamic Content and Depletion of Oxytocin . 235
D. Ablation and Lesion Studies ... 236
E. Selective Inactivation of Oxytocin ... 238
F. Blocking of Oxytocin Release with Ethanol ... 238
III. Direct Evidence of a Role for Oxytocin ... 241
Circulating Levels of Oxytocin during Parturition ... 241
IV. Control of Uterine Sensitivity ... 249
Oxytocin Receptors ... 250
V. Interaction of Oxytocin with Prostaglandins ... 256
VI. Conclusions ... 260
References ... 260

I. Introduction

Recent years have brought greater understanding of the hormonal control of parturition in many species, particularly the small laboratory animals and

Current Topics in Experimental Endocrinology, Vol. 4

ISBN 0-12-153204-6

the large domestic animals. In these species, the withdrawal of progestational hormones is a necessary prerequisite for the conversion of the relaxed pregnant uterus to an actively contracting organ, but in other species the levels of the main regulatory steroids of pregnancy do not change significantly at the time of parturition. The human and most primates belong to the latter group. Fetal adrenal activation, the event that leads to the decrease in maternal progesterone levels in sheep, goat, and cow (Liggins *et al.*, 1977; Thorburn and Challis, 1979) does not seem to be of critical importance for the timing of parturition in pregnant women and other primates (Peterson, 1983). Uterus-activating agents may therefore be responsible for the conversion of the pregnant uterus to the contracting parturient uterus in primates. Both oxytocin and prostaglandins are involved in the mechanism of parturition, but there is no agreement on their relative importance and the actual role of both oxytocin and prostaglandins in the activation of uterus needs to be elucidated.

Oxytocin is the most potent of all agents known to elicit uterine contractions. The threshold concentration for stimulation of the estrogenized rat uterus *in vitro* is 5 to 30 μU/ml (Fitzpatrick and Bentley, 1968) and about 50 to 100 μU/ml for term pregnant human myometrium *in vitro* (Fuchs and Fuchs, 1963). Expressed in molar concentrations, these values correspond to 1 to 6 $\times$ 10^{-11} and 1 to 2 $\times$ 10^{-10} M, respectively, ED_{50} being 3.2 $\times$ 10^{-9} M in rat uterus preparations (Walter and Wahrenkrug, 1976). No other uterus-stimulating agent approaches this oxytocic potency on the basis of either weight or molar strength. The parturient human uterus *in vivo* is even more sensitive to oxytocin than isolated strips *in vitro;* the effective plasma levels are estimated to be less than 10 μU/ml (2 $\times$ 10^{-11} M) (Saameli, 1963). The potency of oxytocin *in vivo* is especially striking in comparison to other uterus-activating agents. Thus, $PGF_{2\alpha}$ has about 1/150 to 1/500 of the potency of oxytocin on rat uterus *in vitro* (Mozler *et al.*, 1974), and only about 1/2500 of the potency of oxytocin *in vivo* (Fuchs, 1974). In addition, oxytocin causes little or no stimulation of smooth muscles outside the reproductive organs, except at much higher concentrations. At high concentrations, oxytocin exerts some antidiuretic action on the kidney, has an insulin-like effect on glucose metabolism in the adipocytes of certain species (Mirsky and Perisutti, 1962), and may affect memory processes in the brain (DeWeid, 1978).

The great potency of oxytocin has made the measurement of the circulating oxytocin levels very difficult, and until recently most evidence for a physiological role of oxytocin in the mechanism of labor was circumstantial. In the following we shall review both the indirect and direct evidence for a role of oxytocin in the initiation and maintenance of labor in various species.

II. Indirect Evidence of a Role for Oxytocin

A. Effects of Exogenous Oxytocin

1. Uterine Contractions

Oxytocin induces uterine contractions that cannot be distinguished from those observed during parturition in women (Caldeyro-Barcia and Poseiro, 1959) as well as in various animals (Fuchs, 1978). The subtle differences described by Johnson *et al.* (1970), Seitchik and Chatkoff (1976), and others are probably due to the fact that by necessity oxytocin-induced activity must be studied on a uterus which is quiescent before stimulation and therefore not maximally sensitive, and that the infusion rates are higher than the physiological secretion rates. The threshold for stimulation of uterine contractions at the time of delivery is only 0.25 to 0.5 mU/minute (Theobald, 1963), whereas in the last three weeks before parturition it is 12 to 14 mU/minute on the average (Saameli, 1963). The uterus of all species becomes increasingly sensitive to oxytocin as gestation progresses, and in many there is a rather sudden increase in sensitivity shortly before parturition, as reviewed by Fuchs (1978). In pregnant women a gradual increase in oxytocin sensitivity takes place during gestation, reaching a maximum in the fortieth week (Caldeyro-Barcia and Poseiro, 1959; Hendricks and Brenner, 1964), with a further rise in sensitivity shortly before parturition (Theobald, 1963, Caldeyro-Barcia and Theobald, 1968). A recent study of women at risk for preterm labor indicated that women who subsequently did deliver before term had a higher sensitivity to oxytocin than normal women at corresponding stages of gestation. At the time of preterm delivery, the uterine oxytocin sensitivity was as high as during term parturition (Takahashi *et al.,* 1980).

2. Induction of Labor

In all species studied labor can be induced with oxytocin only near the time of the spontaneous onset of labor. In most mammals the uterine cervix provides an obstacle to be overcome before the fetuses can be expelled. An "unripe" cervix is not dilated by strong contractions caused by an infusion of oxytocin, and after cessation of infusion uterine activity returns to preinfusion levels, whereas with a "ripe" cervix contractions stimulated by oxytocin infusion cause marked progress in cervical dilatation and the first stage of labor begins (Caldeyro-Barcia and Poseiro, 1959; Husslein *et al.,* 1981). Labor often continues by itself without need for further oxytocin infusion. Since exertion of maximal force against a closed cervix could result in uterine or cervical rupture, the uterine contractile activity must increase gradually, as is observed in women before and during normal spontaneous labor. The pattern of uterine contractions during labor in women, sheep, and goats can be mimicked by slow intravenous infusions of oxytocin. In certain species such as the rabbit and the cat, rapid expulsion of the young is necessary to avoid asphyxia, and in these animals the cervix offers very little resistance to dilation. Rapid injections of large amounts of oxytocin (250–500 mU) produce a similar pattern of uterine activity as seen during spontaneous delivery in rabbits (Fuchs, 1964a; Fuchs and Dawood, 1980).

Oxytocin is the only substance that consistently induces delivery in rats and rabbits at term. Prostaglandins of the E and F series, as well as norepinephrine and other biogenic amines, fail to induce delivery in pregnant rats at term when oxytocin is effective (Fuchs, 1972). In rabbits, injections of $PGF_{2\alpha}$ are much less effective than oxytocin in inducing delivery at term (Matsumoto *et al.,* 1971; Fuchs and Dawood, 1979). In pregnant women, on the other hand, prostaglandins E_2 and $F_{2\alpha}$ are as effective as oxytocin for the induction of term labor, and at mid-gestation prostaglandins are much more effective than oxytocin for the induction of uterine contractions and abortion (Burnhill *et al.,* 1962; Karim, 1975).

The failure of oxytocin to interrupt gestation in women and in most other mammals has been considered evidence against an important role for oxytocin in parturition. However, the relative refractoriness of the pregnant uterus to oxytocin prior to term can be considered an important biological adaptation to protect the fetus against premature expulsion as a result of inappropriate oxytocin secretion.

B. Effects of Endogenous Oxytocin

1. Induction of Uterine Contractions and Labor

Delivery can be induced by stimulation of endogenous oxytocin secretion. Thus, in women labor can be induced by suckling which elicits the release of oxytocin (Augusto, 1965). In rabbits (Lincoln, 1971) and in rats (Boer *et al.,* 1975), electrical stimulation of the posterior pituitary lobe, the neural stalk, or the neurohypophysiotropic area of the hypothalamus caused expulsion of the young when performed near term. Stimulation of the same areas in lactating animals induced milk ejection, indicating that the treatment did cause the release of oxytocin. Recordings of uterine contractions during parturition have been used to monitor oxytocin release (Fuchs, 1964a,b, 1966; Fuchs and Poblete, 1970), but the evidence from such experiments is not conclusive, due to the nonspecific nature of uterine contractions. However, simultaneous recordings from both horns of the bicornuate uterus of rats and rabbits provide evidence for the humoral nature of the uterine stimulant during labor, since both horns are activated at the same time. This is also observed when one of the horns is not pregnant, thus excluding local factors emanating from the products of conception (Fuchs, 1973). Recordings made from myometrial tissue explants grafted into the ear of pregnant rabbits have very convincingly confirmed the humoral nature of the uterine stimulus during parturition in rabbits, since even nervous influences are eliminated by this procedure (Wagner, 1975).

2. Induction of Milk Ejection during Labor

Milk ejection has been observed during labor in pregnant women who were still lactating from a previous pregnancy (Gunther, 1948; Sica-Blanco *et al.*, 1959). The mammary gland is a relatively specific target organ to oxytocin and has therefore been used to monitor oxytocin release during parturition. Whereas Cross (1958) found evidence for the release of oxytocin in rabbits, Boer (1976) in rats and Cobo *et al.* (1968) in women failed to observe milk ejection during labor, except in a few instances. This has been considered strong evidence against the involvement of oxytocin in parturition in women. However, the sensitivity of mammary gland is not maximal until postpartum (Guillof, 1970), and is critically dependent on the degree of filling of the ducts (DeNuccio and Grosvenor, 1974; Boer, 1976). In women, milk secretion does not start until postpartum and the amount of colostrum present in the glands may be insufficient for adequate filling of the ducts. Moreover, stress (Cross, 1955; Boer, 1976), catecholamines, (Cross, 1958; Vorherr, 1969) and $PGF_{2\alpha}$ (Vorherr and Vorherr, 1979) can inhibit the milk ejection response to oxytocin, and vaginal dilatation also was found to interrupt ongoing milk ejection reflexes in lactating rats (Lincoln *et al.*, 1978). Since all of these inhibitory factors are present during labor, the measurement of oxytocin release using mammary gland responses as an index of oxytocin release is not a reliable method during parturition. The failure to detect significant milk-ejecting activity during spontaneous labor therefore does not rule out the secretion of oxytocin.

C. *Pituitary and Hypothalamic Content and Depletion of Oxytocin*

During gestation the content of neurosecretory material in the hypothalamoneurohypophysial neurosecretory system (HNS) increases (Malandra, 1956; Vazquez, 1970; Swaab and Jongkind, 1970), and the content of pituitary oxytocin rises, reaching maximum levels shortly before parturition (rats: Kumaresan *et al.*, 1979; guinea pigs: Burton and Forsling, 1972). The rise in hormone content during gestation is specific for oxytocin; the vasopressin content does not change, at least not in guinea pigs.

During parturition, the oxytocin content of the pituitary gland drops significantly in all species studied (rats: Fuchs and Saito, 1971; Kumaresan *et al.*, 1979; mice: Fuchs and Dawood, 1980b; guinea pigs: Burton and Forsling, 1972). The depletion is specific for oxytocin in guinea pigs, whereas in rats the content of both oxytocin and vasopressin falls during normal delivery, although at different rates (Fuchs and Saito, 1971). The pituitary content of oxytocin and vasopressin is already reduced at the end of the first stage of labor, with a further drop during the expulsive phase of labor, suggesting a sustained release throughout the course of labor (Fuchs and Saito, 1971; Kumaresan *et al.*, 1979). However, the activation of the HNS during parturition need not be causally related to the labor contractions but could be a nonspecific response to the stress of labor, rather than the cause of it. Depletion of pituitary oxytocin and vasopressin has been observed in animals undergoing chronic stress (Tyler, 1961); however, acute stress tends to inhibit the release of vasopressin (Keil and Severs, 1977) and oxytocin (Cross, 1955; Boer, 1976). The depletion of vasopressin during labor may in fact be a stress response, since it occurs both in spontaneous and oxytocin-induced labor, while oxytocin depletion is observed only during spontaneous labor (Fuchs and Saito, 1971). In parturient women, vasopressin seems also to be released in response to stress, since urinary excretion of antidiuretic activity is much reduced in women given spinal anesthesia for pain relief (Cobo *et al.*, 1968). Vasopressin does not seem to be essential for parturition, since the Brattleboro rats are able to deliver spontaneously. These rats have a genetically defective neurosecretory system which is unable to synthesize vasopressin, but have a normal or even increased capacity to secrete oxytocin (Valtin *et al.*, 1965). Similarly, spontaneous labor and normal delivery have often been described in women who suffer from diabetes insipidus. Many of these patients have been able to breastfeed their infants, indicating that the neurosecretory defect only involves the vasopressin-secreting neurons. In one study, oxytocin was actually detected in the maternal blood during parturition (Sende *et al.*, 1976), confirming the fact that oxytocin and vasopressin are secreted by separate neurons.

D. Ablation and Lesion Studies

1. Ablation of the Neurohypophysis

Selective removal of the posterior pituitary has rarely been achieved. In most studies the entire pituitary or part of it was removed; this has had a variable effect on parturition, depending on the species and the time of the operation. In pregnant women, section of the stalk or hypophysectomy during pregnancy has been associated with normal parturition. In animals, no effect on parturition was detected in some species (Allan and Wiles, 1932; Pencharz and Long, 1933; Smith, 1932, 1946), while in others the removal of the hypophysis was associated with severe dystocia, prolonged parturition, and fetal death (Firor, 1933). Because of the unusual regenerative capacity of the HNS tract, the severed stalk is rapidly organized into a miniature neural lobe (Billenstein and Leveque, 1955; Moll and DeWied, 1962; Daniel and Prichard, 1970) which contains significant amounts of neurohypophysial hormones (Dogterom and Van Wimersma, 1977) and is capable of releasing hormones upon appropriate stimuli. Thus, the milk ejection reflex was normal in rabbits after transection of the pituitary stalk (Donovan and vander Werff ten Bosch, 1957) and in rats 10–12 days after hypophysectomy (Bintarningsih *et al.,* 1958). Low stalk section failed to produce diabetes insipidus in human patients (Hays, 1976). Ablation studies are therefore inconclusive.

2. Hypothalamic Lesions

Hypothalamic lesions involving the nuclei concerned with oxytocin secretion have led to severe impairment of parturition in most experimental animals (Fisher *et al.,* 1938; Dey *et al.,* 1941; Nibbelink, 1961) although apparently normal deliveries were observed in some instances (Gale and McCann, 1961). However, islands of magnocellular nuclei with similar characteristics as those found in the paraventricular (PVN) and supraoptic nuclei (SON) are situated between those nuclei and within the optic chiasma (George, 1978). These cells appear to be activated by the same stimuli as those in the PVN and SON (George, 1976), and lesion studies are also subject to some doubt as to the completeness of the lesion.

3. Hypothalamic Paraventricular Unit Activity during Parturition

The extracellular electric activity of magnocellular neurons in the paraventricular nucleus of pregnant rats has been recorded during parturition in anesthetized and unanesthetized rats (Boer and Nolten, 1978; Summerlee, 1981). These neurons were antidromically identified as oxytocinergic or vasopressinergic, the activation of which is known to cause the release of posterior pituitary hormones. A significant increase in the level of the spontaneous activity of both types of neurons was found during labor, this was observed before any overt signs of abdominal contractions or delivery. The authors also found that the firing pattern of these neurons changed in the course of labor to a tonic form from the intermittent and burst-like pattern seen in cyclic or lactating rats. In addition, bursts of accelerated discharge were seen before the delivery of either fetuses or placentas. These electrophysiological changes in the oxytocin and vasopressinergic neurons are a clear indication of their activation during spontaneous labor and provide evidence to suggest the release of both oxytocin and vasopressin during parturition.

E. Selective Inactivation of Oxytocin

Administration of antiserum against oxytocin to pregnant or lactating rats is reported to suppress lactation without any apparent effect on parturition, suggesting that oxytocin is not essential for parturition in rats (Kumaresan *et al.,* 1971). However, a different interpretation is possible. During parturition large amounts of oxytocin (about 300 mU/rat) are released within a relatively limited time, as judged by the depletion of the posterior pituitary content (Fuchs and Saito, 1971; Kumaresan *et al.,* 1979), whereas during lactation, small amounts of oxytocin (1–2 mU) are released intermittently every 4–10 minutes, over most of the day (Wakerley and Lincoln, 1972). Oxytocin may therefore be released in excess during parturition and the antibody may not have time to bind to all the released oxytocin molecules before they are taken up by the high affinity uterine receptors, the circulation time from brain to uterus being only about 10–15 seconds.

F. Blocking of Oxytocin Release with Ethanol

Ethanol blocks vasopressin release in response to osmotic stimuli and to certain pharmacologic stimuli, such as nicotine (Van Dyke and Ames, 1951). Ethanol also inhibits oxytocin release in response to the suckling stimulus and to pharmacologic stimuli such as acetylcholine (Fuchs and Wagner, 1963). The inhibition is dose dependent, but even a high concentration of ethanol fails to block the stimulatory effect of certain strong stimuli such as hemorrhage or intraarterial injections of hypertonic NaCl (Ginsburg, 1968). In rabbits (Fuchs, 1966) and rats (Fuchs, 1973), the administration of ethanol delays the onset of labor and causes a marked impairment of the process of parturition. Expulsion of the young is not completely prevented; it is associated with considerably reduced uterine activity and achieved mainly by abdominal straining efforts (Figs. 1 and 2). The effect of ethanol on uterine activity is overcome by exogenous oxytocin. These results indicate that oxytocin is essential for the initiation and maintenance of normal labor, at least in rabbits and rats. Besides oxytocin alternative means for the stimulation of uterine contractions do exist which probably come into play in the absence of

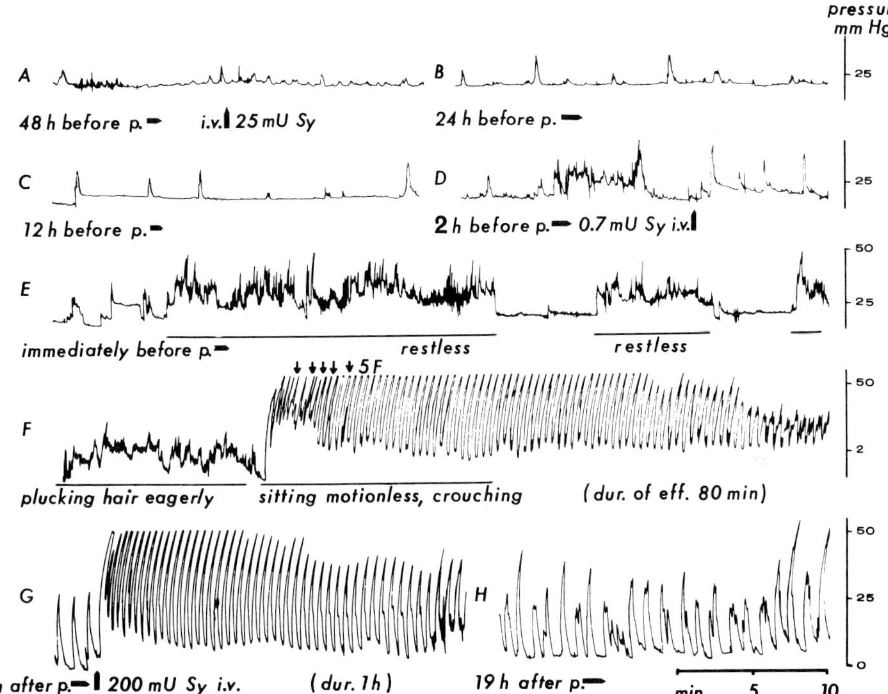

Fig. 1. Uterine activity of a pregnant rabbit in the last 48 hours prior to (A, B, C, D, and E) and during parturition (F). For comparison, the response to 250 mU synthetic oxytocin (Sy) is shown, injected iv shortly after parturition (G). p, Parturition; each arrow indicates the expulsion of a single fetus; duration of parturition: 5 minutes. (From Fuchs, 1964a).

oxytocin. However, parturition is then abnormal and results in a high proportion of dead or damaged offspring.

In the human, ethanol was shown to block the milk ejection .eflex and the release of oxytocin, while the response of the uterus and the mammary gland to exogenous oxytocin was retained, suggesting that the inhib·tion was central, and not peripheral (Wagner and Fuchs, 1968). These results were confirmed by Cobo (1973). The levels required for complete inhibition were high (0.3%); with lower alcohol levels (0.1 to 0.2%) a partial inhibition was observed. Ethanol ingestion during labor caused uterine contractions to cease when blood concentrations of 0.15 to 0.18% were reached (Fuchs *et al.*, 1967). The effect was seen in both preterm and in term labor but the inhibition during term labor was only transient at these dose levels. During

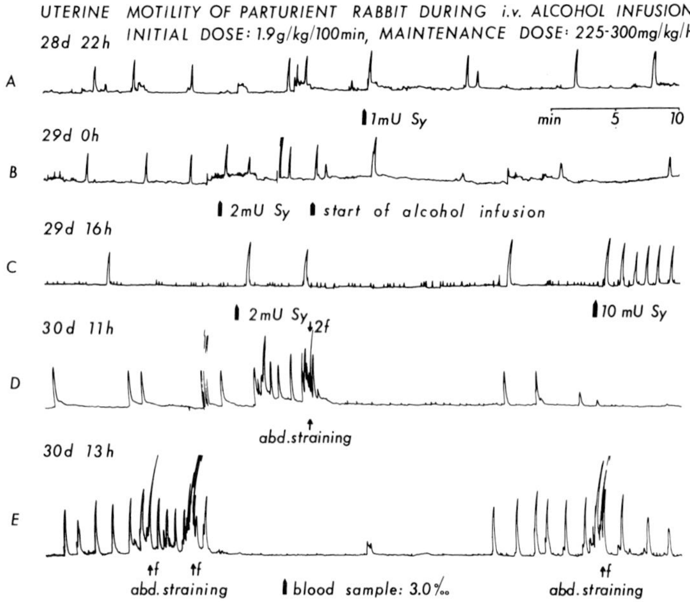

Fig. 2. (A–E) The influence of ethanol on uterine activity of a pregnant rabbit at term and during parturition, which was delayed and of abnormally prolonged duration: 2 hours, 30 minutes. (From Fuchs, 1966, by permission.)

preterm labor, on the other hand, the inhibitory effect persisted in the majority of patients, even after the discontinuation of the alcohol administration. More than 500 patients have been treated with ethanol infusions and the results have been very consistent, preterm labor being arrested in about 65% of the patients (Fuchs *et al.*, 1979). Contrary to the report of Karim and Sharma (1971), we have not observed any effect of ethanol on prostaglandin-induced contractions (Fuchs, 1977; Lauersen *et al.*, 1973) and we therefore attribute the effect of ethanol to its inhibitory effect on oxytocin release; however, a slight effect on the myometrium itself cannot be excluded, as pointed out by Mantell and Liggins (1970) and confirmed by us (Lauersen *et al.*, 1981).

We have recently measured blood oxytocin levels in patients treated with ethanol for the prevention of preterm labor (Fig. 3). Plasma oxytocin decreased initially in all patients consistent with the effect on uterine contractions. In patients in whom the treatment was successful, plasma oxytocin remained low; in treatment failures plasma oxytocin rose in spite of continuous ethanol infusion (Fuchs *et al.*, 1982d). These experiments confirm the inhibitory effect of ethanol on oxytocin release and indicate that oxy-

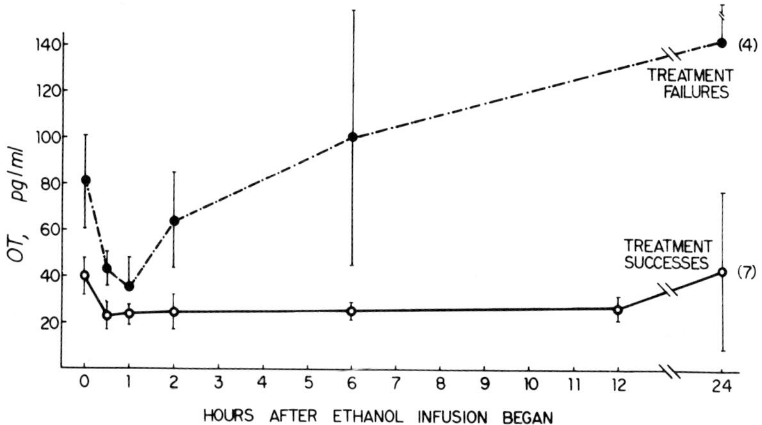

Fig. 3. Influence of ethanol on blood oxytocin (OT) levels in patients treated for threatened preterm labor. OT levels decreased initially in all patients but returned to high levels in treatment failures in spite of continued ethanol administration. Initial levels were higher in treatment failures than in patients in which preterm birth was averted. (From Fuchs *et al.*, 1982d.)

tocin participates in the initiation and maintenance of uterine contractions during preterm labor, if not during term labor.

III. Direct Evidence of a Role for Oxytocin

Circulating Levels of Oxytocin during Parturition

1. Measurement by Bioassays

Until recently, only bioassays were available for the measurement of oxytocin. The amounts needed to perform the assay range from 50 to 250 μU per assay necessitating the use of relatively large volumes of blood from which oxytocin has to be extracted and concentrated prior to assay. Serial samples could usually be obtained only from cattle and other large animals. With these methods oxytocin was detected in the jugular vein plasma of cows, sheep (Fitzpatrick and Walmsley, 1965) goats, (Folley and Knaggs, 1965), and rabbits (Fuchs, 1964b; Haldar, 1970) during the second stage of labor, while in goats Irving *et al.* (1971) found oxytocin also during the first stage of labor. In the jugular plasma of parturient women high levels of oxytocin were also detected during the second stage (Coch *et al.*, 1965), while during the first stage the levels were low. There was a great concentration gradient between the jugular vein and peripheral vein oxytocin levels, demonstrating the pituitary origin of the circulating oxytocin. These findings confirmed that oxytocin is released during parturition, but a major discharge of oxytocin appeared to be limited to the second stage of labor.

2. Measurement by Radioimmunoassay

a. Human Oxytocin Levels. Radioimmunoassay (RIA) techniques have increased the sensitivity of the assays and made measurements in serial samples more feasible. However, difficulties of specificity plagued even the early RIAs (Chard, 1972). With the presently available antibodies against oxytocin it is still necessary to extract oxytocin from biological fluids prior to assay. Unextracted human pregnancy plasma contains oxytocinase and other proteolytic enzymes which are inactivated by the extraction procedures.

During pregnancy the levels of immunoreactive oxytocin are usually low, mean levels being in the range of 10–30 pg/ml (Dawood *et al.*, 1978a,b, 1979a; Sellers *et al.*, 1981), but occasionally higher levels are found, indicating that the release of oxytocin is not inhibited during pregnancy. Whether a rise in plasma oxytocin occurs in late gestation is still open to dispute. Kumaresan *et al.* (1974) found a steady rise in plasma oxytocin throughout the second half of gestation with maximum levels of about 350 μU/ml near term. These high levels are not physiological and are probably due to the use of unextracted plasma for the assay. The data reported by others (Dawood *et al.*, 1979a; Sellers *et al.*, 1981) also show a rising trend in the plasma levels, but the increase during gestation is not significant (Table I).

The levels measured during labor by different authors vary considerably. Gibbens and Chard (1976) expressed their results as a proportion of positive results and found that the frequency of positive values increased during labor, reaching a maximum during delivery. Kumaresan *et al.* (1974) and Vasicka *et al.* (1977) found very high levels both during pregnancy and labor but no increase in labor values in comparison to the levels in late pregnancy, whereas Sellers *et al.* (1981) found very low levels and no increase during labor (Table I).

We have consistently found oxytocin in the peripheral blood of pregnant women during spontaneous labor at term (Dawood *et al.*, 1978a,b, 1979a; Fuchs *et al.*, 1982c) as well as preterm labor (Fuchs *et al.*, 1982d) (Table I). Mapa (1982) has confirmed our results. In cross-sectional studies as well as in serial samples taken during the first stage of labor, mean plasma oxytocin concentrations were significantly higher than in late pregnancy before the onset of labor (Fuchs *et al.*, 1982a,d) (Table II). The levels often increased further during the second stage (Fig. 4). The release of oxytocin during

Table I
Oxytocin Levels during Pregnancy and Labor

Stage of pregnancy and labor	Oxytocin (pg/ml)[a] Kumaresan *et al.* (1974)[b]	Dawood *et al.* (1978, 1979a)	Sellers *et al.* (1981)	Fuchs *et al.* (unpublished)
First trimester	139 ± 20.8	17.3 ± 2.1	—	—
Second trimester	148 ± 13.0	28.9 ± 4.7	7.5	—
Third trimester	243 ± 14.6	32.6 ± 29.0	15.0	17.1 ± 4.9
Term, no labor	328 ± 28.8	21.3 ± 5.3	10.3 ± 1.2	18.4 ± 5.9
Labor, early first stage	—	—	7.4 ± 1.0	32.3 ± 9.2
Labor mid first stage	362 ± 20	40.3 ± 9.8	—	43.5 ± 14.1
Labor late first stage	—	—	9.3 ± 2.0	62.5 ± 17.0
Labor second stage	180 ± 22	123.9 ± 23.6	8.6 ± 1.8	—
Labor third stage	164 ± 24	64.5 ± 13.1	—	85.4 ± 18.2
Umbilical artery	190 ± 24	114.8 ± 18.3	90 ± 15	101 ± 28
Umbilical vein	120 ± 20	37.5 ± 5.5	40 ± 8	55.1 ± 10.9

[a] Values are from cross-sectional studies and are means ± SEM.
[b] Data converted to pg/ml by assuming that 1μU equals 2 pg.

pregnancy as well as labor appears to occur in a pulsatile fashion (Dawood *et al.*, 1979; Gibbens *et al.*, 1972).

To determine the circulating oxytocin levels at which uterine contractile activity is induced, as well as to validate our RIA, we have measured the levels of circulating oxytocin during infusions of oxytocin for the induction of labor (Table III; Fuchs *et al.*, 1982c). During infusion of 1–3 mU/minute the concentration of plasma oxytocin was not significantly raised over values found in late pregnancy, and were similar to those observed in very early spontaneous labor. With increasing infusion rates, plasma oxytocin rose in a dose-dependent manner. When labor was induced by exogenous oxytocin,

Table II
Oxytocin Levels during Spontaneous Labor[a,b]

Stage of labor	Cervix (cm)	Oxytocin (pg/ml)
Term, no labor	≤2	19.9 ± 3.1
Early first stage	≤4	47.2 ± 7.6[c]
Mid first stage	5–6	46.3 ± 7.8[c]
Late first stage	7–8	43.0 ± 6.6[c]
Fully dilated	10	45.8 ± 13.8[d]

[a] From Fuchs *et al.* (1982c).
[b] Values are means ± SEM, measured serially in 17 women.
[c] Difference from controls is significant, $p < 0.05\alpha_2$.
[d] Difference from controls is significant, $p < 0.05\alpha_1$.

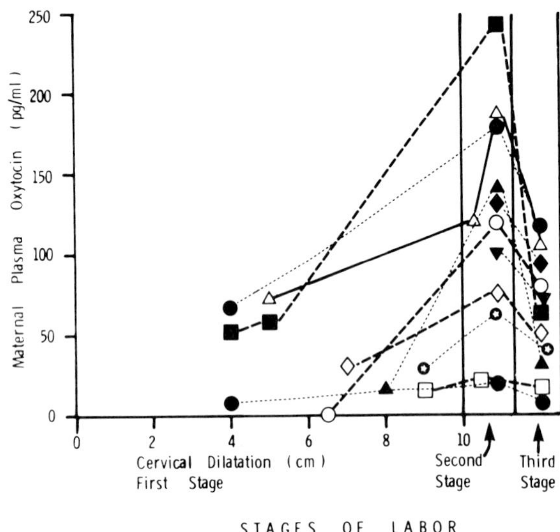

Fig. 4. Blood oxytocin levels in serial samples taken during the first stage of labor, at crowning of the fetal head and at the expulsion of the placenta in 11 patients. (From Dawood *et al.*, 1978, by permission).

uterine contractions were elicited at the rate of 1–3 mU/minute, and active labor was maintained at infusion rates of 4–8 mU/minute. Infusions of 10–16 mU/minute resulted in levels seen during the expulsive stage of spontaneous labor. Thus, concentrations of 2×10^{-11} *M* suffice to initiate contractions of the human uterus at term. During active spontaneous labor, the

Table III

Oxytocin Levels during Infusion of Oxytocin for Induction of Labor[a,b]

Infusion rate (mU/minute)	Oxytocin (pg/ml)
0	17.4 ± 3.9
1–3	21.1 ± 6.4
4–6	49.1 ± 10.9[c]
7.9	58.9 ± 9.9[c]
10–16	110.2 ± 25.7[c]

[a]From Fuchs *et al.* (1982c).

[b]Values are means ± SEM, measured serially in 15 women.

[c]Differences from control values significant, $p < 0.05\alpha_2$.

observed levels of endogenous oxytocin were similar to the concentrations seen during the infusion of 4–8 mU/minute. Our data are in very good agreement with the estimates of Saameli (1963), who calculated plasma levels from the infusion rates and the observed latency of the uterine response. The similarity between oxytocin levels during oxytocin infusions and spontaneous labor indicates that the levels observed during the first stage of labor are sufficient to stimulate the human uterus during labor.

b. Oxytocin Levels in Animals. Oxytocin has been measured by radioimmunoassay in the maternal circulation of goats (McNeilly *et al.*, 1972), cows (Schams *et al.*, 1979), mares (Allen *et al.*, 1973), guinea pigs (Burton *et al.*, 1974), miniature pigs (Taverne *et al.*, 1979), baboons (Dawood *et al.*, 1979b), and rats (Fuchs and Raghavan, 1981). The levels in these species were low during the first stage, rising to maximum during the expulsive phase, indicating that the pattern of oxytocin secretion follows a similar course as in parturient women. In pregnant rats, oxytocin infusions of 1 mU/minute did not increase plasma oxytocin significantly over late pregnancy values, while infusions of 2 or 5 mU/minute increased the plasma concentrations in a dose-dependent manner (Fuchs and Raghavan, 1981). A different pattern of oxytocin release was found in rabbits in which plasma oxytocin rose to maximal levels at the onset of labor and declined thereafter in accordance with its metabolic clearance rate (Fuchs and Dawood, 1980a; Fig. 5). A second rise in plasma oxytocin was often seen but unrelated to the expulsion of individual fetuses. The changes in plasma oxytocin during delivery in rabbits were similar to levels observed after iv injections of about 250 mU synthetic oxytocin (Fuchs and Dawood, 1980a; Fig. 6).

So far, rabbit is the only species in which there is clear evidence that a discharge of oxytocin initiates labor. In rabbits uterine activity and plasma oxytocin increase simultaneously at the onset of labor (Fig. 7), and labor can be induced by a single 20 second train of electric stimulation of the neurohypophysis (Lincoln, 1971). In species other than rabbits, the rate of oxytocin secretion appears to be maximal during the passage of the fetus through the cervix and vagina, and the liberation of oxytocin therefore may be triggered by the stretching of these tissues, as demonstrated in sheep and cattle (Hays and Van Denmark, 1953; Roberts and Share, 1969; Peeters and Houvenaghel, 1973). However, the possibility that labor in women and rats is precipitated by earlier much smaller discharges of oxytocin is suggested by the similarity between oxytocin levels during spontaneous early labor and slow infusions of oxytocin, and by the recorded activation of the hypothalamic, oxytocinergic nuclei during the first stage of labor (Section II,D,3). The studies in other animals do not exclude such a possibility because sampling intervals have not been adequate to detect oxytocin secretion in small quantities during the first stage of labor.

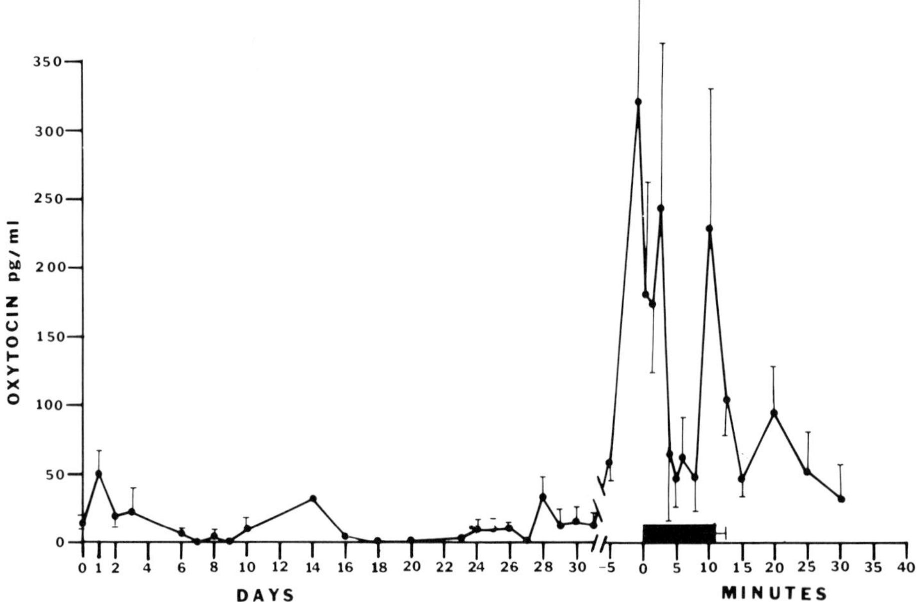

Fig. 5. Blood oxytocin levels during parturition in rabbits. Serial samples were collected before any signs of labor were observed, and with 0.5–2 minute intervals after simultaneous recordings of intrauterine pressure changes indicated that labor contractions had started. (From Fuchs and Dawood, 1980a, by permission.)

c. *Oxytocin Levels in Fetal Circulation.* Fetal cord blood collected at delivery has a high concentration of oxytocin and vasopressin (Chard *et al.*, 1970). There is general agreement that the concentration in the umbilical artery is higher than in the umbilical vein (Chard *et al.*, 1971; Kato and Torige, 1974; Kumaresan *et al.*, 1975; Dawood *et al.*, 1978b; Sellers *et al.*, 1981) (Fig. 8). Moreover, the umbilical arterial oxytocin levels appeared to be higher than maternal peripheral venous levels when measured after spontaneous vaginal or emergency abdominal delivery (Table I). It should be pointed out, however, that the maternal and fetal blood samples have rarely been taken simultaneously, the maternal sample usually being taken somewhat earlier and perhaps before the final discharge of oxytocin. In one study in which maternal blood was collected at delivery, the maternal venous and fetal arterial levels did not differ significantly (Kumaresan *et al.*, 1975). Because of the rapid changes in plasma oxytocin levels at the time of delivery a comparison of oxytocin concentrations in the two circulations is difficult. The significant positive arteriovenous difference in the umbilical circulation indicates, however, that oxytocin in fetal blood is of fetal origin. The extrac-

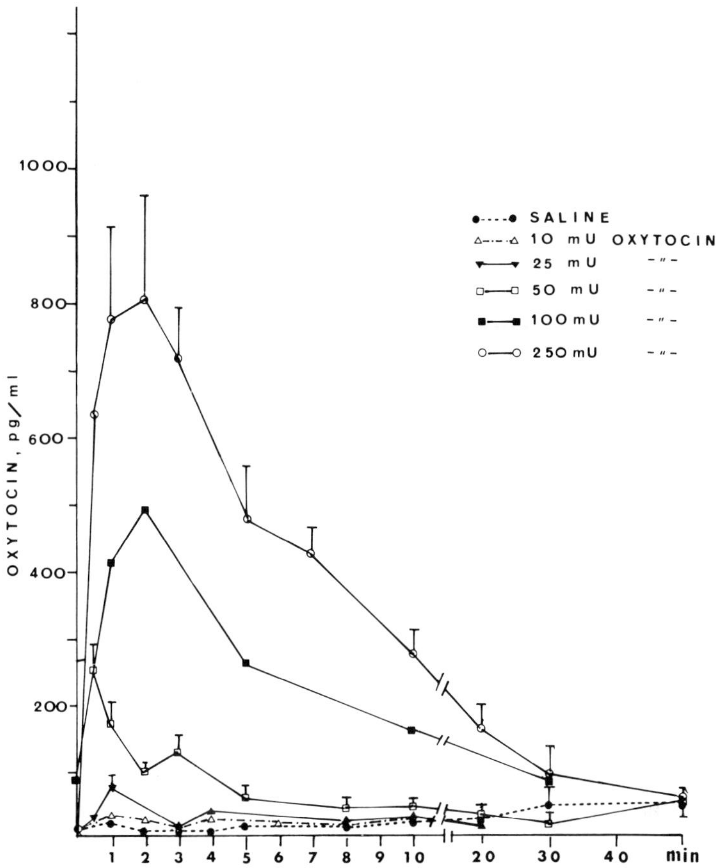

Fig. 6. Oxytocin levels in rabbits following iv injection of various doses of synthetic oxytocin. (From Fuchs and Dawood, 1980a, by permission.)

tion of oxytocin from fetal blood by the placenta suggests either a rapid inactivation of oxytocin or a transport through the placenta. Placental tissue is a rich source of aminopeptidases that also can degrade oxytocin and the fate of oxytocin during its diffusion through the placental barrier is not known. However, when oxytocin is infused into the mother for the induction of labor, the arteriovenous difference in the cord blood at delivery is reversed (Figs. 8 and 9), indicating that oxytocin can pass the placenta from mother to fetus without degradation (Dawood *et al.,* 1978b). After injections of oxytocin into the fetal circulation of pregnant baboons *in utero,* the maternal oxytocin levels rose suggesting that passage of undegraded oxytocin from fetus to mother is possible (Dawood *et al.,* 1979b). A passage of oxytocin

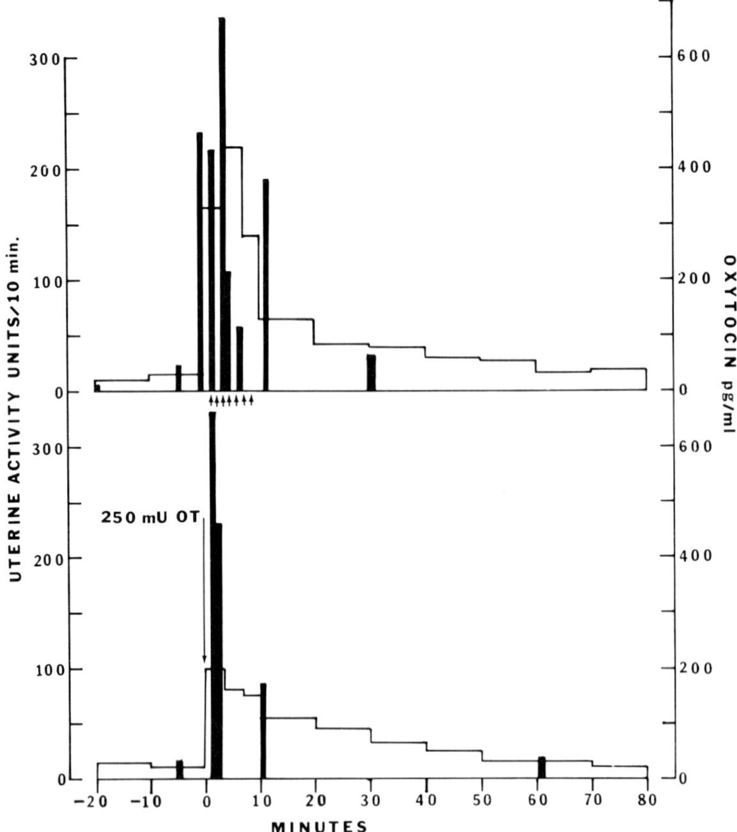

Fig. 7. Comparison of blood oxytocin levels (black columns) and uterine activity (expressed in Montevideo units) during spontaneous parturition (top panel) and injection of 250 mU of synthetic oxytocin (bottom panel) iv in rabbits. (From Fuchs and Dawood, 1980a, by permission.)

through the placenta in both directions was also demonstrated in guinea pigs (Burton *et al.,* 1974) and in sheep (Noddle, 1964), although conflicting results were reported in the ewe by Glatz *et al.* (1980). From the mean arteriovenous difference of 80 pg/ml during spontaneous vaginal delivery and a fetal blood flow through the placenta of 75 ml/minute the maximal transfer of oxytocin can be calculated to be about 3 mU/minute, an amount sufficient to stimulate uterine contractions at term.

The umbilical oxytocin levels are increased both at spontaneous vaginal delivery and at abdominal delivery performed during labor. The stimulus for the increased fetal oxytocin secretion during labor is therefore not the

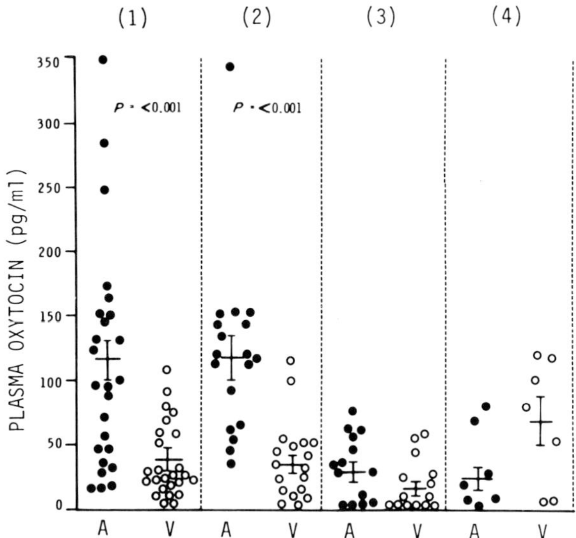

Fig. 8. Oxytocin levels in umbilical artery (closed circles) and vein (open circles) at delivery, grouped according to the mode of delivery. (1) Spontaneous vaginal; (2) emergency abdominal; (3) elective abdominal; (4) abdominal following failed OT induction. (From Dawood *et al.*, 1978b, by permission.)

pressure on the head during the passage through cervix and vagina. Recent reports have shown that abdominal compression is a very potent stimulus for vasopressin release (Husain *et al.*, 1979); whether it will also stimulate oxytocin release is not known. We have found that fetal oxytocin levels are raised even at an early stage of labor, namely, in patients in whom labor has started while waiting for admission to the operating room for an elective cesarean section (Fig. 9). In this group of patients the mean maternal oxytocin level is not significantly increased, and fetal oxytocin may therefore be more important for the initiation of labor than maternal oxytocin.

Amniotic fluid contains measurable amounts of oxytocin at term; the concentration rises during labor from 13.6 ± 6.7 pg/ml before the onset of labor to 48.1 ± 12.4 pg/ml after the onset of labor (Dawood *et al.*, 1979a).

IV. Control of Uterine Sensitivity

The uterine sensitivity to oxytocin changes during gestation in all animals so far studied, reaching maximal levels shortly before or at parturition. The

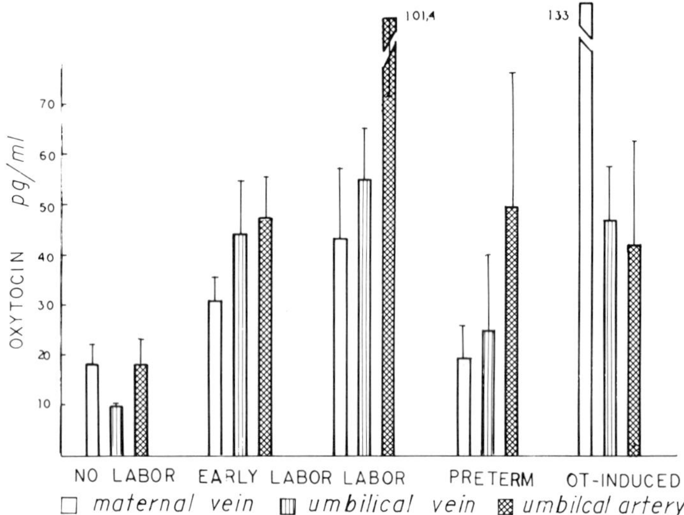

Fig. 9. Comparison of maternal (open columns) and fetal oxytocin levels at delivery by Cesarean section. Umbilical artery, crosshatched columns; umbilical vein, hatched columns. Elective section, no labor; elective section at the onset of labor; emergency section after active labor; emergency section after failed induction with oxytocin. (From Fuchs *et al.*, unpublished.)

uterine response to oxytocin is at least partially regulated by ovarian or placental steroids, although species variations exist that so far defy a unifying concept. In many species progesterone inhibits the uterine response to oxytocin and progesterone withdrawal is necessary for the onset of labor. By contrast, no decrease in plasma progesterone occurs prior to delivery in pregnant women, other primates, guinea pigs, and in certain marsupials, nor is a rise in plasma estrogens observed in the immediate peri-parturient period. A progesterone withdrawal theory cannot therefore account for the sensitization of the uterus to oxytocin in these species, and other factors must contribute to the increased oxytocin sensitivity at term.

Oxytocin Receptors

1. Myometrial Receptors

Soloff *et al.* in a series of papers, summarized in 1977, have demonstrated the presence of specific binding sites for oxytocin and characterized the binding sites with respect to affinity and specifity. The binding affinity of various oxytocin analogs correlated in general with their potency as agonists or antagonists, and factors that affected the binding of oxytocin affected the biological response in the same way. Because of these correlations, it may be assumed that these binding sites represent true receptors, the binding to which constitutes the first step in oxytocin action. Crankshaw *et al.* (1978) have further purified the fraction containing the myometrial receptor proteins, and located the oxytocin receptors on the plasma membrane of the smooth muscle cells of the uterus.

The physiological significance of the receptors was ascertained by correlating the uterine response to oxytocin with the number of myometrial oxytocin receptors measured in the same uteri after the oxytocin sensitivity tests were concluded. The threshold dose and the magnitude of the response to oxytocin were well correlated with the concentration of oxytocin binding sites (Fuchs *et al.,* 1982e), supporting the assumption that these binding sites serve a true receptor function and mediate the biological action of the hormone (Fig. 10).

In pregnant rats the number of oxytocin receptors rises sharply at the time of parturition (Soloff *et al.,* 1980) (Fig. 11), and parallels the observed changes in oxytocin sensitivity (Fuchs and Poblete, 1970). This increase in oxytocin receptor concentration may sensitize the rat uterus to the low circulating oxytocin levels at term, thus triggering labor contractions. We have recently measured oxytocin receptor concentrations in human uterus at various stages of gestation and at term (Fuchs *et al.,* 1982a). The results are shown in Table IV. The receptor concentration was low in the nonpregnant myometrium and rose dramatically during gestation. The main increase in

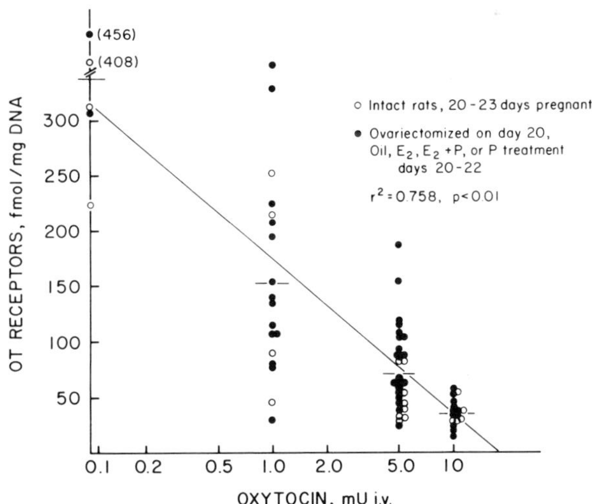

Fig. 10. The threshold dose for the stimulation of uterine contractions measured in pregnant rats correlated with myometrial oxytocin receptor concentrations measured in the same rats after the oxytocin sensitivity tests were completed. (From Fuchs *et al.,* 1982e.)

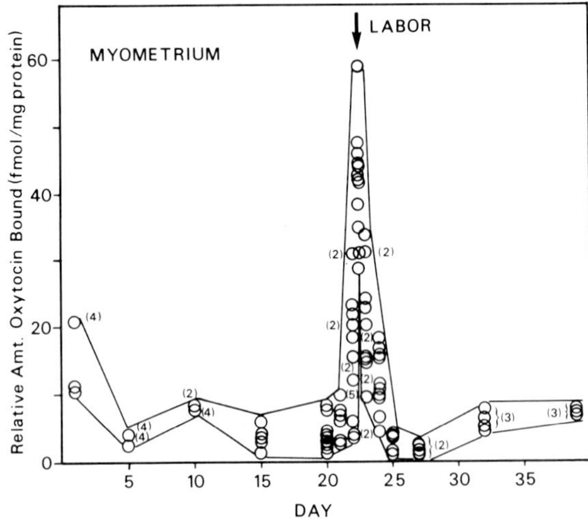

Fig. 11. The myometrial oxytocin receptor concentrations measured in intact pregnant rats in late pregnancy, at term, and during and after parturition. (From Soloff *et al.*, 1979, by permission.)

receptor concentration occurred during the second half of gestation; at 13–17 weeks gestation, the increase was still very moderate. The myometrial oxytocin receptor concentration was maximal in early term labor and significantly higher than in myometrium obtained before the onset of labor.

Table IV
Oxytocin Receptors in Human Myometrium[a,b,c]

	n	fmol/mg DNA	K_d (nM)
Nonpregnant	(14)	27.6[d] ± 7.9	—
Pregnant			
13–17 weeks	(5)	171.6[e] ± 67.4	2.4
28–36 weeks preterm labor	(8)	2353 ± 358	1.62 ± 0.27
37–43 weeks before labor	(6)	1391[g] ± 180	1.57 ± 0.21
37–43 weeks	(5)	3468[f] ± 886	1.30 ± 0.10
37–43 weeks advanced labor	(7)	257[e] ± 104	1.40 ± 0.23

[a]From Fuchs *et al.* (1982a).
[b]Values are means ± SEM.
[c]All samples were obtained from transverse low flap incision.
[d-g]Values with different superscript are different (Student's t test) $p<0.05$.

The receptor density in the myometrium during preterm labor (28–35 weeks) was also higher than in late pegnancy before the onset of labor.

We also found that the receptor concentrations were not evenly distributed over the entire uterus. The upper segment had a high oxytocin receptor concentration, whereas the lower part had a low one, the cervix having the lowest. The receptor concentrations in various parts of two pregnant uteri are shown in Fig. 12. The distribution was similar in preterm and term pregnant uterus, as well as in nonpregnant human uterus (Fuchs and Soloff, unpublished). Scatchard analyses indicated that the affinity of the receptors was uniform in all parts of the uterus, with no significant differences between the different stages of gestation (Table IV). The K_d values varied between 1 and 2 n*M*.

The increase in oxytocin receptors during gestation parallels the increase in uterine oxytocin sensitivity (Caldeyro-Barcia and Poseiro, 1959; Caldeyro-Barcia and Theobald 1968). The high receptor concentrations during preterm labor are in agreement with the findings of Takahashi *et al.* (1980) that the oxytocin sensitivity of women who deliver preterm is as great as in term deliveries. Because of the rise in tissue receptor concentration it is not necessary for circulating oxytocin levels to increase to initiate the biological action of oxytocin. The rise in myometrial oxytocin receptor concentration at the time of parturition adds support to the long disregarded view that oxytocin plays a role in the triggering of labor contractions in pregnant women.

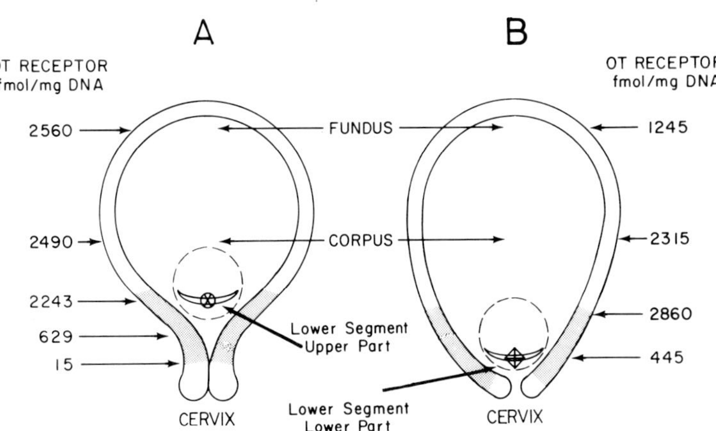

Fig. 12. The concentration of oxytocin receptors in various parts of pregnant human uterus measured in a preterm (A) and a term (B) patient in whom the uterus had to be removed for medical reasons. Shading indicates the lower segment. (From Fuchs *et al.*, 1982g.)

2. Decidual Oxytocin Receptors

In addition to the myometrium, specific oxytocin receptors were found in the endometrium of nonpregnant uteri and in decidua removed from pregnant uteri (Fuchs *et al.,* 1982a). Their concentration was similar to or even higher than that in the myometrium, rising to a maximum at the time of term or preterm labor (Table V). Only decidual parietalis had high receptor levels; decidua vera scraped from the placental rim had a low concentration of oxytocin binding sites. The affinity of the decidual and the myometrial oxytocin receptors was very similar: K_d values varied from 1 to 2 nM with no significant differences between different gestational ages. Decidual cells are not contractile cells and the function of the oxytocin receptors in decidua is therefore obscure. We have suggested that these receptors mediate an interaction between oxytocin and the prostaglandin synthetase system of the decidual cells; this novel aspect of oxytocin function is discussed in Section IV.

3. Regulation of Oxytocin Receptor Concentrations

Many peptide hormones regulate their own receptors by an incompletely understood process called "down-regulation." It has been suggested that the low receptor concentration in samples taken from the lower segment during active labor (Section III,1) may be due to a down-regulation by endogenous oxytocin secreted during labor (Sakamoto *et al.,* 1980). However, the receptor concentrations measured in the upper segment showed no evidence of

Table V
Oxytocin Receptors in Human Decidua and Endometrium[a,b]

	n	fmol/mg DNA	K_d (nM)
Nonpregnant			
Endometrium	(6)	24.9 ± 5.9	—
Pregnant			
17 weeks	(1)	629	1.4
28–36	(8)	3673 ± 947	1.75 ± 0.35
37–43 weeks before labor	(6)	1510 ± 382	2.25 ± 0.35
37–43 weeks early labor	(3)	3177 ± 1426	—
37–43 weeks advanced labor	(2)	786	2.0

[a]From Fuchs *et al.* (1982a).
[b]Values are means ± SD.

down-regulation during labor, and the apparent decrease in receptor numbers in the lower segment can be ascribed to the anatomical changes occurring in this part of the uterus during labor (Section III,1). Moreover, infusions of large amounts of oxytocin to pregnant rats did not influence the number of oxytocin receptors in the myometrium, militating against a possible down-regulation by oxytocin of its own receptors (Fuchs *et al.*, 1982e).

The influence of ovarian hormones on oxytocin receptors has been studied in rats (Alexandrova and Soloff, 1980b; Fuchs *et al.*, 1982e) and rabbits (Nissenson *et al.*, 1978). Estrogen increased the number of oxytocin receptors in both species, but had no significant influence on the affinity of the receptors. Progesterone prevented the estrogen-induced increase in receptor numbers in both species and prevented the acute increase seen after ovariectomy in pregnant animals (Fuchs *et al.*, 1982e) (Fig. 13). In intact pregnant rats, the concentration of oxytocin receptors was well correlated with nuclear estradiol receptor concentrations (Alexandrova and Soloff, 1980b). This was also the case in ovariectomized estradiol-treated pregnant rats, and progesterone treatment caused a decrease in the number of both oxytocin receptors and nuclear estradiol receptors (Fuchs *et al.*, 1982e). In rabbits,

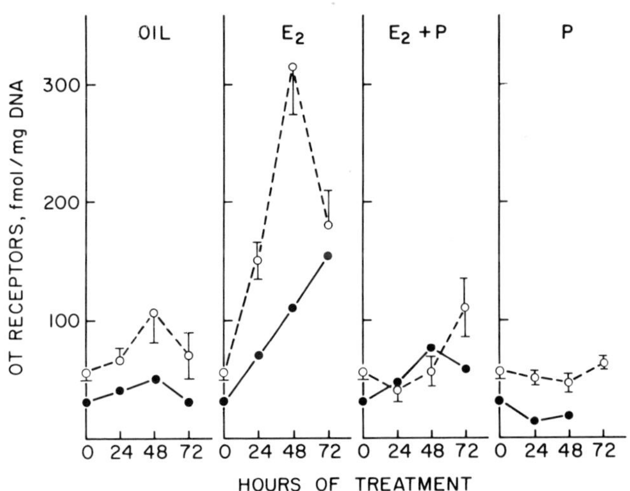

Fig. 13. Influence of estradiol (E_2) and progesterone (P) on myometrial receptor concentrations in pregnant rats ovariectomized on day 20 of gestation, and treated with either oil, estradiol-17β (5 μg/rat/day), E_2 and P (5 mg/rat/day), or P alone. The OT receptor concentrations were measured 24 and 48 hours after ovariectomy, and are expressed as fmol/mg DNA. (From Fuchs *et al.*, 1982e.)

cycloheximide prevented the estradiol-induced increase in oxytocin receptors, suggesting that the effect of estrogen involves the synthesis of new receptor proteins (Nissenson *et al.,* 1978). The turnover rate of receptors is probably relatively fast, judging by the decline in receptor numbers following parturition or ovariectomy.

The regulation of receptor numbers in the human uterus is less clear, since oxytocin receptors increase in the face of high or increasing progesterone levels. Measurement of estrogen receptors in pregnant human uterus has not clarified the issue; the total number of nuclear estradiol receptors was found to be the same or lower than in nonpregnant uteri and even the number of occupied receptors was not higher than in proliferative myometrium (Giannopoulos *et al.,* 1980). This may be due at least partially to technical difficulties since the nuclear receptors in human myometrium are particularly unstable and difficult to measure.

Stretch and distension of the uterine wall induce uterine growth in intact as well as in ovariectomized animals and it improves cell to cell communication. Stretch may also influence oxytocin receptors as suggested by a greater response to oxytocin in a distended uterine horn than in its unstretched contralateral counterpart (Csapo *et al.,* 1963; Fuchs, 1973). In ovariectomized pregnant rats, stretch had a synergistic effect with estrogen on myometrial oxytocin receptor concentration (Fuchs *et al.,* 1982f), but an effect of distension did not manifest itself in intact rats at term (Alexanderova and Soloff, 1980c). In face of the rather constant endocrine milieu found in women at term, it is an attractive hypothesis that the rapidly increasing volume of the human uterus contributes to the rise in oxytocin receptor levels at term by a stretching mediated mechanism.

V. Interaction of Oxytocin with Prostaglandins

Prostaglandins participate in the process of parturition in many species although their exact role in myometrial activation is not fully understood. Most convincing evidence for the importance of prostaglandins in parturition has been obtained in sheep, goats, and cattle (Liggins *et al.,* 1973; Thorburn and Challis, 1979), but there is ample evidence for the involvement of uterine prostaglandins in parturition also in women (Turnbull *et al.,* 1979) and rhesus monkeys (Novy, 1977). In comparison to oxytocin, prostaglandins have a wide range of biological activities and they can therefore influence the length of gestation and the onset of parturition in a variety of ways. These may involve (1) direct stimulation of myometrial contractions; (2) mediation or potentiation of oxytocin release; (3) inhibition of progesterone synthesis in the corpus luteum or placenta; and (4) vascular effects on fetal or placental haemodynamics. Only the first two items need concern us here.

Prostaglandins (PG) of the E and F series are uterine smooth muscle stimulants. Their action on the uterus is modified by ovarian hormones, but the influence of estrogen and progesterone on uterine prostaglandin sensitivity is much less marked than their effect on oxytocin sensitivity. In some species, estrogen and progesterone have opposite effects on the uterine responsiveness to prostaglandins and oxytocin. In rat progesterone enhances the uterine response to PGEs and PGFs while estrogen treatment suppresses the response (Fuchs, 1974). In rabbits progesterone treatment diminishes the uterine response to $PGF_{2\alpha}$ although to a lesser degree than that to oxytocin (Porter and Behrman, 1972). In human uterus, prostaglandins of E and F type can induce contractions at any stage during gestation, indicating that progesterone does not inhibit the response (Karim, 1975). Somewhat larger doses of PGs are required in early and mid-gestation than in late gestation to elicit contractile activity, and the PG sensitivity rises in parallel with the increase in progesterone and estrogen levels.

The levels of PGE or PGF do not rise significantly in peripheral plasma during parturition, probably due to their rapid inactivation in the lungs, but uterine vein levels of prostaglandin F increase in many species during labor (Liggins *et al.,* 1973; Thorburn and Challis, 1979). In women, the plasma levels of the more stable metabolite, 15-keto-13,14-dihydro $PGF_{1\alpha}$ (PGFM) rise during labor (Green *et al.,* 1974; Mitchell *et al.,* 1978), and both PGE and PGF rise in amniotic fluid during labor (Karim and Devlin, 1968; Keirse, 1975). In spite of intensive investigation no rise has been detected in any of these levels before the onset of labor, and there has been no information on the nature of the stimulus that elicits the rise in prostaglandins during human labor.

Cyclooxygenase inhibitors such as indomethacin, naproxen, and meclofenamate suppress uterine contractions in nonpregnant and pregnant women (Wiqvist, 1979) and in rhesus monkey (Novy, 1978), suggesting a role for endogenous prostaglandins in the generation of uterine contractile activity in primates. These inhibitors also suppress the contractions of uterine strips *in vitro* and diminish the response to oxytocin (Vane and Williams, 1973). Some but not all the effects of indomethacin are reversed by PGE_2 or $PGF_{2\alpha}$ (Anderson *et al.,* 1981; Northover, 1977), indicating that the drug may have an action of its own separate from its inhibitory effects on cyclooxygenase activity. Contrary to findings *in vitro,* oxytocin-induced contractions of rat or sheep uterus *in vivo* were not significantly suppressed by indomethacin treatment, although PG synthesis was severely reduced (Fuchs *et al.,* 1976; Roberts and McCracken, 1976). Chan (1980) has provided further evidence for the independence of oxytocin-induced contractions and prostaglandin production.

Several reports in the literature suggest that oxytocin may cause prostaglandin release from the uterus. In heifers and sheep, oxytocin increased the concentration of PGF in the uteroovarian venous effluent (Sharma and Fitzpatrick, 1974; Mitchell *et al.*, 1975). In sheep, the oxytocin-induced increase in uterine PGF originates entirely from the endometrium in which significant numbers of oxytocin receptors were found (Roberts *et al.*, 1976). In pregnant rats, oxytocin increased uterine PGF production (Chan, 1980) and prostacyclin production (Bamford *et al.*, 1980) *in vitro*. Several reports also indicate that release of PGF is stimulated directly by oxytocin and not by uterine contractions (Roberts and McCracken, 1976; Chan, 1980; Husslein *et al.*, 1981). In pregnant women, oxytocin infusions result in increased plasma PGFM levels (Green *et al.*, 1974; Husslein *et al.*, 1981). This increase was observed only when uterine contractions resulted in progressive cervical dilatation and delivery; in patients in whom induction failed, plasma PGFM levels did not rise even though oxytocin did elicit contractions (Fig. 14) (Husslein *et al.*, 1981). The generation of prostaglandins seems therefore essential for the propagation of uterine contractions although they do not seem necessary for oxytocin-induced contractile activity per se. This lends

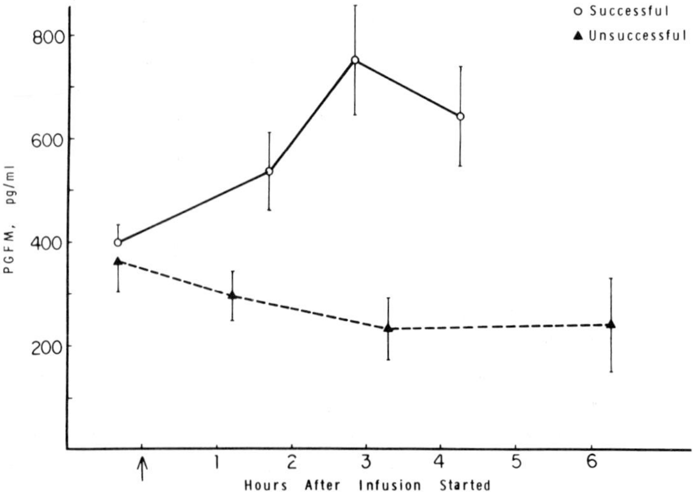

Fig. 14. Plasma concentrations of 15-keto-13,14-dihydro $PGF_{2\alpha}$ (PGFM) in 15 women before and during oxytocin infusions for the induction of labor at term. Open symbols represent levels in 9 women in whom the induction was successful, and closed symbols represent the levels in 6 women in whom induction failed. Values are ± SE. (Adapted from Husslein *et al.*, 1981.)

support to the proposal of Garfield that prostaglandins participate in gap junction formation (Garfield *et al.,* 1980).

The findings of oxytocin receptors in decidua parietalis led us to examine this tissue as a possible site for stimulation of prostaglandin release by oxytocin. Decidua and the fetal membranes are especially rich in arachidonic acid containing phospholipids within the uterus (Schwarz *et al.,* 1975) and possess an active prostaglandin synthetase complex (Willman and Collins, 1976). Experiments carried out in our laboratory with decidual tissue *in vitro* demonstrated that oxytocin increased the production of PGE and PGF in the decidua but had no influence on myometrial PGE and PGF production (Fuchs, *et al.,* 1981, 1982a). Oxytocin increased the PGE production also in amnion, but had no significant effect on PGF production in this tissue. (Fig. 15). Both basal and oxytocin-stimulated PGE and PGF production in decidua were greater in tissues removed during labor than before labor, whereas their production in amnion decreased during labor (Fuchs *et al.,* 1982a,b). So far the evidence implicating oxytocin receptors in the stimulation of PG production by oxytocin is only inferential. In a few instances oxytocin receptors were measured in samples obtained from patients with cesarean section after failed induction. The levels were lower in both myometrium and decidua, but the number of measurements is too small to permit any conclusions. Further studies are needed to prove this assumption.

The coupling of oxytocin receptors and the phospholipase–cyclooxygenase complex in the decidua may be the crucial event that precipitates labor in women. Decidual cells are accessible to oxytocin of both maternal and fetal origin, fetal oxytocin reaching the decidua by diffusion from the amniotic fluid via the intercellular canaliculi traversing the amnion and the

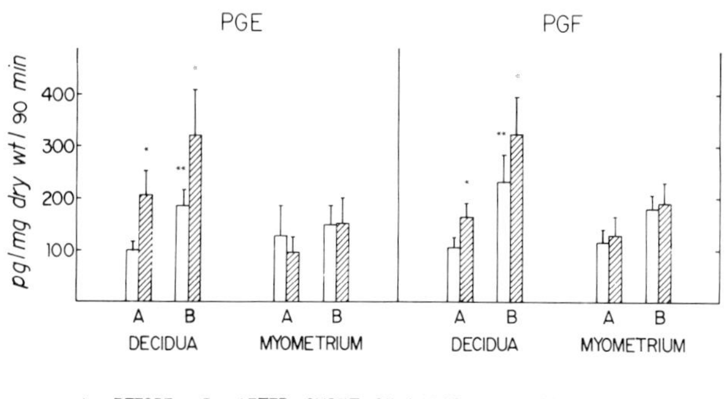

Fig. 15. PGE and PGF production in uterine tissues *in vitro* in the presence (hatched bars) and absence (open bars) of oxytocin. Samples of human decidua and myometrium were obtained before (A) and after (B) the onset of labor. (From Fuchs *et al.* 1982a, by permission.)

chorion (Minh *et al.,* 1980). As mentioned in Section II,A,3, a rise in fetal oxytocin has been demonstrated in early labor (Fuchs *et al.,* 1982a). Oxytocin originating from the fetal pituitary could thus be the signal for the increased prostaglandin production during labor. The released prostaglandins diffuse to the adjacent myometrium and enhance the oxytocin-induced contractions, making them synchronous and propagated. Such a sequence of events is compatible with the observation that both ethanol and cyclooxygenase inhibitors can prevent preterm labor.

VI. Conclusions

The hypothesis that oxytocin from the maternal or fetal neurohypophysis triggers the onset of labor has not been in favor for a long time. As pointed out in this article, evidence against the role of oxytocin in parturition has often been based on inadequate methodology or misinterpretation of the results. Careful analysis of the collective data supports the view that oxytocin plays an important role in both initiation and maintenance of human labor. The low blood levels found in early labor are compatible with physiological secretion rates, and are comparable to values found during infusions of exogenous oxytocin for induction of labor. Because the threshold to oxytocin stimulation decreases at the time of parturition due to increases in tissue receptor numbers, the circulating oxytocin levels need not rise to provide the trigger for the labor contractions. The proposed dual role for oxytocin in the mechanism of labor, namely, the stimulation of myometrial contractions and the stimulation of prostaglandin release from the decidua and fetal membranes, provides a unifying concept for the divergent opinions which consider *either* prostaglandins *or* oxytocin as the activator of the parturient human uterus.

Acknowledgment

Supported in part by Grant 6-219 from the March of Dimes Birth Defect Foundation and the O. W. Caspersen Foundation.

References

Alexandrova, M., and Soloff, M. S. (1980a). *Endocrinology* **160,** 730–735.
Alexandrova, M., and Soloff, M. S. (1980b). *Endocrinology* **160,** 736–738.
Alexandrova, M., and Soloff, M. S. (1980c). *Endocrinology* **106,** 739–743.
Allan, H., and Wiles, P. (1932). *J. Physiol.* **75,** 23–28.

Allen, W. E., Chard, T., and Forsling, M. (1973). *J. Endocrinol.* **57,** 175–176.
Anderson, G. F., Kawaratayashi, T., and Marshall, J. M. (1981). *Biol. Reprod.* **24,** 359–372.
Augusto, N. (1965). *Dissertation Fac. Med.,* University of Ribeirao Preto, São Paulo, Brasil.
Bamford, D. S., Jogee, M., and Williams, K. I. (1980). *Br. J. Obstet. Gynaecol.* **87,** 215–218.
Billenstein, D. C., and Leveque, T. F. (1955). *Endocrinology* **56,** 704–717.
Bintarningsin, W. M., Lyons, R., Johnson, R. E., and Li Choh, H. (1958). *Endocrinology* **63,** 540–548.
Boer, K. (1976). Dissertation, University of Amsterdam.
Boer, K., and Nolten, J. W. L. (1978). *J. Endocrinol.* **76,** 155–163.
Boer, K., Lincoln, D. W., and Swaab, D. F. (1975). *J. Endocrinol.* **65,** 163–176.
Burnhill, M. S., Gaines, J. A., and Guttmacher, A. (1962). *Obstet. Gynecol.* **20,** 94–99.
Burton, A. M., and Forsling, M. (1972). *J. Physiol. (London)* **221,** 6P.
Burton, A. M., Illingworth, D. V., and Challis, J. R. G. (1974). *J. Endocrinol.* **60,** 499–506.
Caldeyro-Barcia, R., and Poseiro, J. J. (1959). *Ann. N. Y. Acad. Sci.* **75,** 813–830.
Caldeyro-Barcia, R., and Theobald, G. W. (1968). *Am. J. Obstet. Gynecol.* **102,** 1181.
Chan, W. Y. (1980). *J. Pharmacol. Exp. Ther.* **213,** 575–579.
Chard, T. (1977). *In* "Endocrinology of Pregnancy" (F. Fuchs and A. Klopper, eds.), 2nd Ed. pp. 271–293, Harper, New York.
Chard, T., and Boyd, N. R. H . (1971). *Nature (London)* **234,** 352–354.
Chard, T., Boyd, N. R. H., Forsling, M., McNeilly, A., and Landon, J. (1970). *J. Endocrinol.* **48,** 223–234.
Cobo, E. (1973). *Am. J. Obstet. Gynecol.* **115,** 817–821.
Cobo, E., De Bernal, M. M., Quintero, C. A., and Cuadrado, E. (1968). *Am. J. Obstet. Gynecol.* **101,** 479–489.
Coch, J. A., Brovetto, J., Cabot, H. M., Fielitz, C. A., and Caldeyro-Barcia, R. (1965). *Am. J. Obstet. Gynecol.* **91,** 10–17.
Crankshaw, D. J., Branda, L. A., Matlib, M. D., and Daniel, E. E.(1978). *Eur. J. Biochem.* **86,** 481–486.
Cross, B. A. (1955). *J. Endocrinol.* **12,** 29–37.
Cross, B. A. (1958). *J. Endocrinol.* **16,** 261–276.
Csapo, A., Erdos, T., DeMattos, C. R., Gramass, E., and Moscovitz, C. (1963). *Nature (London)* **207,** 1378–1379.
Daniel, P. M., and Prichard, M. L. (1970). *Acta Endocrinol. (Copenhagen)* **64,** 696–704.
Dawood, M. Y., Raghavan, K. S., Pociask, C., and Fuchs, F. (1978a). *Obstet. Gynecol.* **51,** 138–148.
Dawood, M. Y., Wang, C. F., Gupta, R., and Fuchs, F. (1978b). *Obstet. Gynecol.* **52,** 205–209.
Dawood, M. Y., Ylikorkala, O., Trivedi, D., and Fuchs, F. (1979a). *J. Clin. Endocrinol. Metab.* **49,** 429–433.
Dawood, M. Y., Lauersen, N. H., Trivedi, D., and Fuchs, F. (1979b). *Acta Endocrinol. (Copenhagen)* **91,** 704–718.
DeNuccio, D. J., and Grosvenor, C. E. (1971). *J. Endocrinol.* **51,** 437–446.
Dey, F. L., Fisher, C., and Ranson, S. W. (1941). *Am. J. Obstet. Gynecol.* **42,** 459–472.
Dogterom, J., and Van Wimersma Greidanus, T. B. (1977). *Neuroendocrinology.* **24,** 108–118.
Firor, W. M. (1933). *Am. J. Physiol.* **104,** 204–215.
Fisher, G., Magoun, H. W., and Ranson, S. W. (1938). *Am. J. Obstet. Gynecol.* **36,** 1–15.
Fitzpatrick, R. J., and Bentley, P. B. (1968). *In* "Handbook of Experimental Pharmacology" (B. Berde, ed.), Vol. 23, pp. 190–285. Springer-Verlag, Berlin and New York.
Fitzpatrick, R. J., and Walmsley, C. R. (1965). *In* "Advances in Oxytocin Research" (J. H. M. Pinkerton, ed.), pp. 51–73. Pergamon, Oxford.

Folley, S. J., and Knaggs, G. S. (1965). *J. Endocrinol.* **33,** 301–315.
Fuchs, A.-R. (1964a). *J. Endocrinol.* **30,** 217–227.
Fuchs, A.-R. (1964b). *Excerpta Med. Int. Congr. Ser.* **83,** 753–758.
Fuchs, A.-R. (1966). *J. Endocrinol.* **35,** 125–134.
Fuchs, A.-R. (1972). *Fertil. Steril.* **26,** 410–416.
Fuchs, A.-R. (1973). *In* "Memoirs of the Society for Endocrinology" (A. Klopper and J. Gardner, eds.), Vol. 20, pp. 163–185. Cambridge Univ. Press, London and New York.
Fuchs, A.-R. (1974). *Am. J. Obstet. Gynecol.* **118,** 1093–1098.
Fuchs, A.-R. (1977). *In* "Endocrinology of Pregnancy" (F. Fuchs and A. Klopper, eds.), 2nd Ed. pp. 294–326. Harper, New York.
Fuchs, A.-R., and Dawood, M. Y. (1979). *Endocrine Soc. Annu. Meet., Anaheim,* **A353,** 161.
Fuchs, A.-R., and Dawood, M. Y. (1980a). *Endocrinology* **107,** 1117–1126.
Fuchs, A.-R., and Dawood, M. Y. (1980b). *Soc. Gynecol. Invest. Annu. Meet., Denver,* **A305,** 182.
Fuchs, A.-R., and Fuchs, F. (1963). *J. Obstet. Gynaecol. Br. Commonw.* **70,** 658–664.
Fuchs, A.-R., and Poblete, V. F., Jr. (1970). *Biol. Reprod.* **2,** 387–400.
Fuchs, A.-R., and Raghavan, K. S. (1980). *In* "Advances in Experimental Medicine: A Centenary Tribute to Claude Bernard" (H. Parvez and S. Parvez, eds.), pp. 403–428. Elsevier, Amsterdam.
Fuchs, A.-R., and Saito, S. (1971). *Endocrinology* **88,** 574–578.
Fuchs, A.-R., and Wagner, G. (1963). *Acta Endocrinol.* **44,** 593–605.
Fuchs, A.-R., Smitasiri, Y., and Chantharaksri, U. (1976). *J. Reprod. Fertil.* **48,** 321–340.
Fuchs, A.-R., Fuchs, F., and Husslein, P. (1981). *Am. J. Obstet. Gynecol.* **141,** 694–697.
Fuchs, A.-R., Fuchs, F., Husslein, P., Soloff, M. S., and Fernström, M. J. (1982a). *Science* **215,** 1396–1398.
Fuchs, A.-R., Fuchs, F., Husslein, P., and Weksler, B. B. (1982b). *Endocrine Soc. Annu. Mtg. San Francisco,* Abstr. 1306.
Fuchs, A.-R., Goeschen, K., Husslein, P., Rasmussen, A., and Fuchs, F. (1982c). *Am. J. Obstet. Gynecol.* (in press).
Fuchs, A.-R., Husslein, P., Dawood, M. Y., Micha, J., and Fuchs, F. (1982d). *Am. J. Obstet. Gynecol.* (in press).
Fuchs, A.-R., Periyasami, S., Alexandrova, M., and Soloff, M. S. (1982e). *Endocrinology* (submitted).
Fuchs, A.-R., Periyasami, S., and Soloff, M. S. (1982f). *Endocrinology* (submitted).
Fuchs, A.-R., Soloff, M. S., Fernström, M. J., Husslein, P., and Fuchs, F. (1982g). *Am. J. Obstet. Gynecol.* (submitted).
Fuchs, F., Fuchs, A.-R., Poblete, V. F., Jr., and Risk, A. (1967). *Am. J. Obstet. Gynecol.* **99,** 627–637.
Fuchs, F., Fuchs, A.-R., Lauersen, N. H., and Zervoudakis, A. (1979). *Dan. Med. Bull.* **26,** 123–129.
Gale, C., and McCann, S. M. (1961). *J. Endocrinol.* **22,** 107–117.
Garfield, R. D., Kannan, M. D., and Daniel, E. E. (1980). *Am. J. Physiol.* **238,** C-81–85.
George, J. M. (1976). *Science* **193,** 146–148.
George, J. M. (1978). *Science* **200,** 343–343.
Giannopoulos, G., Goldberg, P., Shea, T. B., and Tulchinsky, D. (1980). *J. Clin. Endocrinol. Metab.* **51,** 702–710.
Gibbens, G. L. D., and Chard, T. (1976). *Am. J. Obstet. Gynecol.* **126,** 243.
Gibbens, G. L. D., Boyd, N. R. H., and Chard, T. (1972). *J. Endocrinol.* **53,** 14.
Ginsburg, M. (1968). *In* "Handbuch der experimentelle Pharmacologie" (B. Berde, ed.), Vol. XXIII, pp. 286–371.

Glatz, T. H., Weitzman, R. E., Nathanielsz, P. W., and Fischer, D. W. (1980). *Endocrinology* **126,** 1006–1011.
Green, K., Bygdeman, M., Toppozada, M., and Wiqvist, N. (1974). *Am. J. Obstet. Gynecol.* **120,** 25–31.
Guillof, E. (1970). *Proc. Meeting Lat. Am. Assoc. Human Reprod., 4th, Punta del Este, Montevideo,* Abstract.
Gunther, M. (1948). *Br. Med. J.* **1,** 567.
Haldar, J. (1970). *J. Physiol. (London)* **206,** 723–730.
Hays, R. L., and VanDemark, N. L. (1953). *Endocrinology* **52,** 634–637.
Hays, R. M. (1976). *N. Engl. J. Med.* **295,** 659–665.
Hendricks, C. H., and Brenner, W. T. (1964). *Am. J. Obstet. Gynecol.* **90,** 485–492.
Husain, M. K., Manger, W. M., Rock, T. W., Weiss, R. J., and Frantz, A. G. (1979). *Endocrinology* **104,** 641–664.
Husslein, P., Fuchs, A.-R., and Fuchs, F. (1981). *Am. J. Obstet. Gynecol.* **141,** 688–693.
Irving, G., Jones, D. E., and Knifton, A. (1971). *Res. Vet. Sci.* **12,** 472–473.
Johnson, W. L., Depp, R., and Hunter, C. A., Jr. (1970). *Am. J. Obstet. Gynecol.* **107,** 268–273.
Karim, S. M. M. (1975). "Advances in Prostglandin Research: Prostaglandins and Reproduction, pp. 149–228. MTP, Lancaster.
Karim, S. M. M., and Devlin, J. (1967). *J. Obstet. Gynaecol. Br. Commonw.* **74,** 230–234.
Karim, S. M. M., and Sharma, S. D. (1971). *J. Obstet. Gynaecol. Br. Cwlth.* **78,** 251–254.
Kato, H., and Torige, T. (1974). *Endocrinol. Jpn.* **21,** 81–87.
Keil, L. C., and Severs, W. B. (1977). *Endocrinology* **100,** 30–38.
Keirse, M. J. N. C. (1979). *In* "Human Parturition: New Concepts and Developments" (M. J. N. C. Keirse, A. B. M. Anderson, and J. Bennebroek Gravenhorst, eds.), Boerhaave Series for Medical Education, Vol. 15, pp. 101–142. Leiden Univ. Press, Leiden.
Kumaresan, P., Kagan, A., and Glick, S. M. (1971). *Nature (London)* **230,** 468–469.
Kumaresan, P., Anandarangam, P. B., Dianzon, W., and Vasicka, A. (1974). *Am. J. Obstet. Gynecol.* **119,** 215–223.
Kumaresan, P., Han, G. S., Anandarangam, P. B., and Vasicka, A. (1975). *Obstet. Gynecol.* **46,** 272–274.
Kumaresan, P., Subramanian, M., and Anandarangam, P. B. (1979). *J. Endocrinol. Invest.* **2,** 65–70.
Lauersen, N. H., Raghavan, K. S., Wilson, K. H., Fuchs, F., and Niemann, W. H. (1973). *Am. J. Obstet. Gynaecol.* **114,** 912–918.
Lauersen, N. H., Wilson, K. H., and Fuchs, F. (1981). *J. Reprod. Med.* **26,** 547–550.
Liggins, G. C., Grieves, S. A., Kendall, J. Z., and Knox, B. S. (1973). *Recent Prog. Horm. Res.* **29,** 111–150.
Liggins, G. C., Fairclough, R. J., Grieves, S. A., Foster, C. S., and Knox, B. S. (1977). *CIBA Found. Symp.* (N. S.) **47,** 5–30.
Lincoln, D. W. (1971). *J. Endocrinol.* **50,** 607–618.
Lincoln, D. W., Tribollet, E., and Dreifuss, J. (1978). *J. Endocrinol.* 7lP–72P.
McNeilly, A. S., Martin, M., Chard, T., and Hart, I. C. (1972). *J. Endocrinol.* **52,** 213–214.
Malandra, B. (1956). *Z. Zellforsch.* **46,** 594–610.
Mantell, C. D., and Liggins, G. C. (1970). *J. Obstet. Gynaecol. Br. Commonw.* **77,** 976–981.
Mapa, M. K., (1982). Ph. D. Dissertation, University of Chandigarh, India.
Matsumoto, K., Sasada, M., and Sakai, T. (1971). *Oyo Yakuri* **5,** 741–956.
Minh, H. N., Douvin, D., Smadja, A., and Orcel, L. (1980). *Eur. J. Obstet. Gynecol. Reprod. Biol.* **10,** 213–224.

Mirsky, A., and Perisutti, G. (1962). *Endocrinology* **71,** 158.
Mitchell, M. D., Flint, A. P. F., and Turnbull, A. C. (1975). *Prostaglandins* **9,** 47–56.
Mitchell, M. D., Flint, A. P., Bibby, J., Brunt, J., Arnold, J. M., Anderson, A. B. M., and Turnbull, A. C. (1978). *J. Clin. Endocrinol. Metab.* **46,** 947–951.
Moll, J., and DeWied, D. (1962). *Gen. Comp. Endocrinol.* **2,** 215–228.
Nibbelink, D. W. (1961). *Am. J. Physiol.* **200,** 1229–1232.
Nissenson, R., Flouret, G., and Hechter, O. (1978). *Proc. Natl. Acad. Sci. U.S.A.* **75,** 2044–2048.
Noddle, B. A. (1964). *Nature (London)* **203,** 414.
Northover, B. J. (1977). *Gen. Pharmacol.* **8,** 293–296.
Novy, M. J. (1978). *Advn. Prostaglandin Thromboxane Res.* **4,** 285–300.
Pencharz, R. I., and Long, J. A. (1933). *Am. J. Anat.* **53,** 117–140.
Peeters, G., and Houvenaghel, A. (1973). *J. Endocrinol.* **58,** 53–66.
Peterson, R. E. (1983). *In* Endocrinology of Pregnancy (F. Fuchs and A. Klopper, eds.), 3rd Ed. Lippincott, New York (in press).
Porter, D. G., and Behrman, H. R. (1971). *Nature (London)* **232,** 627–628.
Roberts, J. S., and McCracken, J. A. (1976). *Biol. Reprod.* **15,** 457–463.
Roberts, J. S., and Share, L. (1969). *Endocrinology* **84,** 1076–1081.
Roberts, J. S., McCracken, J. A., Gavagan, J. E., and Soloff, M. S. (1976). *Endocrinology* **99,** 1107–1114.
Saameli, K. (1963). *Am. J. Obstet. Gynecol.* **85,** 186–192.
Sakamoto, H., Den, K., Yamamoto, K., Arai, T., and Kawai, S. (1979). *Endocrinol. Jpn.* **26,** 515–522.
Schams, D., Schmidt-Pole, B., and Kruse, V. (1979). *Acta Endocrinol.* **92,** 258–270.
Schwarz, B. E., Schultz, F. M., MacDonald, P. C., and Johnston, J. M. (1975). *Am. J. Obstet. Gynecol.* **45,** 564–568.
Seitchik, J., and Chatkoff, N. (1976). *Obstet. Gynecol.* **48,** 436–441.
Sellers, S. M., Hodgson, H. T., Mitchell, M. D., Anderson, A. B. M., and Turnbull, A. C. (1981). *Br. J. Obstet. Gynaecol.* **88,** 725–729.
Sende, P., Pantelakis, N., Susaki, K., and Bashore, R. (1976). *Obstet. Gynecol.* **48,** 38–41.
Sharma, S. C., and Fitzpatrick, R. J. (1974). *Prostaglandins* **6,** 97–106.
Sica-Blanco, Y., Mendez-Bauer, C., Sala, N., Cabot, H. M., and Caldeyro-Barcia, R. (1959). *Arch. Gynecol. Obstet. (Montevideo)* **17,** 63–72.
Smith, P. E. (1932). *Am. J. Physiol.* **99,** 345–348.
Smith, P. E. (1946). *Anat. Rec.* **94,** 497–499.
Soloff, M. D., Schroeder, B. T., Chakraborty, J., and Pearlmutter, A. F. (1977). *Fed. Proc. Fed. Am. Soc. Exp. Biol.* **36,** 861–866.
Soloff, M. S., Alexandrova, M. and Ferustrom, M. J. (1979). *Science* **204,** 1313–1315.
Summerlee, A. J. S. (1982). *J. Physiol. (London)* **327,** 43.
Swaab, D. F., and Jongkind, J. F. (1970). *Neuroendocrinology* **6,** 133–145.
Takahashi, K., Diamond, F., Bieniarz, J., Yen, H., and Burd, I. (1980). *Am. J. Obstet. Gynecol.* **136,** 774–779.
Taverne, M. A. M., Naaktgeboren, C., Elsaesser, F., Forsling, M. L., van der Weyden, G. C., Ellendorff, F., and Smidt, D. (1979). *Biol. Reprod.* **21,** 1125–1134.
Theobald, G. W. (1963). *In* "Modern Trends in Obstetrics" (R. T. Keller, ed.) pp. 87–103. Butterworths, London.
Thorburn, G. D., and Challis, J. R. G. (1978). *Physiol. Rev.* **59,** 863–918.
Turnbull, A. C., Anderson, A. B. M., Flint, A. P. F., Jeremy, J. Y., Keirse, M. J. N. C., and Mitchell, M. D. (1971). *Ciba Found. Symp. (N. S.)* **47,** 427–452.
Tyler, C. (1961). *Arch. Int. Pharmacol.* **131,** 301–308.

Valtin, H., Sawyer, W. H., and Sokol, H. W. (1965). *Endocrinology* **77**, 701–706
Van Dyke, H B., and Ames, R. G. (1951). *Acta Endocrinol. (Copenhagen)* **7**, 110–121.
Vane, J. R., and Williams, K. J. (1973). *Br. J. Pharmacol.* **48**, 629–639.
Vasicka, A., Kumaresan, P., Han, G. S., and Kumaresan, M. (1977). *Am. J. Obstet. Gynecol.* **130**, 263–273.
Vazquez, R. (1970). *Am. J. Anat.* **19**, 247–266.
Vorherr, H. (1969). *Acta Endocrinol. (Copenhagen)* **138**, 5–38.
Vorherr, H., and Vorherr, U. F. (1979). *Endocrinology* **104**, 989–995.
Wagner, G. (1975). *Acta Endocrinol. (Copenhagen)* **79**, 767–777.
Wagner, G., and Fuchs, A.-R. (1968). *Acta Endocrinol. (Copenhagen)* **58**, 133.
Wakerley, J. B., and Lincoln, D. W. (1972). *Nature (London) New Biol.* **233**, 180–181.
Walter, R., and Wahrenkrug, M. (1976). *Pharmacol. Res. Commun.* **8**, 81–89.
Willman, E. A., and Collins, W. P. (1976). *Br. J. Obstet. Gynaecol.* **83**, 786–789.
Wiqvist, N. (1979). *In* "Human Parturition: New Concepts and Developments" (M. J. N. C. Keirse, A. B. M. Anderson, and J. Gravenhorst, eds.), Boerhaave Series, Vol. 15, pp. 189–200. Leiden Univ. Press, Leiden.

THREATENED ABORTION

Rodney P. Shearman

DEPARTMENT OF OBSTETRICS AND GYNECOLOGY
UNIVERSITY OF SYDNEY
AND
DIVISION OF OBSTETRICS AND GYNECOLOGY
ROYAL PRINCE ALFRED HOSPITAL
SYDNEY, AUSTRALIA

I. Definition 268
II. Incidence 268
III. Natural History 268
A. Progression to Spontaneous Abortion 269
B. Subsequent Prematurity 269
C. Fetal Abnormality 270
IV. Etiology 271
Maternal Factors 271
V. Clinical Features 273
A. Differential Diagnosis 275
B. Other Aids to Diagnosis 277
VI. Management 282
A. Prevention 282
B. Treatment 282
VII. Threatened Abortion and the Intrauterine Device (IUD) 284
References 285

Current Topics in
Experimental Endocrinology, Vol. 4

ISBN 0-12-153204-6

I. Definition

Any definition should be finite. There are immediate difficulties in defining threatened abortion, as the definition of abortion varies between countries. In many countries, a birth is defined as the expulsion of a fetus of more than 400 g and/or more than 20 weeks menstrual age; an abortion is the expulsion of products of conception that does not meet the definition of birth. Partly because of these difficulties, there are widely conflicting data on subjects of fundamental importance such as incidence and outcome. The definition used here is the same as that used by Johannsen (1970): "Threatened abortion is defined as hemorrhage from the uterus in association with an intrauterine pregnancy prior to 20 weeks gestation, with the cervix incompletely effaced and the os closed, and irrespective of whether or not uterine contractions are occurring."

In a book that has an endocrinological bias this definition has the advantage that it excludes the predominantly mechanical problem of threatened abortion and the incompetent cervix.

II. Incidence

Of those pregnancies that reach the level of clinical consciousness, the quoted incidence of threatened abortion varies between 2.4 and 20% (Editorial comment, 1980). The figure of 16% quoted by Hertig and Livingstone (1944) is still widely used in the literature, perhaps because age has given it a patina of acceptability and authenticity. None of these figures match very well with the usually quoted incidence of spontaneous abortion of 15% (Shearman 1980), figures based on clinical data and a total implantation loss of 43%, based on endocrinological data (Grudzinskas *et al.,* 1981). It should be recognized that no uniformly accepted figures of the incidence of threatened abortion exist. There are, however, good figures on the numbers of women who deliver a viable fetus who had a threatened abortion during that pregnancy. In a very carefully documented group of nearly 8000 private patients, Correy (1980) found an incidence of 6.6% of threatened abortion before the sixteenth week of pregnancy dated on menstrual age, but there are no figures in this study to indicate those women who had a threatened abortion and then proceeded to abortion.

III. Natural History

Almost all women who suffer from bleeding in the first half of pregnancy will have several concerns. "Will I miscarry?," "Will the baby be premature?." "If I do not miscarry will the baby be abnormal?" There is no evidence that therapeutic intervention has any effect on the ultimate outcome. Because of this one might expect that the natural history of this common problem would be well documented but it is not. Almost all the available data come from those women admitted to hospital; for example in Britain "In general, admission to hospital for threatened abortion is confined to women with heavy or prolonged bleeding" (Editorial Comment, 1980). The same criteria for hospital admission apply in most other countries so that data based on hospital studies will be heavily biased toward those most likely to abort since there is a relationship between the amount of bleeding and ultimate outcome (Mantoni and Pedersen, 1981).

A. Progression to Spontaneous Abortion

In a study of 266 patients admitted to hospital with threatened abortion, Johannsen (1970) found that 50.8% proceeded to spontaneous abortion. Of those women who ultimately aborted, this occurred within 1 week in 43.7% and within 1 month in 80% of the total aborting. Eriksen and Philipsen (1980) found 35% of patients admitted to hospital with threatened abortion proceeded to abort. Spontaneous abortion in 80% of patients admitted to hospital with threatened abortion has been reported by Evans and Beischer (1970) while in another Australian study, 35% aborted (Ho and Jones, 1980). Joupilla *et al.* (1979) found that 50% of admitted patients aborted. In a small but careful study, Mantoni and Pedersen (1981) found a relationship between the amount of bleeding, assessed by ultrasonic measurement of uterine hematoma size and outcome. Hematomas of less than 35 ml had, in general, a good prognosis, while those larger than 50 ml had a very poor prognosis. The quoted incidence of progression to abortion ranges, therefore, between 35 and 80% of hospital population studies, suggesting almost certainly that this relates to the original criteria for admission rather than to differences in the behavior of the total population.

On purely clinical grounds only two factors of prognostic significance emerge—abortion is more likely when the bleeding occurs early in pregnancy; abortion is more comon when the bleeding is heavy. It is unfortunate that there are no data on risk in all women with threatened abortion as there is no information on the natural history of this condition that includes women with threatened abortion who were not admitted to hospital.

B. Subsequent Prematurity

In Correy's study of almost 8000 patients, 487 of 524 women with threatened abortion delivered after the thirty-eighth week, an incidence of prematurity that is, in fact, less than the Australian national incidence of prematurity. It is probably significant that all of his patients were private patients. Social class undoubtedly has a major impact on the total incidence of premature labor and the same increased risk is seen in relation to social class in women with threatened abortion (Johannsen, 1970). Correy's study apart, there is a near concensus that threatened abortion is followed by a significant increase in premature delivery and/or birth of small for dates infants. Nineteen percent of Johannsen's patients delivered prematurely. The largest study relevant to this problem is that of Funderburk *et al.* (1980). The total population consisted of 25,387 consecutive deliveries. Prematurity occurred in 12.7% of women with a history of threatened abortion (5.4% in controls), low birth weight, defined as less than 2500 g in 17.4% (6.9%), and very low birth weight, defined as less than 1501 g in 8.9% (1.3%). These are not trivial figures. In this study, the main clinical clue to an increased risk was a history of heavy bleeding.

C. *Fetal Abnormality*

While some studies have shown an increase in the incidence of congenital abnormality, more recent and substantial data have, fortunately, not confirmed this. While an abortion is disappointing for a couple who want a baby and a premature baby a cause of substantial concern (perhaps less now than it used to be, with continuing improvement in survival), the birth of a baby with a major malformation is a tremendous blow. Correy (1980) found 1.9% of major malformations in patients with a history of threatened abortion and a figure of 0.9% in controls, significant at only the 5% level. Funderburk *et al.* (1980) found 2.7% of subsequent births to be associated with fetal abnormality compared with 1.6% in controls and this difference was not significant.

Any clinician faced—as they often are—with a discussion about the risk of congenital malformation is in a "no win" situation. No pregnancy carries with it a guarantee of fetal normality. The patient who has had a threatened abortion cannot be told there is no risk of fetal abnormality, but she may be told, with reasonable confidence, that her risk is no greater than if she had not suffered this episode of bleeding.

In summary, about 50% of women admitted to hospital with threatened abortion will ultimately abort. Of those who do not, there is a substantially greater risk of delivering an immature or small for dates baby but no greater risk of delivering an abnormal fetus. Suggestions (Editorial Comment, 1980) that the live born and surviving infant from a pregnancy complicated by threatened abortion faces a greater risk of psychomotor retardation or psychological abnormality remain to be confirmed. Given the great difficulties in studies of this type, no clinician should hold his breath awaiting the outcome.

IV. Etiology

There are no data in the confused, confusing, and controversial problems of the etiology of threatened abortion that satisfy Koch's postulate! In a volume dealing with experimental endocrinology, it would be nice to produce evidence that endocrine deficiency or imbalance caused abortion. The quickest and simplest way to dispose of this suggestion would be to say that no such evidence exists and that is undoubtedly the case. The reasons for reaching this conclusion will be discussed later in Section V,2. If one excludes such causes of bleeding as cervical carcinomas or trauma (Section V,A,5) there seems to be general agreement that threatened abortion is due to bleeding from early separation of a normal or abnormal trophoblast. But what causes the bleeding?

Maternal Factors

1. General

A poor socioeconomic environment provides an equally poor background for reproductive efficiency and this is seen just as much in threatened abortion (Johannsen, 1970) as it is in a high perinatal mortality, increased risk of prematurity, and greater risk of congenital malformation in socially disadvantaged women. Cigarette smoking and alcohol intake increase the risk, but knowledge of relationship, if any, to other commonly used drugs is meager or nonexistent.

Any maternal infection that causes a high fever, whether this be influenza, pneumonia, or typhoid fever, increases the risk of both threatened and incomplete abortion. Concurrent fetal infection—rubella, cytomegalovirus, toxoplasmosis—further and substantially increases the risks. The possible role of chorioamnionitis due to *Mycoplasma hominis* or *Lysteria monocytogenes* is no less obscure now than it was a decade ago. An acute concurrent infection in a woman who is threatening to abort will be evident on clinical grounds, even although the precise cause of the infection may not be clear on clinical grounds alone.

2. Maternal Occupation

With one exception, there is no good evidence that maternal occupation is causally related to the risk of threatened spontaneous abortion. The exception is exposure to an environment of anesthetic gases, best documented in female anesthetists, female dentists, and nursing staff in the same environment. This anxiety first surfaced in a study from Russia (Vaisman, 1967) where more than 50% of all pregnancies in female anesthetists were reported to end in abortion. Vessey and Nunn (1980) have summarized and analyzed critically all data to that date. Despite valid criticisms of the methods of data collection (largely questionnaires) and the inadequacy of controls, Vessey and Nunn conclude that there is an additional risk of about 40% of abortion, and given the earlier data in this article an even greater excess of threatened abortion. The material analyzed came from Russia, the United Kingdom, and the United States and the most likely cause seems to be exposure to high concentrations of nitrous oxide and possibly, also, halothane. Accepting that most operating theatres and dental surgeries do not have adequate scavenging systems and also accepting that there are no hard data that such systems are protective, Vessey and Nunn (1980) conclude that "On present evidence, a theatre nurse or female anesthetist becoming pregnant or wishing to become pregnant should be advised to avoid working in an environment contaminated with anesthetic gases."

3. Chromosomal Aneuploidy

There is no longer any doubt that aneuploidy of the conceptus is one of the major causes of early spontaneous abortion and, therefore, of the preceding threatened abortion (Carr, 1971). Earlier studies indicated that between 25 and 50% of all first trimester abortions are associated with aneuploidy of the conceptus, particularly trisomy of the D group and X monosomy. For every infant live born with Turner's syndrome, 10 will abort and in this particular group there is a relationship to young maternal age, while trisomy and triploidy increase with advancing maternal age. The introduction of banding techniques has further increased this association to about 60% of early abortions and 55% overall (Lauritson, 1976). For most women this is an isolated "act of God," a nondysjunctional problem of that particular ovum or that particular sperm. However, in couples with recurrent abortion there is a balanced translocation in 3.25% which increases the risk of recurrence very substantially (Tsenghi *et al.*, 1976).

4. Other Maternal Conditions

While most of these relate to recurrent abortion, each in turn will cause threatened abortion in an index pregnancy. A full review will be found in Shearman (1980).

Of uterine abnormalities, cervical incompetence is not, by definition, relevant to this article. However, two uterine abnormalities—one congenital, the other acquired—are relevant.

Varying degrees of Müllerian malfusion may be present in any woman threatening to abort. These are rare in the total population and it would be meddlesome to seek them in a woman who has an isolated threatened abortion, whether it proceeds to abortion or not; but if the clinician is dealing with a patient with a history of recurrence, further investigation is warranted. In many texts it seems to be customary to include all degrees of Müllerian malfusion as possible etiological factors in abortion. However, I have been impressed that in the women I have seen, the only congenital uterine malformation that recurs with any frequency in relationship to abortion is that of the septate uterus. More extensive degrees of malfusion such as the truly double uterus, while sometimes causing difficulties during labor or delivery, have not appeared in my own experience to increase the risk of abortion, although premature labor may undoubtedly occur. Radiology still forms the basic step in diagnosis, but laparoscopy/hysteroscopy may be necessary to distinguish a septate uterus from the reproductively more benign bicornuate uterus.

Intrauterine synechiae will be usually suspected in a woman with the appropriate history presenting with secondary amenorrhea. In these women obliteration of the endometrial cavity is total, but partial obliteration is both more common and clearly related to an increased risk of abortion. The diagnosis may be suspect on hysterosalpingography, but should be confirmed, and treated, by hysteroscopy.

Immunological causes of abortion should also be considered in patients with a history of recurrence. Jones (1976) has found a high incidence of abortion, as well as relative infertility in women with sperm immobilizing antibodies. Otherwise covert systemic lupus erythematosis will be found in a substantial minority of women with a poor reproductive history as long as it is looked for. In this particular group, those who demonstrate a lupus Type III coagulation inhibitor, which is both IgG and IgM, are at particular risk of abortion. Appropriate assays for antinuclear factor, DNA binding, and assay of lupus inhibitor should be part of the investigation of recurrent abortion. However, it is doubtful if the expense of these assays is justifiable in a patient with a simple and single episode of threatened abortion unless there are other clinical features to make one suspect the diagnosis.

V. Clinical Features

The clinical diagnosis of threatened abortion will be entertained in a woman, presumed to be less than 20 weeks pregnant, who presents with vaginal bleeding with or without crampy pains and in whom the cervix is closed and uneffaced. The bleeding may be little more than a brown "show," bleeding like that of a normal period, or less frequently, heavier bleeding associated with the passage of clots. Heavy bleeding carries a poor prognosis. A further clinical sign that is helpful is the presence or severity of nausea. Clinically there is a good correlation between continued morning sickness and continuation of pregnancy. A patient who has experienced no nausea, or alternatively, having experienced it indicates that it has improved with the onset of bleeding has a much poorer prognosis. This almost certainly relates to the endocrine associations that precede abortion, discussed in Section V,B,2.

Clinical evidence of severe blood loss should suggest another diagnosis such as incomplete abortion or ruptured tubal pregnancy. Cardiovascular decompensation is exceptionally rare in threatened abortion, although tachycardia may be present due to understandable and related maternal anxiety.

Threatened abortion is not associated with abdominal tenderness unless there is significant retroplacental bleeding in a pregnancy between 14 and 20 weeks. If such tenderness is present the prognosis for an intrauterine pregnancy is poor. If abdominal tenderness is present, particularly with rebound and the uterus is not palpable abdominally then ruptured ectopic pregnancy, a twisted or ruptured ovarian cyst, or criminal interference should be considered. In those countries where legal abortion is available, illegal interference has almost, thankfully, disappeared. In countries where abortion is illegal, attempted induced abortion should always be kept in mind, particularly if the patient has a fever. An increased temperature almost never occurs in a patient with a simple uncomplicated threatened abortion. There are, however, special problems in the patient with a threatened abortion with an intrauterine device *in situ* and this is discussed in Section VII.

On vaginal examination the cervix will be closed. The uterine size should be evaluated. If it is of the expected size the prognosis is improved. If it is bigger, trophoblastic disease should be considered (and twins and wrong dates). If it is smaller the patient may have a missed abortion or may prove to have an episode of dysfunctional uterine bleeding (or wrong dates). A small uterus with bleeding and tenderness on cervical movement may be associated with ectopic pregnancy. In frank cases of ectopic pregnancy the diagnosis is rarely in doubt, but a chronic ectopic can fool even the most experienced clinician.

Vaginal examination must include inspection with a speculum and a good light. Cervical carcinoma may present as a threatened abortion; coital trauma causing injury to the vaginal vault or bleeding from a vascular area of erythroplakia will not be noted unless looked for. Exceptionally rarely, a cervical pregnancy may be seen. In about 50% of patients, threatened abortion will become inevitable and then incomplete. Apart from the clinical clues already described, endocrine and biophysical methods to be discussed in Section V,B, may be very helpful in diagnosis and prognosis.

A. Differential Diagnosis

As well as threatened abortion, bleeding during the first 20 weeks of apparent pregnancy may be due to (1) dysfunctional bleeding, (2) inevitable or incomplete abortion, (3) hydatidiform mole, (4) ectopic pregnancy, (5) local causes, including carcinoma of the cervix, and (6) missed abortion.

1. Dysfunctional Bleeding

Any experienced clinician will be aware how often an episode of dysfunctional bleeding is confused with threatened or incomplete abortion. Many patients who present with a history of "recurrent abortion" are found to have had recurrent episodes of dysfunctional bleeding if trouble enough is taken to verify histopathology from previous curettages. Clinically most women with dysfunctional bleeding will have a long history of irregular and often heavy menstruation. In the adolescent girl, at least in Australia, a history of 3 to 4 months amenorrhea followed by prolonged vaginal bleeding is far more frequently due to juvenile metropathia than it is to one or other of the varieties of abortion. On clinical examination the cervix will be closed, the uterus will be small while endocrine and ultrasonic investigation will exclude pregnancy; the diagnosis is confirmed by diagnostic curettage if this is thought necessary—a rare event in the adolescent girl.

2. Inevitable or Incomplete Abortion

Apart from the severity of bleeding, inevitable abortion will always be associated with cervical dilatation. Products of conception may be felt in the cervical canal in either inevitable or incomplete abortion. In a patient with an old incomplete abortion, however, the cervix may be closed, but the uterus will be small.

3. Hydatidiform Mole

These women often have very severe morning sickness and the uterus is frequently larger than it should be on dates; but sometimes and just to make life more difficult, the uterus will be smaller. The presence of bilateral ovarian cysts would strengthen the clinical suspicion of this diagnosis, although I have rarely been able to feel these cysts until after the uterus is empty. Ultrasound is of paramount assistance in making or excluding this diagnosis (Section V,B).

4. Ectopic Pregnancy

This remains the great imposter and every clinician has made a mistaken diagnosis in the short run and most clinicians have made the same mistake in the medium haul as well. The classical ruptured ectopic with gross intraperitoneal bleeding is not the problem; the leaking ectopic is. Shoulder pain, faintness, peritonism, and pain on moving the cervix raise the likelihood of ectopic pregnancy. A mass in the fornix increases the probability. Then again, every clinician will sooner or later make this diagnosis and find that he is dealing with a large corpus luteum of pregnancy and a threatened abortion. In some cases of ectopic pregnancy the diagnosis will not be suspected until a revealing ultrasound is obtained and in many other patients, final differentiation will only be made after laparoscopy. A ruptured bleeding corpus luteum cyst is more likely to be confused with an ectopic than with threatened abortion.

Most clinicians will go through their lives without seeing a cervical pregnancy. The clinical presentation may be identical to an "ordinary" threatened abortion, but once seen on inspection of the cervix, neither the appearance nor the frightening clinical course will ever be forgotten (Shearman and Parkin, 1977).

5. Local Causes, Including Carcinoma of the Cervix

Unless adequate inspection through a speculum is a routine part of clinical assessment, this cause of vaginal bleeding will be missed. Very rarely, bleeding from a ruptured vaginal vault will be so massive that transfusion and suture under anesthesia are required. A vascular area of erythroplakia may be differentiated from carcinoma by colposcopy. Cervical carcinoma (the age-specific incidence of which continues to drop in most developed countries) will be confirmed by biopsy where there is clinical suspicion. Here, generally, management of the malignancy will take priority over the pregnancy.

6. Missed Abortion

Classically, most of these women suspected clinically will have a long history of bleeding, often slight, and a uterus that is either absolutely smaller than it should be or is observed over a week or more to diminish in size.

Other evidence of pregnancy such as breast tenderness and enlargement and nausea will have regressed. More recently it has become evident that many women with a short history of bleeding and some with no bleeding at all have a dead, or nonviable embryo ("blighted ovum"). While clinical evidence may be sufficiently firm to make a diagnosis, most physicians now prefer additional endocrine or more particularly ultrasonic evidence of embryonic death before emptying the uterus.

B. Other Aids to Diagnosis

1. Biophysical Methods

The development and refinement of ultrasonics has made a substantial impact in many areas of obstetrics and gynecology. Originally introduced to reduce the use of X rays in pregnancy, ultrasound can now go into places where X rays cannot. The simplest and earliest use of ultrasound relevant to this article was the use of audible Doppler effect whereby fetal heart movements translated into audible sound could be demonstrated fairly readily after the twelfth week of pregnancy. Progressive refinement of grey scale scanning and real time ultrasound has proved to be immensely valuable in the assessment of some patients with vaginal bleeding in the first 20 weeks of pregnancy. In very early pregnancy, the mean diameter of the gestational sac can be measured readily and shortly afterward crown–rump length (Fig. 1), then biparietal diameter may be assessed. With adequate real time equipment, fetal heart movements can be detected from the earliest weeks of pregnancy.

Hunter and Picker (1977) applied these methods to patients with threatened abortion and developed a high degree of prognostic discrimination. In a careful study of 93 patients with threatened abortion with a successful outcome, Jouppila *et al.* (1979) made a positive diagnosis of fetal life in 35% at 8 weeks gestation, 83% at 9 weeks gestation, and 100% at 10 weeks gestation. In 50 patients with an anembryonic sac (blighted ovum) the empty sac was demonstrated at the first examination in all patients (Fig. 2). The ultrasonic findings were confirmed histologically in each case. The diagnostic accuracy in 14 patients with incomplete abortion and missed abortion (12 patients) was 100%. In the latter group evidence of fetal echo patterns will be seen in the absence of fetal life signs. In their hands, ultrasonography was usually suggestive rather than diagnostic of ectopic pregnancy, but pictures of startling clarity showing an empty uterus and ectopic gestational sac may be obtained. In patients with an apparent threatened abortion, the typical

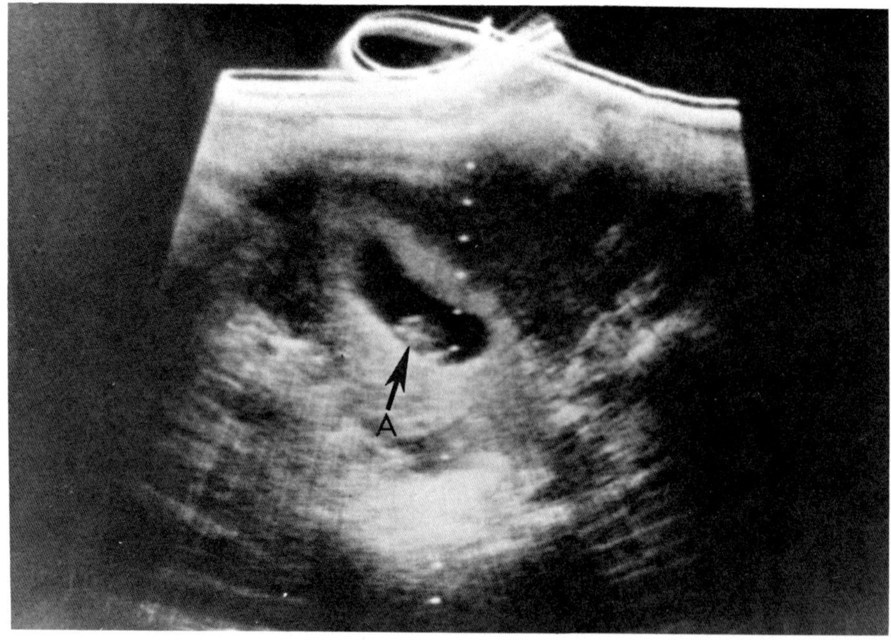

Fig. 1. Intrauterine pregnancy, 8 weeks gestation. A, Normal embryo.

ultrasonic appearances of hydatidiform mole are diagnostic in all cases even in that minority with a concurrent fetus. Eriksen and Philipsen (1980) studied 97 patients with a threatened abortion between 6 and 20 weeks and obtained similar results—100% accuracy in the diagnosis of blighted ovum at the first ultrasound examination and the same accuracy in determining absence of fetal heart movements after 9 weeks gestation.

2. Hormonal Indices

The history of hormonal intrarelationships in threatened and recurrent abortion is long and complex. In a text devoted to endocrinology it would be nice to say that it had also been rewarding, but unfortunately it has not. Far too often investigators have found a pattern of low or falling hormone levels in patients who subsequently aborted and made the grave error that the first caused the second, rather than being both simply related to the fundamental cause of ultimate abortion. These findings became embedded in the folklore of abortion. For historical reasons and particularly because many physicians still believe, emotionally rather than intellectually, that there is such a causal relationship, the evidence in this area warrants careful examination.

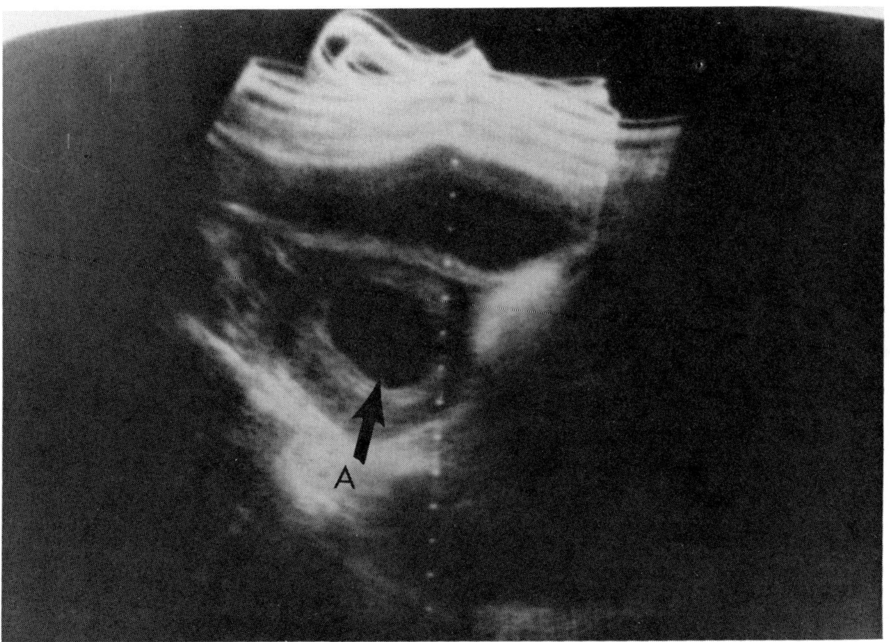

Fig. 2. Intrauterine anembryonic sac (blighted ovum).

a. Progesterone and its Metabolites The majority of spontaneous abortions occur between 9 and 12 weeks of pregnancy. Since the human corpus luteum goes into decline—but not complete retirement—during the eighth week of pregnancy and following Corner's classical purification of progesterone from the corpus luteum, the events were seen to be causally related by many people and this unleashed a mass of uncritical thinking and writing unmatched in almost any other area of medicine.

The first objective evidence of a *relationship* between threatened and subsequent abortion and low levels of pregnanediol, using a method of assay that fulfilled all reliability criteria, was published by Shearman in 1959 (Fig. 3). These five women were part of a group being followed serially throughout pregnancy to delineate normal levels of pregnanediol excretion. Assays on each of these five, who ultimately aborted, began before there was any bleeding or other objective evidence of disturbance in the pregnancy. In discussing these results I wrote:

> Since there appears to be a correlation between placental progesterone content and urinary pregnanediol, it is reasonable to say that in some cases of abortion there is an associated fall in progesterone production preceding, in some cases by weeks, the onset of bleeding. However,

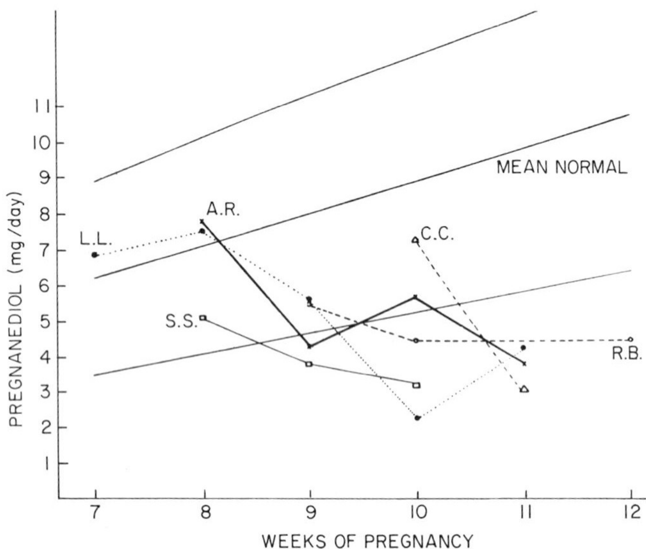

Fig. 3. Urinary excretion of pregnanediol in five cases of first trimester abortion. The normal mean and range are shown by the parallel lines. (From Shearman, 1959, courtesy *J. Obstet. Gynaecol. Br. Emp.)*

it is impossible to say yet whether these patients abort because the progesterone secretion falls or whether the factor responsible for the abortion also causes the fall in progesterone secretion.

Further work showed that while abortion rarely occurred with normal levels of pregnanediol, in 80% of patients with low or falling levels of pregnanediol there was spontaneous restoration of levels to normality with continuation of pregnancy (Shearman and Garrett, 1963).

Assays of serum progesterone have been no more helpful. In their study of 97 patients with threatened abortion, Eriksen and Philipsen (1980) showed that 30 patients with low levels of progesterone aborted, but 21 with low levels did not; 4 patients with normal levels aborted. Even with a blighted ovum, 28% of patients had normal levels of progesterone at the time of first assay (Jouppila *et al.*, 1979). Measurements of 17-hydroxyprogesterone are no more helpful (Batzer, 1980).

b. Estrogens. Earlier studies of the urinary excretion of either total estrogens or estriol (Klopper and Macnaughton, 1965; Brown *et al.*, 1970) showed the same pattern as that seen with urinary pregnanediol—low or falling levels before abortion.

Jouppila *et al.* (1979) found that plasma estradiol levels were below the normal distribution in 32% of patients with threatened abortion who proceeded to term and low levels were found in 92% of patients with a blighted ovum. Put another way, 23% of patients with threatened abortion and low levels of estradiol went to term while 21% of patients with normal levels aborted. This is not exactly a high index of discrimination. Similar results were found by Eriksen and Philipsen (1980).

c. Human Chorionic Gonadotropin (hCG). Theoretically, hCG should have advantages over progesterone and estrogens as it is unique to trophoblast, and over 17-hydroxyprogesterone, which is not produced at all by trophoblast. Using immunoassay for the whole molecule of hCG, Brody and Carlstrom (1962) showed that low levels of hCG invariably preceded spontaneous abortion. Mishell and Davajan (1966) found similar results, as did Nygren *et al.* (1973). The development of assays for the β-subunit of hCG might have been expected to help further, but the results have been less uniform (Batzer, 1980). Jouppila *et al.* (1980) found low levels of β-hCG in only 7% of patients with threatened abortion who proceeded to term. But in 50 patients with threatened abortion and a blighted ovum, 34% of initial assays were within the normal range, although all decreased after the eleventh week. Excellent longitudinal data have been published by Mellows *et al.* (1980). One hundred and twenty-five patients were studied and all were initially normal. Thirty-nine patients who developed threatened abortion went on to have successful pregnancies and hCG levels were the same as those found in women who did not bleed at all. Thirty-two other patients with threatened abortion proceeded to abort. While the average levels of hCG were reduced, there was substantial overlap with normal pregnancies. The authors conclude that "this precludes the use of hCG estimation prognostically in the management of threatened abortion."

d. Human Placental Lactogen (hPL). In theory this hormone has advantages in this clinical situation. It is unique to trophoblast and has a very short half life of 29 minutes (Batzer, 1980). Changes in production rate will, therefore, be followed rapidly by changes in body fluid levels. However, unlike hCG, levels in early pregnancy rise very slowly. Reviewing evidence to that date, Batzer (1980) indicates that single assays are not helpful, but serial assays do have prognostic significance. In a further study, Biswas *et al.* (1980) found that all of 25 patients with threatened abortion and low levels of hPL went on to abort, while all of 27 patients with threatened abortion and normal levels of hPL had a normal outcome. They conclude that "abnormal hPL levels during a bleeding episode are an accurate means of predicting outcome of pregnancy."

e. Pregnancy-Specific β_1-Glycoprotein (SP-1). Like a bitch whelping at every bound, the human placenta continues to be the source of "new" peptides. Obviously, they are not new, only newly discovered, and whether or not they will ultimately fulfill the definitional criteria of a hormone remains to be seen. Inevitably they have been studied in relationship to pregnancy outcome. For technical and historical reasons most attention, to date, is available on SP-1. Jandial *et al.* (1978) found that assays of SP-1 were of no more value than other chemical measurements. Somewhat different findings were published by Ho and Jones (1980). All of 19 patients with threatened abortion whose pregnancies proceeded normally had normal levels of SP-1, 5 with missed abortion or blighted ovum had low levels of SP-1. However, normal levels were also found in 35% of pregnancies which subsequently aborted.

What then do all of these endocrinological associations mean? In terms of etiology nothing. In essence, most but not all women with threatened abortion who proceed to abort will have low and/or falling levels of any fetoplacental hormone you may care to measure. This is a reflection of the tortured trophoblast and has nothing to do with the etiology of ultimate abortion. The correlation between clinical outcome and single assays of any of these hormones is too poor to use in clinical management, but serial assays, in association with clinical features and ultrasound, are of use in some women.

VI. Management

A. Prevention

Where known causes are few, prophylaxis is difficult. Women planning pregnancy should be advised not to smoke and not to drink alcohol. Female anesthetists, theater nurses, dentists, and dental assistants exposed to nitrous oxide (and/or halothane) should be advised to change their environment before attempting conception. Advice about smoking and alcohol may, for behavioral reasons, fall on stony ground. Environmental changes for those exposed to anesthetic gases may be impossible for economic reasons. It is not yet known whether improved scavenging techinques to reduce ambient levels of volatile anesthetics will alter the outlook in terms of general principle, but this makes a lot more sense than asking a theater nurse or female anesthetist or dentist to give up work.

B. Treatment

If knowledge of prophylaxis is meager, knowledge related to effective treatment is nonexistent. The saga begins when the pregnant woman, up to that time normal, begins to bleed. Should she stop work? Should she be put to bed? If so should this be at home or in hospital? To stop work may be a financial disaster for the single parent or for the family dependent on two incomes and no one could say with any honesty that it effects the ultimate outcome. Bedrest at home does not cost anything, but may be socially disruptive if there is no one else to care for children. Admission to hospital is always expensive, either directly to the patient or to the wider community, depending on the system of health care. Given the frequency of threatened abortion, the total costs of management of the problem are enormous, which would be easier to justify if medical intervention made any difference to the outcome. We live in a real world where physicians look after the total patient, and it is unwise to ignore the affective component of threatened abortion. For the woman who really wants a child, bleeds, and aborts at home, she will inevitably think that the outcome may have been different if she had gone to bed or been admitted to hospital. For the same woman admitted to hospital who ultimately aborts, the costs of the hospital bed and investigations may be rationalized along the lines that "everything possible was done." This may not be good news for the mandarins who control a nation's health services, but it is not necessarily bad medicine. It will be a sad day for society if science ultimately replaces completely old fashioned tender loving care. Fortunately in many, if not all societies, there is still room for both.

Lacking any real guidelines, the clinician must make his initial decisions on emotional rather than intellectual grounds. If there is no pain and if the amount of bleeding is slight then bed rest at home may be advised. If there is any pain or bleeding is heavier than that of a normal menstrual loss, or if there is maternal anxiety for whatever reason, the patient may be better in bed, in hospital. Physical examination should be complete and must include adequate speculum examination. Full differential diagnosis described in Section V,A is mandatory. In most cases of threatened abortion there is no clinical doubt of the diagnosis and the physician should not be afraid of relying on his clinical skills alone. Where real doubt exists other investigations described above from hormone assays, ultrasound, to laparoscopy may be needed to resolve the doubt. However, let us assume that a firm diagnosis of threatened abortion has been reached. First the patient must be reassured; she should be told that there is about a 50% chance that the bleeding will settle and the pregnancy proceed. She can be reassured that there is no increased risk of fetal abnormality if the pregnancy continues, but should be told that there is a slightly increased risk of prematurity and/or retarded intrauterine growth. She needs to know this because of the implications it has for the management of the rest of the pregnancy.

If the patient is still anxious and concerned an anxiolytic drug such as diazepam may be used for 1 or 2 days; but many women prefer to avoid medication if possible, even if there is no evidence that the drug, in this case diazepam, is teratogenic.

It should be evident that I am a therapeutic nihilist as far as hormone therapy is concerned. We showed (Shearman and Garrett, 1963) in a double blind study that progestins made no difference to the outcome of pregnancy in patients with a history of habitual abortion and similar findings with different progestins were subsequently published by Goldzieher (1964) and Klopper and Macnaughton (1965). Fuchs (1963, quoted by Johannsen, 1970) in a survey of the literature reached the same conclusions regarding progestins and threatened abortion. The abuse of drugs in this area is long and often sad, some of the compounds being actively harmful. Stilbestrol was widely used for threatened abortion in the 1940s and 1950s with no good effect and has left a legacy of young women with adenosis and a poor reproductive potential and young men with oligospermia because of their intrauterine exposure to this stilbene derivative. The 19 nor-steroids caused a mini-epidemic of nonprogressive virilism of the female fetus in the 1950s, while medroxyprogesterone acetate (Depo-Provera) was first used as a systemic contraceptive when it became evident that women given the drug for "pregnancy support" usually had months of anovulatory amenorrhea either postpartum or after abortion.

In many patients, further investigations will not be needed. The threatened abortion will progress to inevitable and incomplete abortion or will resolve and the pregnancy continue. If the bleeding persists for more than a couple of days or if there is doubt about viability of the pregnancy then further investigations are very helpful but not essential. Pregnancy, whether it ends in the delivery of an infant or abortion, is finite with the very rare exception of a missed abortion that may stay *in utero,* if untreated, for months or even years. But for the patient, waiting can be both nerve-racking and expensive. Of all investigations, ultrasound is the most helpful. Demonstration of an empty or collapsed sac by B-mode scanning or of a dead fetus on real time is definitive and can be followed by suction curettage without unnecessary delay. In very early pregnancy, before 8 or 9 weeks, even ultrasound in other than the very best units may be misleading or inconclusive. If this circumstance prevails, then serial measurements of β-hCG, hPL, or progesterone probably offer the best endocrinological discriminants, but a single assay should never form the sole basis for a clinical decision.

VII. Threatened Abortion and the Intrauterine Device (IUD)

The woman who conceives with an intrauterine device *in situ* is in a class all of her own. By definition the pregnancy is unplanned, but it is a mistake to assume that all unplanned pregnancies are unwanted. An intrauterine pregnancy with a coexisting IUD carries about a 60% chance of abortion. If the tail of the device is visible it should be removed and the risk of abortion will then be reduced to about 30%.

If the tail of the IUD cannot be seen there is a major problem, not just of increased risk of abortion but of septic threatened and incomplete abortion. This illness is explosive in onset, rapid in its evolution, and carries a high mortality from septicemia. If the tail of the device cannot be seen the patient and her consort should be advised of the risks. If they so wish and there is no legal impediment, termination of pregnancy should be considered.

References

Batzer, F. R. (1980). *Fertil. Steril.* **34,** 1–13.

Biswas, S., Murrey, M., Buffoe, G., Graves, L., Jelowitz, J., and Dewhurst, J. (1980). *J. Obstet. Gynecol.* **1,** 75–77.

Brown, J. B., Evans, J. H., Beischer, N. A., Campbell, D. G., and Fortune, D. W. (1970). *J. Obstet. Gynaecol. Br. Commonw.* **77,** 690–700.

Carr, D. H. (1971). "Advances in Human Genetics" Plenum, New York.

Correy, J. F. (1980). *Asia-Oceania J. Obstet. Gynaecol.* **6,** 49–52.

Editorial Comment (1980). *Br. J. Med. J.* **281,** 470.

Eriksen, P. S., and Philipsen, T. (1980). *Obstet. Gynecol.* **55,** 435–438.

Evans, J. H., and Beischer, N. A. (1970). *Med. J. Aust.* **2,** 165–168.

Funderburk, S. J., Guthrie, D., and Meldrum, D. (1980). *Br. J. Obstet. Gynaecol.* **87,** 100–105.

Goldzieher, J. W. (1964). *J. Am. Med. Assoc.* **188,** 651–654.

Grudzinskas, J. G., Gordon, Y. B., Miller, J. F., and Williamson, E. (1981). *Aust. N. Z. J. Obstet. Gynaecol.* **21,** 56.

Hertig, A. T., and Livingstone, R. G. (1944). *N. Engl. J. Med.* **230,** 797–806.

Ho, P. C., and Jones, W. R. (1980). *Am. J. Obstet. Gynecol.* **138,** 253–256.

Hunter, C., and Picker, R. H. (1977). *Aust. N. Z. J. Obstet. Gynecol.* **17,** 192–196.

Jandial, V., Towler, C. M., Horne, C. W. H., and Abramovich, D. R . (1978). *Br. J. Obstet. Gynaecol.* **85,** 832–836.

Johannsen, A. (1970). *Acta Obstet. Gynecol. Scand.* **49,** 89–93.

Jones, W. R. (1976). *In* "Immunology of Human Reproduction" (J. J. Scott and W. R. Jones, eds.), p. 396. Academic Press, New York.

Jouppila, P., Huhtaniemi, I., and Tapanainen, J. (1979). *Obstet. Gynecol.* **55,** 42–47.

Klopper, A. I., and Macnaughton, M. (1965). *J. Obstet. Gynaecol. Br. Commonw.* **72,** 1022–1028.

Lauritson, J. G. (1976). *Acta Obstet. Gynecol. Scand. Suppl.* **52.**

Mantoni, M., and Pederson, J. F. (1981). *Br. J. Obstet. Gynaecol.* **88,** 47–51.

Mellows, H. J., Bennett, M. J., Brackpool, P., Gordon, Y. B., and Dewhurst, J. (1980). *J. Obstet. Gynecol.* **1,** 7–11.

Mishell, D. R., and Davajan, V. (1966). *Am. J. Obstet. Gynecol.* **96,** 231–239.

Nygren, K. G., Johansson, E. D., and Wide, L. (1973). *Am. J. Obstet. Gynecol.* **116,** 916–922.

Shearman, R. P. (1959). *J. Obstet. Gynaecol. Br. Emp.* **66,** 1–11.

Shearman, R. P. (1980). *In* "Gynecologic Endocrinology" (J. J. Gold, ed.), 3rd Ed., pp. 752–759.

Shearman, R. P., and Garrett, W. J. (1963). *Br. Med. J.* **1**, 292–295.
Shearman, R. P., and Parkin, G. M. (1977). *Aust. N. Z. J. Obstet. Gynecol.* **17**, 105–107.
Tsenghi, C., Metaxotou-Stavridaki, C., Strataki-Benetov, M., Kalpini-Mavrou, A., and Matsaniotis, N. (1976). *Obstet. Gynecol.* **47**, 463–468.
Vaisman, A. I. (1967). *Exp. Khirorgiya* **12**, 44–49.
Vessey, M. P.,and Nunn, J. F. (1980). *Br. Med. J.* **281**, 696–698.

INDEX

C

Cholestasis of pregnancy, prolactin as marker in, 84

E

Endometrium, proteins of, 46–50
Estrogen(s)
  biosynthesis of, 196–197
  control of production, 197–198
    activities of placental enzymes, 208–211
    supply of precursors and, 198–208
  plasma levels, relation to onset of labor, 211–213
Estrous cycle, in marsupials
  corpus luteum, 10–11
  follicle development and ovulation, 8–10
  progesterone levels, 10

F

Fetal abnormality, threatened abortion and, 270–271

H

Histamine, preimplantation period and
  blastocyst and, 60
  as mediator of estrogen action, 59–60
Hormones, in marsupials, measurement of, 6–8
Human chorionic gonadotrophin
  chemistry and biosynthesis, 98–101
    biological properties, 101–103
    immunologic properties, 103–105
  interaction with receptor site
    mechanism of, 121–122
    purification and properties of receptor, 121
  measurement of
    biological pregnancy tests, 105
    do-it-yourself pregnancy tests, 107–108
    hormonal withdrawal tests, 105–107
    immunological tests, 107–108
    radioimmunoassay, 108–109
    radioreceptor assay, 109–110
  role in abnormal conditions, 118–119
    abnormal pregnancies, 119
    cancer, 119–121
  role in early pregnancy, 118
  secretory pattern during reproductive cycle, 110–111
    postimplantation, 113–117
    preimplantation, 111–113
Human placental lactogen
  assay in blood, 179
  biological functions, 174–176
  biological nature, 173–174
  clinical use of, 186–187
  control mechanisms, 176–177
  immunochemical nature, 172–173
  interpretation of biochemical tests of feto-placental function, 180–181
  levels in different biological fluids, 178–179
  maternal levels in complications of pregnancy
    diabetes mellitus, 184
    fetal death, 185
    fetal distress and neonatal asphyxia, 185

Human placental lactogen (*cont.*)
low birthweight infants, 182–183
preeclampsia and hypertension, 183–184
prolonged pregnancy, 186
rhesus isoimmunization, 184–186
threatened abortion, 182
trophoblastic tumors, 181–182
maternal levels in normal pregnancy, 179–180
metabolism and clearance, 177–178
nomenclature, 168
synthesis, 169–172

I

Implantation
morphological aspects of, 37
steroid hormones and, 39–41
time of, 36–37
Infertility lactational, as natural contraceptive, 88
Intrauterine device, threatened abortion and, 284–285

L

Lactation, lactational infertility as natural contraceptive, 88
manipulation of milk production, 86–88
prolactin levels and profiles, 85–86
Lactogenic hormones, placental
in other placental mammals, 169
in other species, 169

M

Marsupials
estrous cycle in
corpus luteum, 10–11
follicle development and ovulation, 8–10
progesterone levels, 10
hormones and measurement of, 6–8
parturition in
corpus luteum and, 23–26
fetus and/or placenta and, 27–28
mammary gland development, 28–29
overview, 22–23
pituitary and, 26–27
pregnancy in
cleavage, 15
conception, 13–14
embryonic diapause, 17–22
maintenance of pregnancy, 15–17
relevant anatomy, 11–12
Milk production, manipulation of, 86–88
Molar pregnancies, prolactin as marker in, 84

O

Ovary, effect of prolactin on, 70–71
Oxytocin
direct evidence for role in parturition, circulating levels during, 241–249
indirect evidence for role in parturition
ablation and lesion studies, 236–238
blocking of release with ethanol, 238–241
effect of endogenous oxytocin, 234–235
effect of exogenous oxytocin, 233–234
pituitary and hypothalamic content and depletion, 235–236
selective inactivation of oxytocin, 238
interaction with prostaglandins, 256–260
Oxytocin receptors, control of uterine sensitivity and, 249–256

P

Parturition
direct evidence for role of oxytocin in, circulating levels during, 241–249
indirect evidence for role of oxytocin in
ablation and lesion studies, 236–238
blocking of release with ethanol, 238–241
effect of endogenous oxytocin, 234–235
effect of exogenous oxytocin, 233–234
pituitary and hypothalamic content and depletion, 235–236
selective inactivation of oxytocin, 238
in marsupials
corpus luteum and, 23–26
fetus and/or placenta and, 27–28
mammary gland development, 28–29
overview, 22–23
pituitary and, 26–27
Placental protein 5, in abnormal pregnancy, 158
chemistry of, 157
function of, 158–159
historical note, 156–157

in normal pregnancy, 157–158
origin of, 157
Preeclampsia, prolactin as marker in, 84
Pregnancy
in marsupials
cleavage, 15
conception, 13–14
embryonic diapause, 17–22
maintenance of pregnancy, 15–17
relevant anatomy, 11–12
prolactin in
amniotic fluid, 76–78
factors influencing production, 79–81
fetal prolactin, 74–76
heterogeneity of prolactin, 79
influence on immune system, 78–79
maternal levels, 71–74
prolactin-secreting tumors and, 88–90
simultaneous development and recognition of, 37–38
Pregnancy-associated protein(s), other, 159–160
Pregnancy-associated plasma protein A
assay of, 149–150
chemistry of, 148–149
function of, 154–155
historical note, 147–148
metabolism of, 151
in normal pregnancy, 151–153
origin of, 150
in pathological pregnancy, 153–154
Pregnancy-associated plasma protein B
chemistry of, 155–156
future studies on, 156
historical note, 155
physiology of, 156
Pregnancy-specific events, influence of prolactin on
fetal lung maturation, 83
osmoregulation, 81–83
Preimplantation period
histamine and
blastocyst and, 60
as mediator of estrogenaction, 59–60
prostaglandins and
endometrial vascular permeability and decidualization, 56–59
luteal function and, 53–56
tissue levels and production, 50–52
Progesterone
biosynthesis of, 213–215
control of production
activities of placental enzymes, 216–217
effect of polypeptides of placental or pituitary origin, 217–218
supply of precursors and, 215–216
plasma levels, relation to onset of labor, 218–219
Prolactin
effect on ovary, 70–71
influence on pregnancy-specific events
fetal lung maturation, 83
osmoregulation, 81–83
levels and profiles, lactation and, 85–86
as marker in pathological pregnancy
molar pregnancies and cholestasis of pregnancy, 84
preeclampsia, 84
in normal pregnancy
in amniotic fluid, 76–78
factors influencing production, 79–81
fetal prolactin, 74–76
heterogeneity of prolactin, 79
influence on immune system, 78–79
maternal levels, 71–74
tumors secreting, pregnancy and, 88–90
Prostaglandins
endometrial vascular permeability and decidualization and, 56–59
luteal function and, 53–56
tissue levels and production, 50–52
interaction with oxytocin, 256–260
Protein(s), endometrial, 46–50

S

Schwangerschaftsprotein 1
chemistry of, 130–133
function of, 146
historical note, 129–130
measurement of, 134–136
metabolism of, 136–137
in normal pregnancy, 137–140
origin of, 133–134
in other animals, 133
in pathological pregnancy, 141–146
Steroid(s), nomenclature, 194–196
Steroid hormones, implantation and, 39–41
Steroid receptors, in uterus, 42–46

T

Threatened abortion
  clinical features, 273–275
    differential diagnosis, 275–277
    other aids to diagnosis, 277–282
  definition, 268
  etiology, maternal factors, 271–273
  incidence of, 268
  intrauterine device and, 284–285
  management
    prevention, 282
    treatment, 282–284
  natural history of, 268–269
    fetal abnormality, 270–271
    progression to spontaneous abortion, 269
    subsequent prematurity, 269–270
Tumors, prolactin-secreting, pregnancy and, 88–90

U

Uterus
  sensitivity, oxytocin receptors and, 249–256
  steroid receptors in, 42–46